PRAISE FOR THE SPORT OF LIFE

"The human body can heal itself through mindfulness. Through his pain prevention education, Dr. Donnie has helped hundreds of people do just that. This book is a must-read."

NICOLETTE RICHER, AUTHOR OF *EAT REAL TO HEAL*

"Dr. Donnie recognizes where treatments like surgery and drugs fall short, offering natural methods of pain recovery that are effective. As a holistic chiropractor myself, I confidently recommend this book to anyone seeking a pain-free life."

DR. KIM MAKOI, AUTHOR OF *BOOZE TO BALANCE*

"When I have a client who is really suffering and motivated to get well, I send them to Dr. Richardson. I've seen him transform my clients from suffering, frustrated, wheelchair-bound accident victims to happy and mobile clients, reclaiming their independence and quality of life. His book is an integral tool to teach anyone how to overcome pain and move with freedom and a joy for exercise."

DEBBIE TOROSI -- INJURY ATTORNEY

"All of my life, physical fitness and well-being have been one of my great loves. After years of being in the gym, I started body-building in my late 20s and continued throughout my 30s before suffering an injury that kept me from lifting no more than 5 lbs without pain. Prepared to try whatever it took, I found Dr. Richardson and his premier body method. Six months later, I was deadlifting and squatting over 200 pounds and bench pressing 55-pound dumbbells again. I have been training with him for 12 years now. His techniques saved my fitness career, and frankly, my life."

TINA SOWERS - CEO COMPLETEFITKID

"When I came to Donnie, I was broken—literally and figuratively. I had just recovered from a broken ankle, but I also had widespread body and lower back pain. He taught me the Premier Body Method, a way of strengthening my core. I was so out of shape, but I strengthened it, and I'm out of pain. I'm kind of amazed. I didn't think I would ever enjoy being active again, but I do."

DUNCAN MACLEOD, PUBLISHER, BOOKS THAT
SAVE LIVES

YOUR LIFE, PAIN-FREE

A DOCTOR'S GUIDE TO HEALING FROM PAIN, STRENGTHENING YOUR CORE, AND LIVING THE SPORT OF LIFE

SPORTS MEDICINE FOR EVERYONE

DONALD JAMES RICHARDSON, DC, CCSP, DACBSP, CSCS

SPORTS MEDICINE SPECIALIST, STRENGTH AND CONDITIONING SPECIALIST

PREMIER
BM BODY METHOD

Published by BTSL/Jim Dandy Publishing
6252 Peach Avenue
Van Nuys, CA 91411
info@jimdandypublishing.com

For bulk orders, special quantities, course adoptions, and corporate sales, please email info@jimdandypublishing.com

ISBN: (print) 978-1963667196, (ebook) 978-1963667202

BISAC: HEA036000; OCC011000; HEA007050; MED093000; HEA009000

Printed in the United States of America

CONTENTS

PART ONE
THE SPORT OF LIFE

PART TWO
THE PREMIER BODY METHOD

PART THREE
HUMAN MOVEMENT EDUCATION

LEVEL I: FULL SPINAL CONTROL

LEVEL II: BASIC FUNCTIONAL HUMAN MOTION

LEVEL III: ADVANCED EXERCISES

APPENDICES

FOREWORD

ALLISON HOELLER - BEAUTY & LIFESTYLE
CREATOR, FOUNDER OF AH MEDIA

Allison Hoeller
Beauty & Lifestyle Creator, Founder of AH Media

The wind catching my mare's mane, the thrill of show jumping—I loved horseback riding as a kid. I lost that childhood love to scoliosis, which brought chronic back pain into nearly every part of my daily life. I never imagined that I could feel better without surgery.

I first came to Donnie to get in shape for my modeling career, but we shifted our focus to managing my scoliosis. We focused on controlled movements with weights—exercises like pushing, pulling, squatting, and deadlifting. The fact that I can even *do* these again is honestly mind-blowing. With his PREMIER Body Method, Donnie taught me that even the smallest movements matter; for example, I have to hold my ribcage differently during certain exercises because of my curved spine. He's taught me how crucial my core is for spinal support—and I carry that with me every day, even at home when I'm picking things up or playing with my niece and nephew.

Donnie's different because he *cares*. He takes the time to explain why your form matters, checks in before every session to see how you're doing, and adjusts the plan if something doesn't feel right.

Today, I live without back pain. I've been hitting my fitness goals, improving my nutrition, and attending spin classes. I can even just sit at a desk for longer periods without discomfort. Donnie's help has lifted a huge weight, literally and figuratively, from my back—and recently, I rode my first horse in seven years.

HOW TO USE THIS BOOK

The Premier Body Method is a human movement education course designed to teach the fundamentals of human physical behavior to improve physical function and performance on every level. This program should be used to improve one's physical ability, regardless of where the individual is starting from. For injured populations, this rehabilitative training strategy will teach you how to rebuild your physical body from the ground up. By going slow and continuing to build one physical piece at a time, you will be amazed at how far you will be able to go physically. For people dealing with chronic pain, in many ways, you may feel as though your physical body has betrayed you. You don't trust your body to be able to do and handle physical efforts anymore. This program will change that. This program will show you step by step that you can do physical things again, even exercise, and be in fantastic physical shape!

For the novice who may be self-conscious or intimidated by exercise and is not sure how or where to begin, this program will take you from the beginner's basics of how the physical body works all the way to a full exercise level. You will be in the best shape of your life, and you will do it in the smartest, safest, and best way possible.

For health and fitness enthusiasts, this program will never take away what you already love to do; it will only enhance and improve it. You will reduce injury and see positive results. Learning to have higher-quality mechanics is the most important aspect of any good exercise fitness program.

For athletes, performance gains depend on how you approach your training. Additionally, gaining a better understanding of how your body functions greatly aids in both injury prevention and enhanced performance.

For youth, this program is essential for teaching us how to use our physical bodies correctly from a young age. This helps reduce the risk of injury and enhances physical abilities as a person grows, develops, and ages, establishing proper physical behavior for the rest of their lives. I cannot tell you how many people I have trained in this manner over the years who have said to me, "I wish someone would have taught me this about my body before I accumulated all these aches and pains." Can you imagine if we were all taught from a young age how to use and care for our physical bodies?

This book can and should be used by all these types of people. Everyone should use it to learn proper movement.

STEP ONE – Read the first part of this book to learn the concepts of how the physical body works. It's much easier and more enjoyable to understand not just what to do but, more importantly, how to do it and, even more importantly, to grasp WHY you are doing something. Simply handing someone a list of exercises and saying, "Do these and you will get better," honestly rarely works. It's not the exercises that improve you physically, but what the exercises represent in terms of how to use your physical body correctly.

STEP TWO – As you acquire the knowledge of how the body works physically, now you must begin to learn how to move this way. Go through each exercise progression in the order in which they are presented in this book. This will begin with the Level One training progressions.

Level One training includes the detailed components of how the body needs to function physically. It is not overly physically demanding (although it can be for some), but is much more mentally challenging in terms of ensuring that the fundamental details are correct and working in harmony.

That said, Level One can sometimes feel a bit tedious for those accustomed to higher-level training. However, I must emphasize that you should not skip or overlook Level One training. The details in this stage are crucial for the success of the more advanced concepts. It's important to pay attention to every detail and every step along the way! You will be happy that you did later on.

We will be building movement throughout this book and the entire Premier Body Method training progressions, so skipping steps will not yield a solid final product. Much like building a house, we must proceed step by step, in the correct order, carefully building each piece to ensure a strong final structure. Once you have mastered the Level One training progressions, you will be ready for Level Two training.

Level Two is going to get more fun now that you'll be back up on your feet, learning the major movement mechanics of the human body. These include hip hinging, squatting, getting up and down, lifting, pushing and pulling, as well as balance and coordination. All these aspects of movement training are essential not just for advancing in exercise and physical performance but, perhaps even more importantly, for the physicality of everyday life.

Follow the Level Two exercise progressions just as you did with the Level One training progressions, building step by step, movement piece by movement piece, until you complete Level Two training. Remember, don't skip steps. Always strive to master the prerequisites before moving on to the next steps. All training progressions have been arranged in a specific order to help you develop your physical body in the most efficient way possible. Once you have mastered the Level One and Level Two training progression, it is time to step it up to Level Three training.

In **Level Three**, things will start to progress more significantly now. You will begin as you did in Levels One and Two, moving through the Level Three exercise training progressions with more advanced exercises. Toward the end of Level Three, the basic exercise, strength, and conditioning strategy will be introduced and incorporated into the mix as you start to combine everything you have learned into a real exercise and/or strength and conditioning routine, depending on your fitness level and physical abilities acquired so far. Remember to continue building piece by piece, step by step, until you achieve this Level Three full exercise training status. From this point, you will be able to take the knowledge you have gained and the physical skills you have developed and apply them to any form of exercise you choose or continue to progress to higher levels of strength, conditioning, and athletic performance.

The best way to go through the Premier Body Method training program is in person with a qualified practitioner, therapist, or trainer. However, since that may not be practical for everyone, the next best option for progressing through this book on your own is to visit PremierBodyMethod.com. The website offers a comprehensive online course with training videos to guide you through the entire program. The online course mirrors the book step by step, providing video instruction to give you a thorough understanding of how to perform each detail for all the movements and exercises presented throughout the PBM program. Premier Body Method is here to help you achieve your physical goals every step of the way.

Steps for Success:

- 1. Read this book for a conceptual understanding of how the physical body functions.
- 2. Follow the exercise progressions step by step through Level One training. Master Level One before moving to subsequent training levels.
- 3. Follow the exercise progressions step by step through

Level Two training. Master Level Two before moving to Level Three.

- 4. Follow the exercise progressions step by step through Level Three training. At the end of Level Three, you will be at a basic exercise training level.
- 5. Follow along online at PremierBodyMethod.com with one of our online courses to enhance your training experience and results.
- 6. Continue advancing to other and more challenging forms of exercise with the knowledge you have gained and the physical skills you have developed.

PREFACE

I used to work as the rehabilitation director for an orthopedic sports medicine clinic in Newport Beach, California. My boss was the head medical director and owner of this clinic. He was a brilliant doctor, but we disagreed on a few big concepts. His philosophy was to avoid training pathology and/or injury at all costs to stop the progression of further damage to the injured area of the body. I agree with this statement, except for the "at all costs" part. I remember one particular situation in which I was teaching a patient correct Hip Hinging and squatting mechanics as part of her rehabilitation process. This patient was suffering from chronic back pain due to repetitive stress caused by having poor mechanics (moving wrong!) throughout most of her life.

It started when she was a young athlete. She was a great athlete, in fact, with a lot of potential, but she had been forced to end her athletic career early because of repeated bouts of back pain. It was not caused by any specific injury or trauma. The pain seemed just to come and go out of nowhere. After her athletic career, she was fine until about her mid-thirties, when her back pain returned off and on. The pain was manageable at first, but it got worse and more frequent over the years. The woman received help from doctors, chiropractors, and physical and massage therapists. They were able to provide temporary relief but did not fix the problem. She eventually came to our clinic.

I know what you're thinking. This is going to be some miraculous, feel-good story about how I finally fixed this woman's problem, and then the rest of this book will tell you how I did it. I wish that were the case, but it's not. We could not cure this suffering woman, either.

At our clinic, we began rehabilitation with this woman, but we ran into a problem when it came time to teach her "Hip Hinge," the proper hip-hinging and squatting movements. My boss decided to discontinue the portion of her rehab program that involved the teaching and training of hip-hinging and squatting mechanics because he said it would just aggravate her pathology. He was technically correct since continual hip hinging and squatting would likely have caused this patient more pain. However, he may not have been right about the bigger picture.

It was improper hip-hinging mechanics throughout this person's life that led her to destroy her back in the first place. And it is easy for the know-it-all doctor to simply say this person can no longer perform a Hip Hinge. In an ideal world, I would completely agree with this solution, but we do not live in an ideal world. We live in the real world. In this real world, we don't always get to just completely avoid anything we want. Sure, this patient can avoid doing the exercise of a Hip Hinge or squat while at the gym, but what happens when this person has to stand up from a chair, get in and out of her car, on and off her bed, or even get up from the toilet? All of these daily life tasks are forms of hip-hinging mechanics.

You see, life demands specific physical abilities. In the real world, this woman needs to improve her hip-hinging mechanics, even if there is a small cost while improving (learning) the movement. Since life dictates that she must Hip Hinge, she is better off knowing how to do it the best way possible rather than continuing with the same horrible mechanics that got her into this mess in the first place and will continue to degenerate her further if not changed. This situation is not ideal, but I'd rather accept reality and take the lesser of two evils than be unrealistic.

It comes down to choosing between using your physical body

correctly or not. Unfortunately for this poor woman, she never had that choice. She never had a choice because she was never taught how to use her body correctly, at least not until it was too late. See, her mechanics were so poor for so long that she used up her body's physical structures by constantly going beyond her physical capability limits due to her lack of knowledge of how to move correctly. The gas tank for her lower back was completely empty. Because of this, she destroyed her physical structure beyond her body's ability to recover and repair the damage. Her lower back just had nothing left.

This woman, like so many people out there, will probably be in pain for the rest of her life. Worse, she was only 40 years old when I met her! That is a long way to go with debilitating pain. She has two small children and a husband at home. The continued pain will limit her ability to play and care for her children. It will limit her work and financial contribution to her family. It will most likely put stress on her relationship with her husband. It will create feelings of resentment and sadness. She will miss out on activities with her friends. She will miss out on many of life's joys that we take for granted (until it is too late.) She will turn to chronic pain, sleep, and anti-depressant medications. She will become more and more sedentary, which will cause her overall health to decline rapidly. She will develop depression, have a poor quality of life for almost half of her life, and most likely die prematurely in both physical pain and mental anguish.

I want the world to know that this story, while all too common, is not inevitable. This story is only a reality because it happens to so many of us, but it does not need to be. Back pain, knee pain, hip pain, shoulder pain...the list goes on and on. The vast majority of this pain is degenerative in nature and caused by repetitive stress. Many of us consider it a normal part of life, writing it off as, "Oh, I am just getting old," or "I'm a competitive athlete training really hard, so of course I'm going to have to deal with some pain." Well, I am here to tell you it is not normal. It is common, yes, but not normal. Musculoskeletal pain is not a normal part of life. It is something you acquire. Sometimes, you do it to yourself, and it can be prevented (or at least the risk reduced). It comes down to simply learning how to take care of your physical body correctly. It is not that difficult, either. It is just something you have to learn, preferably before the damage is done. The problem is most people don't understand it until pain forces them to do so. But by this time, it is usually too late to a certain extent. Think of it like brushing your teeth. How many people's teeth had to fall out of their heads until we realized it might be a good idea to brush our teeth starting as young children fifty years earlier?

My goal is not to force everyone to exercise, be healthy, and train like an Olympic champion. My ultimate goal is to give the world a choice: a choice between a high-quality, happy, healthy, pain-free life or a poor-quality, depressing, unhealthy, painful one. We are talking about physical pain, yes, but really, we are talking about so much more. We are talking about quality of life in all respects. In my mind, the choice is obvious. See, life is a sport. To win, you have to prepare your body correctly.

SOMEONE ONCE ASKED ME: "WHO IS YOUR IDEAL PATIENT?"

I am a doctor, but ideally I would rather treat clients, not patients. Let me explain. Usually, patients come to me only after an injury occurs or, worse, when they have chronic pain for no reason apparent to them. I would much prefer these people to come to me before these injuries and chronic conditions got out of hand and, more importantly, before they had acquired true structural damage to their bodies. It makes me sad and frustrated to think about how many people could have avoided the painful conditions I see and treat every day if they only knew how to use their bodies correctly.

My ideal client is someone who grasps this fact and is interested in reducing the risk of injury, preserving the body's structures, and enhancing physical performance. It is someone who realizes that physical fitness is a vital nutrient to the body and wants to learn how to physically control and take care of the body in the best way possible. Human Movement Education is what really makes the difference. As I see it, life is a sport. If you want to be good at it, you have to prepare your body properly.

As an analogy for this program, Michael Jordan was one of the best basketball players to ever live. To get that good, he did not just go out and shoot hoops all day. He did a hundred things before he even got onto the court, which prepared his body and allowed him to be so good at basketball when it came time to play. He lifted weights, did agility drills, conditioned his body, studied the game by breaking it down into components and watching game film, did skill drills, ate right, and studied the playbook. He was doing unbelievable amounts of preparation aside from actually playing basketball, so by the time he did play, he was incredibly well prepared for it. He did all these things because being good at his sport required certain types of preparation. Life is no different. Life demands specific physical requirements, so to be good at 'The Sport of Life,' you must prepare your body correctly.

PART ONE
THE SPORT OF LIFE

ABOUT THE SPORT OF LIFE

ONE HUNDRED MILLION!

A ccording to the Institute of Medicine (IOM), this is the number of people in the United States suffering from musculoskeletal pain. That's nearly one out of every three Americans. To put it another way, that's more than diabetes, cancer, heart disease, and stroke – *combined*! [1, 3, 4, 5].

SIX HUNDRED BILLION!

Dollars, that is. This is the estimated yearly cost of pain to American society. It's hard to make sense of such a large number, but we can start to understand how serious pain is when we realize that for every dollar that obesity costs us, pain costs Americans *four dollars* [1, 2, 6, 7, 8]. The amount we spend on pain is equivalent to every single person in the country paying $2,000 every single year because of pain. Just under half of the $600 billion estimate amount goes towards tremendous healthcare costs, such as pain medications, doctor's visits, and physical and occupational therapy. Loss of productivity in the American work-force is even higher, with an estimated yearly loss of three hundred thirty-six billion dollars due to missed work and poorer work ability as the result of chronic pain. The financial costs alone are a strain on society. [1, 2, 4, 8, 9]

The financial costs are staggering, but the human costs are worse. The $600 billion annual price tag does not include the emotional, mental, and personal damage caused by physical pain. The impact on quality of life is astounding. Of the 100 million Americans suffering from pain, two-thirds say their pain dramatically affects their overall enjoyment of life. More than three-quarters report depression as a result of their pain. Worse yet, an estimated 86% of pain sufferers report an inability to sleep due to their pain. Physical pain affects our quality of life on an epic scale. [1, 4, 11]

The list of people affected by pain goes on and on, extending from the person suffering from pain to that person's family, friends, and beyond. These are not just any people. These people are the people you know. These people are you.

Another result of pain is the alarming use and misuse of painkillers, antidepressants, alcohol, and other drugs (legal and illicit) related to pain. The Centers for Disease Control and Prevention (CDC) reported in 2010 that 12 million Americans over the age of 12 were addicted to prescription painkillers. This figure doesn't include the millions of non-addicted people taking prescription painkillers for a pain-related condition as part of a treatment and therapy program. Beyond addiction and dangerous side effects, there's another problem. The drugs aren't working! Basically, none of these medications are fixing any of the problems. They are only covering them up. [10]

The first main issue with the use of medications as the answer for pain conditions is that their repeated use causes countless side effects and other physiological problems. The second main problem with medication as the answer to physical pain is the fact that these medications are artificially inhibiting one of our body's main protective mechanisms, pain. [10, 12, 13] Pain gets a bad rap because it is uncomfortable, but pain is actually an essential part of our lives. Pain lets us know when something is wrong. So when you artificially cover up your pain, not only are you not fixing the problem, but there is a strong possibility you are continuing to make the problem worse by continuing to hurt and damage yourself without even knowing it. This brings us to the third problem with medications as the answer to our pain: they bring us false hope. Medicines used for physical pain conditions allow users to avoid and deny their problems to the point of no return. When this illusion ends, the person not only still has the physical pain condition, but it is now much worse to the point that the medications can no longer cover it up. It comes along with overall poorer health due to the physiologic side effects from all the continued pain medication consumption. This is clearly not the solution.

How many people do you know who suffer from pain? Yourself? Your parents, spouse, or friends? Some coworkers? We all know someone with back, neck, knee, hip, or shoulder pain. Pain is so commonplace that we just accept it as a part of life.

Back pain is the leading cause of disability in America and world-wide for people under the age of 45. Statistics show that over twenty-six million Americans suffer from back pain. [1, 3, 4, 5] The pain doesn't stop there. The American Academy of Pain Medicine [4, 11] reports that these individuals are "three times more likely to be in fair or poor health and more than four times as likely to experience serious psycho-logical distress as people without low back pain." They're also more likely to have drug addictions.

All this is not even the sad part. We haven't gotten to the worst of it yet. The worst part is that we have not devised a solution for all this suffering. The physical therapy, medical treatments, medications, oper-ations, surgeries, rehabilitation, chiropractor visits, acupuncture, and massages aren't working. The price tag of 600 billion dollars annually is one piece of evidence. Even more telling is that over half of the one hundred million people with chronic pain feel as though they have no control over that pain. [11, 39]

Where have we gone wrong? Have the experts failed us? Should doctors, physical therapists, chiropractors, and other health experts take the blame? I don't think so. We do the best we can; we're actually doing a remarkable job in terms of treatment. That's a key point.

The true failure lies in our understanding of how we have gotten to this point in the first place. We need to consider why we end up in so much physical pain so we can attempt to prevent it and, when it does occur, treat it more effectively. What is the real cause of physical pain? Is it really just a part of life? Is it genetics? Is it aging? Is it nutrition?

I suspect that, yes, all of these likely play a part. However, I have dedicated and spent more than half my life studying the nature of physical pain and injury. Both as a doctor specializing in sports medicine and as an athlete dealing with pain and injury myself, I have come to see one factor far above any other to be the leading cause of physical pain.

Physical pain is a physical problem. It is caused by physically misusing our bodies. Poor biomechanics, how we move, leads to pain. When speaking about physical pain in our bodies, we are speaking about the result of the physical damage we have caused them due to improper biomechanics. Since we each only get one body, this concept seems critical. Correctly moving your body is fundamental in treating and reducing the risk of pain and injury. How you use (move) your body will determine how you feel. [14, 15, 16]

It is really that simple. If you have back pain, it is because you don't understand how to use your back. If you have knee pain, it is because you don't know how to use your knee. Really, if you don't know how to use one area, you don't know how to use the whole thing. The body works as one machine. Either you know how to operate that machine, or you don't. You can't heal pain from Achilles tendinitis just by focusing on your lower leg. The underlying problem is far more likely to result from improper movement in multiple areas of your body.

Since the movement of your entire body affects pain in any part of your body, it really doesn't matter where your pain is. Fixing the movement of your entire body can treat or reduce the risk of damage caused by overworking certain areas of your body.

We need to understand what causes the type of damage we're talking about, whether it's tendinitis, joint pain from osteoarthritis, or another common injury or condition. Musculoskeletal pain occurs when you have pushed an area of your body past its physical ability by incorrectly using your body and placing undue stress on one or more specific parts. You have overworked and damaged certain areas, which are different for different people - and thus, you have pain. [14, 15, 16, 17, 18, 19, 20, 21, 22]

Pain is your body's way of saying, "Hey! Stop making this part work so hard. You already injured it, and you're continuing to wear it down!" If you don't stop, this physical damage will eventually become so great that it will be irreversible. In fact, that is why more than half of treatment, rehab, and physical therapy fail. The damage is already done! The cartilage in your joints has deteriorated, the discs in your back are destroyed, the tendons and connective tissue have become calcified and adhered...the list goes on and on. You can do all the rehab, take all the medications, and complete as much therapy as you want, and it will help some, but the honest truth is you can't reverse the damage you have already done. [23, 24, 25, 26, 27, 28, 29, 30, 31, 32]

What about surgery? It is unquestionably our best attempt to physically restore the damaged and thereby altered structures of the body back to their original state so as to remove the source of pain. However, surgery has two main problems. First, other damage can result when a surgeon cuts deep into your body and moves around to rearrange, cut, stitch, and staple various parts. Although new minimally invasive surgical techniques have improved, collateral damage often occurs. [33, 34, 35, 36, 37, 38]

The second reason surgery commonly fails, even after the damaged structure is repaired, is that the person continues to move and perform activities that had brought him or her to the injured, painful state in the first place. This goes back to the issue of poor biomechanics and the idea of the body moving as a unit. After surgery, the individual's body just returns to damaging itself again, either leading to re-injury of the same body part or a new injury caused by the wearing down of surrounding structures. Surgery is a good option in some cases, but it is far from a cure-all for physical pain conditions and injuries.

Prevention is the only true cure for our pain epidemic. We can reduce the risk of acquiring painful tissue damage by learning proper biomechanics, that is, how to move our bodies correctly [15, 16, 40, 41, 42, 43, 44, 45, 46, 47, 48, 49, 50, 51, 52, 53, 54, 55, 56, 57, 58, 59, 60, 61, 62, 63, 64, 65]. This knowledge needs to be ground into us, just as we learn other health habits like brushing our teeth to prevent decay and washing wounds to prevent infections. We can only do this through teaching each other. It's no different than driving a car. You may have the keys and the car, but you can't use it until you learn how to drive it. Everyone needs to learn how to drive this wonderful machine we call the human body. The exciting thing is that it is really not that hard. It just has to be learned. Just like we learn to read and write, we can learn to use and control our physical bodies.

HOW MANY MORE PEOPLE WILL SUFFER NEEDLESSLY BEFORE LEARNING HOW TO USE OUR BODIES BECOMES PART OF OUR WAY OF LIFE?

WHOM IS THE PREMIER BODY METHOD FOR?

PREMIER:

- Performance Ready
- Educational Movement Integration
- Enhancement and Rehabilitation

The PREMIER Body Method is for everyone. We all live in a world that presents physical challenges, and places stress on our bodies. Understanding how to use our bodies correctly is critical for living a healthy and pain-free life. Proper movement can prevent premature and accelerated degeneration and arthritis [66, 67, 68, 69, 70, 71, 72, 73, 74, 80]. It also allows for higher levels of physical performance [73, 75, 76, 77, 78, 79, 81, 82]. For all these reasons, The PREMIER Body Method is for everyone.

The PREMIER Body Method is for doctors, physical therapists, athletic trainers, sports performance coaches, strength and conditioning coaches, fitness and personal trainers, and anyone else responsible for treating, teaching, and/or training another's physical body. We encourage all practitioners to learn more about human movement and partake in our PREMIER Body Method seminar series designed specifically for practitioners. The certification program can be found online at http://www.PremierBodyMethod.com

The PREMIER Body Method is also for athletes wanting to achieve higher levels of sports performance. "Faster, higher, stronger" may be the goal, but it is only achievable when athletes are healthy and training effectively. Optimizing an athlete's performance requires a deep understanding of how the body works and how to utilize it to its full capacity. This is true in terms of improving performance and athletic skills and reducing the risk of injury [66-82]. In any sport, an improved understanding of the fundamentals of human movement and how to control the human body lifts athletic performance to another level. It is the difference between having a Ferrari with a two-year-old versus Mario Andretti behind the wheel.

The PREMIER Body Method isn't just for elite athletes but also for the millions of weekend warriors and others who want to live an active, healthy, and pain-free life.

Finally, The PREMIER Body Method is for all those suffering from pain and injury. It can be an acute traumatic injury, debilitating chronic pain, or simply those nagging aches and pains that keep you from focusing on your work, going to the gym, or enjoying time playing with your children. Have you ever wanted to do something but felt you couldn't because of your physical ability? Do you want to get back to an active life, go for a walk, run, hike? Do you wish you could still play tennis or basketball with friends? Do you wish you could still play with your children or grandchildren? The PREMIER Body Method is for you. It is for all of us.

The PREMIER Body Method will teach you how to use your body correctly and efficiently so you can stop fighting yourself by continually compensating. Finally, your body can work as a well-oiled machine as it should. Let's get started!

THE BEGINNING IDEAS

T he original idea for the PREMIER Body Method came from my vision of creating a complete system that works at all levels, from rehabilitation through exercise, strength, and conditioning. My unique experience as both a sports medicine doctor and a strength and conditioning sports performance coach allowed me to identify a large gap between basic rehab programs for injured athletes and the higher-level sports performance training these athletes need to achieve. I have had the privilege of working with some of the best orthopedists, sports medicine specialists, Chiropractors, physical therapists, strength and sports performance coaches, and athletes at all levels, all the way to the elite Olympic level. Throughout these experiences, I could not help but notice the vast gap that lay between two superb programs for athletes. Injured athletes received the best rehabilitation care possible, and healthy athletes received the best sports performance training possible. The problem was the lack of attention to intermediate levels, often leading to re-injury of the same condition or a new injury caused by continued mechanical compensation from the original injury [83, 97]. It became evident that this gap needed to be closed to provide a more complete system of progression between these two fields. I wanted to design a training system to bridge this gap, and that is how I got the idea for PREMIER.

Next, I thought about all the people, not necessarily elite-level athletes, who simply want to live a happy, healthy, pain-free life through exercise and physical fitness. I cannot tell you how many times I have had patients come to see me for injuries caused by fitness training. These people always stress that they want to become physically fit and healthy, but the pain caused by trying to do so prevents them from achieving their health and fitness goals. I have personally treated hundreds of patients in this situation. Still, the number pales in comparison to the millions of individuals who have injured themselves with exercise and fitness programs, classes, DVDs, and trainers, who have ended up not with improved long-term fitness but with pain in the back, neck, knee, hip, shoulder, or other places in the body. [84]

If you ask anyone who knows about injury, pain, and exercise, they will say that poor technique and incorrect movement are the most significant factors leading to injury [85, 86]. Once the individual experiences pain, performance declines, and progression stops.

Because injury results from poor technique, it makes sense that a complete yet simple system that teaches proper human biomechanics from the ground up could potentially reduce the risk of such injuries. I am proud to say that the PREMIER Body Method is this system. This idea continued to drive the development of the PREMIER system to not only be the bridge connecting rehab to sports performance but to make The PREMIER system a fully comprehensive program to train human movement mechanics from the most basic level all the way through a level of functional human fitness, and beyond. It is a system thorough enough to progress from injury to high-level function, yet simple enough that you don't have to be a high-level athlete to perform it nor have a doctorate degree to understand it.

INTRODUCTION TO HUMAN MOVEMENT EDUCATION

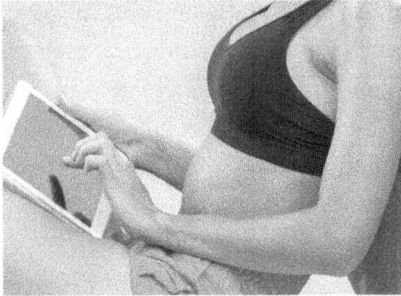

A PROGRESSION TO TEACH HUMAN MOVEMENT.

A PROGRESSION TO CORRECT DYSFUNCTION.

A PROGRESSION TO INCREASE PHYSICAL PERFORMANCE.

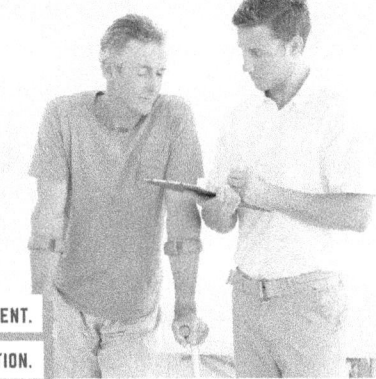

INTRODUCTION TO DYSFUNCTION

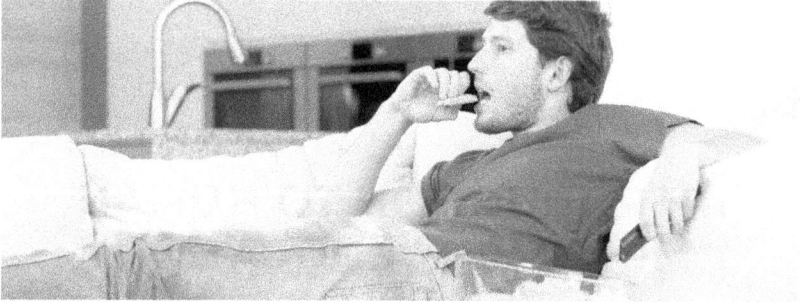

So what happened? How did we go from being a species that walked, ran, and climbed every day to being a population plagued by injuries and pain? Our laziness is one reason. Most of us sit at our computers, watch TV, drive, play video games, and take the elevator. As a result, the balance of our musculature changes. Our hip flexors become adaptively shortened, our abdominals and gluteus become inhibited and weak, and our hip external rotators and lumbar spine erectors become hypertonic ([87, 88, 89, 90]). This is just the tip of the iceberg. Our bodies become mechanically unbalanced, leading to faulty movement and undue extra stress on our joints, ligaments, and tendons. Over time, we develop predispositions to injury, early onset degenerative processes ("arthritis"), and all those chronic aches and pains. The situation has become so commonplace that many believe these pains and dysfunctions are just a normal part of life. How often have you heard you or someone else say, "I'm just getting old," or, "I'm a competitive athlete training really hard, so of course I will have some pain," or, "My body just wasn't born to do this type of exercise." We convince ourselves these problems are normal. They are not! They are common, yes, but not normal. Neuro-musculoskeletal pain is not normal. It is not something you are born with. It is something you have acquired. It is something you did to yourself! You did it because of dysfunctional biomechanics, which directly results from an unbalancing of the neuro-musculoskeletal system. And, you can undo it or, better yet, prevent it.
(15, 16, 40-65, 91)

The explanation above is a simplified description of just one cause of pain. In reality, there are many causes of dysfunction. Acute traumatic injury, chronic repetitive stress, activities of daily living, and athletic training and competition can all cause dysfunctional biomechanical patterns to take hold. Nonetheless, the end result is the same. Faulty mechanics set in and are repeated, and will lead to excessive stress on certain body tissues. Sooner or later, pain and injury may occur.

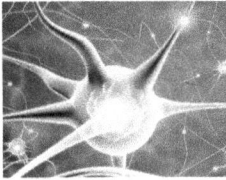

By retraining the neurology that controls the musculoskeletal system, we can teach our bodies to move and function correctly, as they were designed to [73, 74, 75, 78, 81, 82, 86, 87, 88, 92, 93, 94, 95, 96, 97, 98]. The process of rebalancing our neuro-musculoskeletal system can be a long and difficult process for some. It can be very tedious, especially in the beginning, but we must remember that we are training the neurology. This is what rehabilitation is. It is not just exercises to lengthen and strengthen muscles, but, instead, is neurological training to correct motor firing patterns. I believe that all training of the body must be done this way. This includes beginning-stage rehab, elite-level sports performance training, and everything in between. Always remember we are training the neurology. This takes a tremendous amount of focus and concentration. It is the attention and focus on the smallest details, the pursuit to perfect all movements during training, that makes the difference.

KEY CONCEPTS

Before we begin the PREMIER movement education system, we must understand several key concepts regarding how biomechanics and the neuro-musculoskeletal system work. As mentioned, mechanical dysfunction can occur due to various causes, such as muscle imbalance, tight or immobile muscles and connective tissue, or improper joint motion. Too much flexibility or mobility can also be a cause. Some mechanical dysfunction is caused by past injuries, while others are caused by seemingly insignificant amounts of continued repetitive stress from sports training, fitness regimens, or simple daily tasks. Genetic predisposition is another possible cause of dysfunction. There are many possible reasons for mechanical dysfunction, but the approach to preventing and mitigating them is the same. Retraining them for correction will be easier with an understanding of the following key concepts.

THE WHY FACTOR:

The first key concept you must understand is the why factor, as in why do you want to learn this stuff? Why do you want to learn how to use your body correctly? Another way to ask is, what is your motivation?

For many people, the answer is easy. I, for example, have always been obsessed with exercise, human performance, and physical fitness. I love this stuff! Many of you out there feel the same way. You love being active, in shape, and achieving higher and higher levels of physical ability and performance. For all the athletes out there, your 'why' is because you want to become better, stronger, faster, and more efficient and productive in your training and sport. Coaches and others who work with athletes have the same goals. Others find that their motivation is to look and feel good. You want to be lean, hard, and sexy. So, you are motivated by aesthetics. Or, you may want to live longer and have a higher quality of life. These can all be great why factors and fantastic motivators.

But for many others, you don't exactly love exercise. In fact, many of you out there flat-out hate it! So why do it? Why learn this stuff? Well, maybe it is because you are in pain, suffering from an injury or chronic condition. You have to think twice about going hiking with your friends or playing with your children because you simply hurt too much. You have tried everything else, and nothing has worked, so you are hoping this will finally be the answer to your long, terrible battle with pain. This can certainly be a motivating factor at first. However, I have two pieces of advice for you if you are motivated by pain and injury.

The first is to take responsibility. After my career working with so many unfortunate people suffering from pain, I have noticed one single factor differentiating those who succeed in overcoming their pain and those who fail. Surprisingly, it has little to do with the severity of the injury or condition. It is the ability to understand their role in their pain. Those who succeed are those who accept that the pain problem they have is theirs. They caused it, and it is their job, and their job alone, to correct it. Nobody can do it for them. Those who act as victims and don't take responsibility for themselves, those who expect someone else to magically fix it for them, are those who fail to get better. [99, 100, 101, 108]

The second piece of advice for those motivated by pain is to find a deeper motivation. Pain as motivation will only get you so far, especially if you are not even in pain yet. Ask yourself why you want to be pain and/or injury-free. Of course, no one likes to feel pain, and I'm not talking about that obvious answer. I'm talking about what that pain is taking away from you. I have had the pleasure and heartache of seeing, meeting, and working with so many people in my life, and pain steals a lot of important moments and memories. Some of the true costs of pain might be not being able to run around and play with your children or grandchildren, not being able to play that round of golf with your buddies, not being able to go on that evening walk with your significant other, not being able to spend hours at the mall with your girlfriends, not being able to travel on a plane or ride in a car for fear of pain, and not being able work and be a productive member of society and your community. These are wonderful moments and joys that pain will steal from you. Time and time again, I have seen these moments taken away from so many people. Keeping such moments in mind can help you stay motivated to complete The PREMIER Body Method and overcome your condition [Disclaimer #].

It has been one of the true pleasures of my career to watch these simple life joys we all take for granted come back into people's lives, and it has happened through The PREMIER Body Method.

I genuinely want all of us to understand that many of these pleasures don't need to be taken away in the first place. We must have the vision and foresight to look ten, twenty, thirty, forty, fifty years, and even further down the road into the future of our lives, and not take these simple pleasures for granted. It is not easy for someone in their teens or twenties, but imagine being seventy years old and unable to go for a walk outside. Imagine not being able to go to your grandson's baseball game because you can no longer climb the stairs in the bleachers without knee pain. Imagine needing assistance every time you need to get up from a chair, in and out of your bed, or on and off the toilet. It seems so weird and terrible to think about, so we don't, but this is how many of us end up. It doesn't have to be that way. [102, 103, 104, 105, 106, 107, 109, 110]

So the next time you think about why you want to learn about and train your body, think about the why factor. Think about your children and grandchildren. Think about traveling the world with your loved ones. Think about going for that hike or playing that round of golf.

Think about a long, happy life with your family and friends. Think about enjoying all those things we take for granted *before* they are taken away from us. Even if you are not inhibited by pain or decreased functional ability now, it's worth your while to act to prevent pain from coming later. It's no different than brushing your teeth. You brush your teeth every day not because you like scratching bristles against them but because you are smart enough to know that it will help prevent your teeth from falling out a few decades from now [111, 112, 113]. Moving and moving well should be accepted as standard preventive care in life, just like brushing your teeth and putting on sunscreen. So what's the Why Factor? Why move and move well? Because life demands it of us.

SEE, LIFE IS A SPORT, AND JUST LIKE ANY OTHER SPORT, IF YOU WANT TO BE SUCCESSFUL AT IT, YOU HAVE TO TEACH AND TRAIN YOUR BODY TO DO SO.

THE LAW OF 100% MOTION:

Every movement produced by the body has what I like to think of as 100% motion, which is necessary to produce that particular movement. Anything from a full-on sprint to an old man getting up from a chair takes 100% motion to produce the given movement. This 100% represents the workload or stress the body must endure to produce that particular movement. The body naturally divides the given motion between its structures, such as various muscles, tendons, ligaments, joints, cartilage, bones, and fascia. [114, 115, 116, 117, 118, 119, 120, 121, 122, 123, 124, 125, 126, 127, 128]

Let's take a squat as an example. The ankles and their associated musculature and other structures get 10% of the workload necessary to produce this movement, the knees get 20%, the hips 30%, the back 10%, and so on, until 100% is reached, and the movement is produced. Now, let's say that due to prior injury, structural abnormality, or length-strength imbalance, the hip is only able or willing to put out 20% instead of its usual 30%. The Law of 100% Motion states that production of the movement still requires 100%; that 10% deficit in the hip cannot disappear. Other structures must make up for that 10% by taking it on. For example, maybe the knee tries to step up by working harder. Now, instead of the knee performing its expected 20%, it performs 30% of the workload. This would be what we call a compensation pattern. It may work for a while, but eventually, the tissues and structures of the knee will begin to wear down and become overworked and stressed, and sooner or later, pain and/or injury will occur. [129, 130, 131, 132, 133, 134, 135, 136, 137, 138, 139, 140, 141, 142, 143, 144, 145]

Another way to think of this is as Person A and Person B, two partners working on a project together. If Person B were always out taking a coffee break, leaving Person A to do all of the work, Person A might be able to complete the work for a while, but sooner or later, something would happen. Person A could become sick and tired of doing all the work and quit. Or, Person A could have a nervous breakdown from being overworked. Or, Person A might start getting behind on the work. This is exactly how compensation patterns work. [146]

THE NEUROLOGICAL FIRING PATTERN:

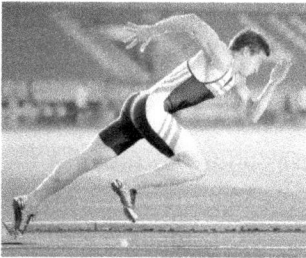

To better understand the musculoskeletal system and the neurology that controls it, we first need to understand how movement occurs on a neurological level. Every movement the body produces has its own unique, eloquent, nearly instantaneous firing pattern. Whether it is an Olympic sprinter running 25+ miles per hour down a track or a 75-year-old woman reaching to get a glass out of her kitchen cupboard, every movement follows a firing pattern. A neurological firing pattern represents the order of electrical signals coming from the central nervous system, down the spinal cord, and out to the peripheral nervous system, telling all of our muscles, joints, ligaments, tendons, blood vessels, and more, what to do, how to do it, and when. It's a complex and carefully orchestrated process. [147, 148]

For example, consider the woman reaching to get the glass out of the cupboard. She lifted her arm to shoulder height, grasped the glass, and then lowered her arm. How many neurological signals did that take? It took much more than can be fit into this book, but here is a summary. To lift her arm, first, all of the scapular stabilizing muscles, upper trapezius, mid trapezius, lower trapezius, serratus anterior, rhomboids, pectoralis minor, and levator scapulae had to stabilize the shoulder blade against the thoracic rib cage. Then all of the rotator cuff muscles, supraspinatus, infraspinatus, teres minor, and subscapularis, had to come on at the precise moment in just the right order to initiate the roll and slide of the humeral head in the glenoid and control the glenohumeral (GH, or shoulder ball and socket) joint. Then, the prime movers, the deltoid, pectoral muscles, biceps, and triceps, go to work to lift the upper extremity. These are just the muscles being activated. Many muscles, such as the latissimus dorsi, are simultaneously inhibited to allow the arm to move up into abduction and flexion without fighting against the opposing muscles [149, 150]. Before all of this, the core muscles, puborectalis, pubococcygeus, iliococcygeus, transverse, oblique, rectus abdominus, quadratus luborum, erector spinae, and other deeper spinal stabilizers, all had to activate in order to keep the body upright as more weight (the arm) is moved further away from the body's center of mass. We will not even get into the lower extremities, but as I'm sure you can guess, the legs are working and receiving signals, too! [151, 152, 153, 154, 155, 156, 157]

That was all just the efferent (neurological signals leaving the central nervous system heading out to the peripheral body) output. Now, think of all the afferent (neurological signals coming from the peripheral body back to the central nervous system) feedback happening during this motion. There is constant proprioceptive and sensory feedback coming from the joints, muscles, tendons, and everything else, telling the brain that the body is safe and not being harmed and that this movement is okay to continue and does not need to be altered. We are talking about hundreds, if not thousands, of neurological signals, occurring in a fraction of a second, in a very specific and well-controlled sequence, to produce this simple motion. The complete list of neuro-muscular events that allowed this lady to lift her arm is even more complex, but you get the idea. [158, 159, 160, 161]

. . .

So, what is biomechanical dysfunction? It occurs because of theloss of control of movement. Neurologically speaking, the motor firing pattern is dysfunctional. In other words, the order of signals is messed up. Perhaps something fires too late, too early, or on time but at the wrong level of strength, causing too much or insufficient contraction, and so forth. So, if the proper order is 1-2-3-4-5-6-7, a dysfunctional motor firing pattern might be 1-3-2-6-5-4-7. The disruption creates holes in the system, causing some structures to be underutilized and forcing other structures to be overworked. This alters the percent of workload and stress endured by these structures as stated by the Law of 100% Motion. Structures forced to take on excess stress will be injured and cause pain. This will then cascade into many other alterations and compensation patterns, which, over time, will create even more dysfunction and pain. It all snowballs from here! [162, 163, 164, 165, 166]

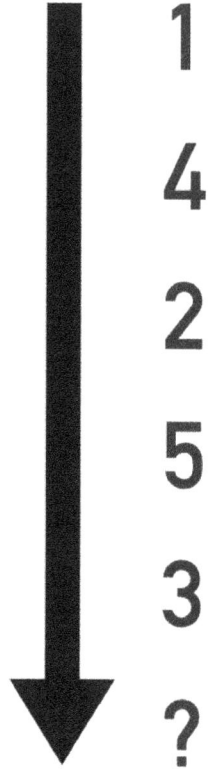

1
4
2
5
3
?

Pain itself can cause an altered firing pattern [167, 168, 169]. The human body will alter its function tremendously to avoid pain. This is another form of compensation, as pain can create a hole in the system. As an example, suppose your movement is completely biomechanically correct to begin with, but at the age of twelve, you sprain your ankle playing basketball. This freak traumatic injury that caused pain has caused you to alter your gait with a limp in order to avoid the pain. Your limp is the obvious compensation. The less obvious one is the underlying movement avoidance your body will remember. Unless you retrain your body correctly, whatever movements your body was performing at the time of injury will be automatically programmed to be avoided in the future from this point on because your body wants to avoid this painful situation from happening again. [170, 171, 172, 173]

You heal soon enough from the ankle sprain, but some neurological and musculoskeletal compensation patterns are retained. In other words, you are left with some holes in the system, which may eventually lead to biomechanical dysfunction down the road.

Sound too complicated and far-fetched? Let's stick with the ankle sprain at age twelve as an example. After the injury heals a few weeks later, this ankle is left with some scar tissue, causing a slightly decreased dorsiflexion (flexing the foot up) range of motion on that side [174, 175, 176]. One of the main compensatory patterns for an ankle with decreased dorsiflexion is an external rotation of the lower leg. This can come from the knee, but since the knee doesn't rotate very easily, the simplest answer for the body is at the hip. So let's say from age twelve to around the age of thirty, this person has been ever so slightly over-activating his/her external rotator muscle group of the hip in order to achieve a slight increase in lower leg external rotation, allowing the ankle to "cheat" since this ankle cannot achieve the proper amount of dorsiflexion. [177, 178, 179, 180]

This compensation pattern worked for eighteen years, from age twelve to thirty. However, during this time, the extra activity of the hip external rotator group, particularly the piriformis, has caused a very minor yet repeated and unbalanced tug and torque on the SI joints in the lower back. The piriformis muscle not only works to rotate the hip joint but also crosses the SI joint in the lower back. Over time, these small repetitive stresses finally add up to take their toll. Now, this person has SI joint (lower back) pain seemingly out of nowhere [181, 182, 183, 184]. This person may choose to seek help at this point from doctors, medications, or other specialists. Hopefully, the specialists will figure out the problem and correct the person's biomechanical dysfunction, starting with the improvement of ankle dorsiflexion. Unfortunately, this is rarely the case.

What if the problem is not figured out, or if the person just decides to live with it? The person can probably get by a few more years, possibly with mild back pain that comes and goes, but the cascade of compensation will continue. This person's mechanics will change and compensate again to avoid the SI joint pain. The core and glutes will become inhibited and dysfunctional, causing more loading stress in the lower back and spine [185, 186, 187, 188, 189, 190]. Now this person is forty and has become more sedentary to avoid continuous lumbar spine facet joint pain. He stops going to the gym and avoids weekend hikes to reduce the chance of aggravating his back pain. Avoidance of physical activity has resulted in the deterioration of physical health. He repeatedly takes over-the-counter pain medications, which have caused physiologic changes in the gastrointestinal tract, liver, and kidneys. Nutritional deficits ensue. Health continues to decline. We will not even get into the emotional and mental detriment caused by chronic pain and continued deterioration of health that begins to take place by the age of fifty and continues for decades. This is all because of a simple ankle sprain at age twelve. Come on, really, that can't be correct, can it? [191, 192, 193]

I see it every day. I am not saying it is just like this for everyone. This is just one of the infinite possibilities for dysfunction. It is a very simple example, but possible – and even likely - nonetheless. Each person has his own dysfunctional path with many factors to consider, but the end result is typically the same; pain, declining health, depression, poor quality of life, and hopelessness.

MOTOR LEARNING:

As we have just seen, motor firing patterns are very complex. You may be surprised to learn that you are not born with your nerves and muscles completely knowing how to execute these complicated firing patterns. While the human body has many innate functions, many of these patterns are actually learned. This concept is known as motor learning or muscle memory. Each movement produced by the body has its own unique firing pattern; this specific firing pattern repeats each time you perform that movement. Neurology learns by repetition. So, the more times a particular firing pattern runs, the more ingrained it will become. [194, 195, 196]

This can be either good or bad, depending on the motion or firing pattern being ingrained. Suppose the movement is biomechanically correct and thus safe for human tissues. In that case, ingraining the pattern is good because your body will automatically be firing in such a way as to prevent excess tissue damage and injury. If the pattern produces inefficient and potentially damaging movement, then ingraining it is bad. Motor learning can just as easily work for or against us.

A CONCEPT FOR CORRECTION

The idea of ingraining neuromuscular firing patterns is fundamental to The PREMIER Body Method. It suggests that when mechanics become dysfunctional, all we have to do is correct the firing pattern. It sounds simple in theory, but how easy is it in practice? There is no quick answer to this question. One approach is to identify the dysfunctional portion of the movement and then correct it. In other words, find the signals in the firing pattern that are out of order from the correct sequence and then retrain them to once again fire in their proper order. This is, in fact, what many good rehabilitation and physical therapy programs currently do. Experts watch movement patterns, assess mechanics, and develop movement-screening systems. This has potential, but as illustrated in our example of the woman lifting her arm to reach a glass, we are talking about hundreds or more signals happening in fractions of a second. So, if you think you can find the one, five, one hundred, or however many signals that are out of the correct sequence just by watching a person move, you are doing better than most, and I can't wait to take your class. [197, 198, 199, 200, 201, 202, 203, 204, 205, 206]

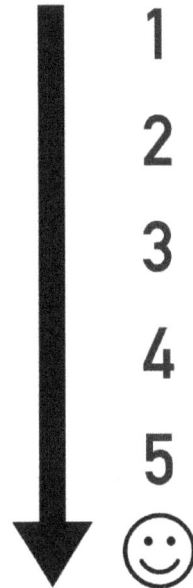

I like to use the building-a-house analogy. Improper firing patterns are like having an old house with many problems. The house has termites in the walls, flooding in the basement, leaks in the roof, cracks in the floors, and broken windows. Is it more effective to try to find, fix, and patch up all of these problems, or should we just start over and build a new house from the ground up?

THE **PREMIER** BODY METHOD IS BUILDING A FUNCTIONAL HUMAN BEING FROM THE GROUND UP THROUGH HUMAN MOVEMENT EDUCATION.

In this method, you do not look for each dysfunction, faulty pattern, and disordered signal. Instead, you build human movement from the beginning so that it is free from dysfunction. Along the way, you will find many holes and dysfunctions in the system. Had you tried to look for specifics, you would have missed many others. In the retraining process, you can find and correct all of them. The same system applies to everyone but becomes specialized for each individual. The system adapts as the trainee progresses through it. Trainees go through the same control and movement exercises, but their specific dysfunctions become evident as they progress and can be repaired or retrained accordingly.

For example, let's say one trainee is performing a bridge movement control exercise. For this person, gluteal activation on the right seems to be faulty. Naturally, this should be one of the main aspects for this individual to focus on during this exercise. Now, take a second trainee performing the same gluteal bridge movement control exercise. The hole in *this* system is this person's faulty pelvic position due to insufficient Core Control. This individual will need to make this aspect of control the focus. Thus, the same movement pattern exercise by name has two completely different focuses for two distinct individuals. The first trainee needs to concentrate on gluteal activation, and the second must focus on pelvic control. In both cases, The PREMIER Body Method identifies each of these people's incorrect movements and the distinct faulty firing patterns that are causing them.

We are training fundamental human movement, the control of that movement, and then the strength and endurance of that control to continue that movement throughout daily life and activity. It's not enough to know the proper way to move; you must also be physically able to do so. This requires a basic level of strength and conditioning.

We are training fundamental human movement from the most basic and primitive level all the way through to large complex human motions such as squatting, pulling, pressing, lifting, running, or jumping. The end goal for most trainees will be to reach a basic level of human function and fitness, which often means uninhibited daily activities and the ability to exercise regularly. For some, the objective will be to reach a higher level of conditioning to perform better as an athlete.

The end stage of the PREMIER Body Method is a basic strength and conditioning workout routine. Each level and each step leading up to this stage is a smaller component necessary to produce the movement to follow at the next level. It is in this way, building from the ground up, teaching components of human biomechanics, building off smaller pieces to larger motions until we reach the large human movement level, that we can rebuild functionally performing people with no more holes in their systems, or at least as few holes as possible.

STRUCTURAL LIMITS:

So far, we have been speaking about a true movement pattern dysfunction as the root cause of the problem. We've identified that neuro-biomechanical imbalance alters the workload of various tissue structures, causing some structures to perform at less than full capacity, thereby forcing other structures to perform beyond normal capacity. Structures performing beyond capacity eventually give out and become damaged, causing pain and injury. [207, 208, 209, 210, 211, 212]

A patient once asked me a very intuitive question: "If these harder-working tissues have to work beyond normal capacity, why don't they just adapt and get stronger to handle the workload? That way, everything would be fine." What a great question and thought! This does, in fact, happen for a time and to a certain extent. However, the human body is all about balance. From homeostasis to length and strength to yin and yang, it is all about balance. As long as you are within the limits of balance, tissues will respond, adapt, change, conform, and grow stronger. When you work out the right way, you get bigger, stronger, and faster. Only when one goes beyond the limits of balance does positive adaptive change become negative deterioration and destruction. [213, 214, 215, 216, 217, 218, 219, 220, 221, 222, 223]

When discussing the limitations of the neuro-musculoskeletal system, we are talking about the structural limits of the tissues. As we are born, grow, and develop, we receive or achieve a specific set of **physical capability limits** [224, 225, 226, 227, 228]. These limits will determine our potential physical abilities, such as how fast, strong, and coordinated we are, how tall we are, how much we weigh, how much endurance we have, what we look like, and so on. These limits are based in large part on the structures and the physiologic processes that create the structures, such as the shape of our bones, how long and thick they are, their contours, where our tendons and ligaments attach, how thick and strong the tensile strength is, etc. [229, 230, 231, 232, 233, 234, 235, 236, 237, 238]. Of course, we all have the same basic anatomy, but we are all individually different. Your femur might be an inch longer than mine; my patellar tendon might attach one inch below the patella, while yours might attach an eighth of an inch closer. We are all slightly different and individualized. This is why some people are bigger, stronger, and faster. These individual anatomical differences shape the boundaries of our physical capability limits.

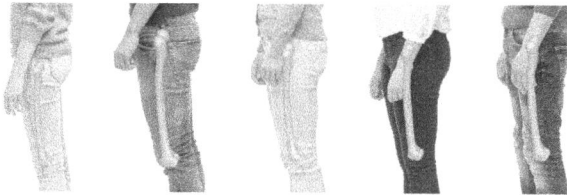

These limits may be enhanced and developed to a certain extent; however, you must stay within the balance of your physical capability limits. Stress, overload, and structural damage are inevitable when one's body structures are pushed beyond the given set limits. [239, 240, 241, 242, 243, 244]

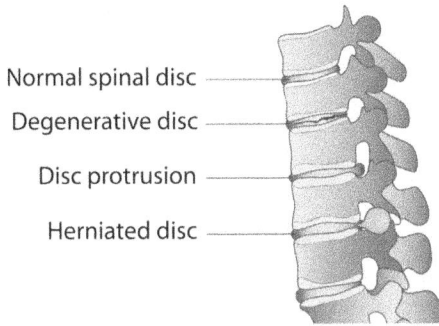

Normal spinal disc
Degenerative disc
Disc protrusion
Herniated disc

As certain structures become damaged, their physical form changes. Fancy medical terms like degenerative disc disease, facet arthropathy, disc bulge or herniation, meniscus tears, labral tears, osteoarthritis, radiculopathy, and nerve impingement are just descriptions of changes to structures of the body. The term 'degenerative disc disease' means that the cartilage and fibrous bands of the discs (annular fibers) between the vertebrae of the spine have begun to deteriorate and break down. Their height, width, elasticity, and rigidity are different. In other words, their structural shape has changed. [245, 246, 247, 248, 249, 250, 251, 252, 253]

Arthritis in your joints is usually due to the wear and tear of your joints' articular cartilage, which cushions and allows for smooth motion in your joints. The shape and structure of this articular cartilage has physically changed in arthritic conditions, mainly osteoarthritis or degenerative joint disease. What is causing this structural change? The change results from repetitive stress on these structures from the workload that movement demands [254, 255, 256, 257, 258, 259, 260, 261, 262, 263, 264]. Think of it like rocks in a river.

JUST AS ROCKS IN A RIVER CHANGE THEIR SHAPE TO BECOME SMOOTHER OVER TIME DUE TO THE STRESS OF THE WATER FLOWING PAST, SO DO THE STRUCTURES OF THE HUMAN BODY CHANGE THEIR SHAPE OVER TIME DUE TO THE STRESS FROM MOVEMENT.

This stress is not necessarily due to high-impact athletic training; it is often the result of normal daily movement in regular daily life.

So, what happens when the structure changes? The answer is that the physical capability limits change because they are based on structure. It does not matter if the tissue change resulted from a chronic biomechanical dysfunction, an instantaneous traumatic injury, or both. I would go so far as to say that it doesn't matter if the limit change came from a congenital structural abnormality. The fact is that the physical structures have changed, so their physical capability limits have changed. [265, 266, 267, 268, 269, 270, 271, 272, 273, 274, 275]

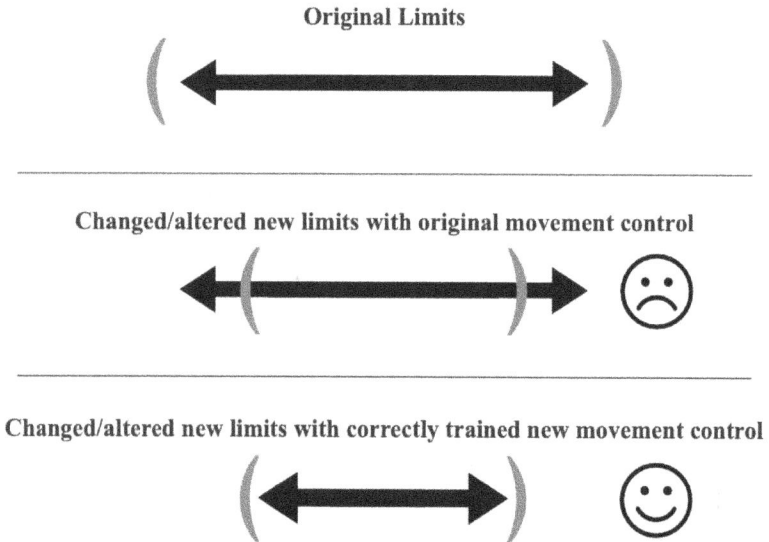

Original Limits

Changed/altered new limits with original movement control

Changed/altered new limits with correctly trained new movement control

The problem with these changes occurs in the control of movement. That's because although physical capability limits have changed, the neurology controlling the movement has not changed to match the new structure. The control still operates within the original or "normal" set of limits, allowing movement to overstep the new limits. Your old movement patterns are placing demands beyond the newly established physical capability limits set forth by your changed, damaged, and altered structures. This means a continual stressing of the limits, the tissues, and continued chronic pain/dysfunction. [276, 277, 278, 279, 280, 281, 282, 283]

A non-injured person can train their body to move correctly within their own unique physical capability limits, decreasing the probability of excessive damage. They can live a happy life with minimal pain. The approach is similar for an injured person. A considerable part of retraining biomechanics from the ground up using this program requires learning the new set of limits given the pathology involved.

THE INJURED PERSON MUST LEARN HUMAN BIOMECHANICS SPECIFIC TO THEIR LIMITS AND STRUCTURAL CHANGES BASED ON INDIVIDUAL PATHOLOGY, ALTERATIONS, AND DAMAGE TO PHYSICAL STRUCTURES.

Let's look at a practical example of this limit concept. We will use the simple spinal condition of L/S facet syndrome, which is caused by overloading the facet joints of the spine [284, 285, 286]. This is usually due to repetitive extension-type movement patterns. If it continues long enough, this repetitive stress on the facet joints can cause facet arthropathy.

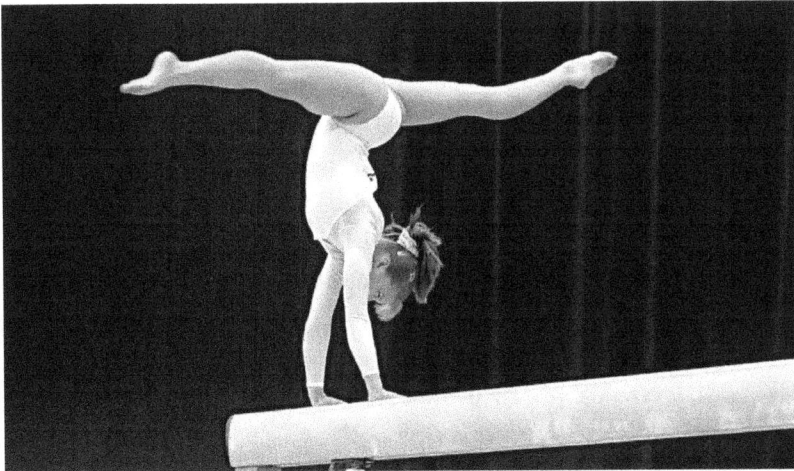

Facet arthropathy is a type of degenerative joint disease (DJD) to the facet joints [287, 288, 289, 290]. DJD is a form of structural change to the joints involved as the body adapts to the excessive stress taken on by those joints, just like the river stone changing shape because of the flowing water. The person with L/S facet syndrome has essentially been performing excessive and repetitive extension patterns for years, and her joints have been worn down. Though she may have originally had 30 degrees of pain-free lumbar spine extension, she may now feel pain in as little as 10 degrees of extension in these joints. Since the structure has changed, the limits the structure can handle have changed [291, 292, 293, 294, 295]. The neurology controlling the movement likely has not changed to an equal extent, so this person's daily movements push her past the new limits of structure and thus continue to stress the tissues, in this case, the facet joints. Pain and damage continue. The problem will remain unresolved and continue to progress until the control of the movement is retrained to allow the movement patterns this person is utilizing to stay within the new structural limits.

The PREMIER Body Method of Human Movement Education is designed to retrain movement, specifically the CONTROL of move-ment, tailored to an individual's acquired structural changes. It is also designed to teach human movement to operate in a tissue-sparing manner. Focusing on functional biomechanics will decrease the likeli-hood of structural changes and adaptations from repetitive stress. This will help preserve the limits of the body's structural capacity. For these reasons, The PREMIER Body Method can be used as an injury preven-tion program. It can also be used as an anti-aging training system by decreasing the probability of structural body damage or degeneration (aging) caused by excessive tissue loading. [1043]

Take a second to imagine if we taught this to each other from the very beginning. We teach everything else: language, reading, writing, and mathematics. Why don't we teach how to move properly around our world? Why isn't this in the primary grade school curriculum? How many of these neuro-musculoskeletal issues could be avoided? How much degenerative joint disease and how many painful arthritic processes could be decreased?

PAIN

Think about how pain affects movement. As mentioned, the human body will go to extraordinary lengths to avoid pain. For example, the body will adopt compensation patterns that alter movement to prevent or minimize pain. On a neuro-musculoskeletal level, this involves inhibition of muscle activation during movements or postures in which pain occurs [296, 297, 298, 299, 300, 301]. The results of compensation patterns during chronic pain syndromes are visible on MRI images, as muscular integrity surrounding pain generators show atrophy. The extent of atrophy depends on the severity and duration of the pain, with greater atrophy seen in cases of longer duration of pain. [302, 303, 304, 305, 306, 307, 308, 309, 310, 435]

In less clinical terms, the body interprets pain as negative and subconsciously works to inhibit or discontinue situations, including movement, that cause pain. Thus, if a particular movement produces pain, the body will program itself to avoid it in the future and adopt a compensatory movement strategy in its place. When teaching human movement, all training must be done free from pain if it is to be productive.

THE OLD FOOTBALL COACH MENTALITY OF "NO PAIN, NO GAIN" IS WRONG!

If you are attempting to train motor learning through pain, the firing pattern will never be thoroughly ingrained because the pain itself will continually inhibit the very movement you are trying to learn. We are trying to teach the body healthy, safe positions and movements. If the trainee feels pain during the position or movement being performed, it is the exact opposite of what we are trying to accomplish.

NEVER TRAIN THROUGH PAIN!

ACTIVE AND PASSIVE TISSUES:

The body needs to create a certain level of force to produce any movement. This force production translates to increased load and stress distributed among the various tissue structures of the body. To effectively train human movement, we need to understand where this loading stress is going. The stress is going to be placed into one of two categories of human tissue: either active structures or passive structures. The active structures are what you are actively in control of --the muscles. The passive structures are all the other structural components, which include the joints, cartilage, ligaments, tendons, bones, fascia, and everything else. Active and passive structures differ in how they respond to the workload or stress.

Muscles are tissues in the active structure category; they respond well to physical stress. Muscles regenerate themselves efficiently and relatively quickly when broken down due to physical stress. They are physiologically designed to do this repeatedly and for our entire lives. The old saying that "Muscles don't age" is true in this respect. Muscles can be broken down and exhausted to a point, and they will recover and regenerate over and over again. Often, the regenerated muscles can become better than they were before! That's the concept of training. Think about it. You work out at the gym and damage your muscles, you're sore for a day or two, and a few days later, you return to the gym stronger than you were before because your muscles have responded to training. Amazing! [311, 312, 313, 314, 315, 316, 317, 318, 319, 320, 321, 322]

In contrast, the tissues in the passive category do not regenerate themselves nearly as well or as fast when broken down due to physical stress. Some of the passive structures, such as certain areas and types of cartilage, will barely regenerate themselves at all. The way I like to think about it is muscles have an unlimited gas tank in terms of longevity if treated correctly. The passive structures have a limited gas tank. Once the tank for the passive structures is empty, that is it. Now you have problems, including degenerative joint disease, degenerative disc disease, disc herniation, nerve pathology, meniscal tears in the knee, labral tears in the hips and shoulders, arthritis, tendinitis, ligament sprains and tears, and many more. [323, 324, 325, 326, 327, 328, 329, 330, 331, 332, 333, 334, 335, 336, 337, 338, 339, 340, 341]

This tells us that we want the force, load, and stress to go on muscles, not passive structures. We need movement to direct the loading stress in favor of the active structures, thus helping to preserve the passive structures as much as possible. The ability to do this creates the distinction between healthy, tissue-sparing, biomechanically correct human movement and unsafe, tissue-wasting, biomechanically incorrect human movement.

WHEN THE FORCES CREATED BY A PARTICULAR MOVEMENT ARE PLACED ON THE ACTIVE STRUCTURES AS MUCH AS POSSIBLE FOR THAT GIVEN MOTION, THEN THE MOVEMENT IS TISSUE-SPARING AND, THUS, BIOMECHANICALLY CORRECT. WHEN THE WORKLOAD PRODUCTION THAT CAN AND SHOULD BE PERFORMED BY THE ACTIVE STRUCTURES IS NOT, AND THEREFORE IS ALLOWED TO TRANSFER INTO LOADING STRESS ON THE PASSIVE STRUC-TURES, THE MOVEMENT IS TISSUE-WASTING AND, THUS, BIOMECHANICALLY INCORRECT AND UNSAFE.

Proper human mechanics should work to take advantage of this distinction in tissue types, not use it against us. By teaching efficient tissue-sparing movement, this program teaches anti-aging mechanics, in which the passive tissues of the body are spared as much as possible. [342, 343, 855, 856, Disclaimer #]

MOVEMENT CONTROL:

Whether you are the average person training to succeed at the sport of life or an elite-level athlete training for a specific sport, the ultimate goal is always to train movement to be more efficient.

You could be training a more efficient squatting pattern so you can stand up and down from a chair without pain [344, 345, 346]. Maybe you are training a more efficient clean-and-jerk pattern so you can jump higher to slam-dunk the basketball in the game [347, 348]. It does not matter; the fundamental goal of all training is to become better, or more efficient, at whatever the goal is. Strength, speed, power, endurance, and agility are all aspects of movement that require control to achieve their full potential. Training the control of movement is the basis of it all.

I like the analogy of having a Ferrari with a two-year-old sitting behind the steering wheel. Here you have one of the most powerful, fast, agile machines on the planet, but with a two-year-old at the controls, it will all go to waste. Now, if we take the two-year-old out and put Mario Andretti behind the wheel, this becomes a very powerful, fast, and well-controlled machine capable of extraordinary performance. Human performance, whether for general life or sport, works the same way. All of the strength, speed, power, endurance, flexibility, and agility in the world are worthless if uncontrolled. We must train the control of movement first, above anything else.

FATIGUE FACTOR:

Fatigue is a critical factor in human movement and exercise. The two basic types of fatigue to understand for this program are muscular fatigue and neurologic fatigue. Understanding the difference between these two types of fatigue is essential to this program.

The first type of fatigue is muscular. This is felt as your muscles become worked. Muscle energy is depleted, lactic acid builds, and a burning or exhausted feeling sets in. With training, you can recover quickly from muscular fatigue. This is the type of fatigue we welcome during training because it will stimulate our bodies to adapt and grow stronger. [349, 350, 351, 352, 353, 354, 355, 356]

The second type of fatigue is neurologic. This is the fatigue responsible for the control, or lack of control, of movement. Once neurologic fatigue sets in, control of the movement being performed will be lost, and thus, the movement pattern will adapt, compensate, and change to a new movement strategy. This may or may not be okay, depending on the alteration of movement. If the compensatory movement is tissue-sparing and biomechanically "safe," then it is fine. However, if the compensatory movement is harmful to body tissues and biomechanically "unsafe," then it is not fine. Imagine a marathon runner towards the end of a race. He is becoming more and more exhausted, and his running mechanics are getting worse and worse. His muscles are fatiguing, yes; however, it is the control over his movement that will create long-term problems for him as his mechanics become compensated. He is suffering from both muscular and neurologic fatigue, but the neurologic fatigue is much more concerning. [357, 358, 359, 360, 361, 362, 363, 364, 365, 366, 367, 368, 436]

In my experience, nearly all compensatory movement during neurologic fatigue is the "unsafe" kind. As this fatigue sets in, neurologic output to the motor points in muscles decreases, causing muscle contraction capacity to reduce and become more difficult to perform. If the muscles cannot produce enough force and power to generate the movement pattern effectively, where is this force and load transferred instead? That's right, if it is not going to the active tissues (muscles), it goes to the passive tissues: joints, cartilage, ligaments, and tendons.

WHENEVER THE WORKLOAD PRODUCTION THAT CAN AND SHOULD BE PERFORMED BY MUSCLES IS TRANSFERRED TO JOINTS, CARTILAGE, LIGAMENTS, OR TENDONS, THE MOVEMENT IS CONSIDERED TISSUE-WASTING AND THUS BIOMECHANICALLY "UNSAFE."

Now, let us apply these concepts to human movement education. As we teach and train movement mechanics, remember that we are training new neurological firing patterns to produce the given movement we want. Training neurological firing patterns will, at some point, create neurologic fatigue for that pattern. Once neurologic fatigue sets in, the firing pattern can no longer be performed, so it will adapt to a new and undesired firing pattern. This will create a different or compensatory movement pattern. Once this change occurs, you are no longer practicing and training the correct firing pattern and biomechanics you want, thus defeating the purpose of training.

IF YOU'RE GOING TO EFFECTIVELY TRAIN HUMAN MOVEMENT MECHANICS, YOU CAN NEVER FORCE PAST NEUROLOGIC FATIGUE.

All of these firing patterns, neurologic signals, and compensatory movements may sound complex, but they are simple from a practical application standpoint. As soon as you reach the point where you can no longer perform the movement with perfect control and, therefore, correct form, you have reached the neurologic fatigue point. If you try to push beyond this point and squeeze a few more reps out, the neurological pattern will change, and thus the movement mechanics will change. You will no longer be practicing what you are trying to learn. Remember, neurology learns through repetition, motor learning, and muscle memory. If you are no longer repeating the correct pattern after neurological fatigue sets in, you are not ingraining the desired pattern. Worse, you are likely ingraining an "unsafe" tissue-wasting pattern

When retraining an injury or pain condition, the pattern I see most trainees revert to after hitting neurological fatigue is the faulty biomechanical movement pattern that created the dysfunction in the first place. When tired, your body will naturally revert to what is most familiar. Continuing to push past the neurologic fatigue point during human movement education will not only be worthless in the sense you are no longer ingraining new, correct patterns, but you will likely reinforce the already very-well-ingrained faulty patterns that first got you in trouble.

DO NOT TRAIN MOVEMENT PAST NEUROLOGIC FATIGUE.

WHAT MUSCLES REALLY DO:

So far, we have been talking about muscles as active structures and key players in proper movement, so let's ensure we understand how they work. Let's briefly discuss how the musculoskeletal system works from a mechanical standpoint. First, what do muscles do? What they do is very simple. They pull on bones. They pull bones together, and they pull bones apart. However, when considering how effective these muscles are at pulling on bones, there are two critical questions. First, do the muscles have a solid foundation from which to pull? Second, from what position/angle are they pulling? [369, 370, 371, 372, 373, 374, 375, 376, 377]

Let's first talk about having a solid foundation from which to pull. Suppose two bones are going to either be pulled together or pulled apart by a muscle. In that case, the pulling can and will happen much more efficiently when one of the bones is held fixed, thus providing a solid foundation for the muscle to pull in order to move the other bone. The fixed bone providing the solid foundation may be relative depending on the body position and the movement taking place. Imagine playing a game of tug of war with a friend of equal size and strength. However, during the first match, you are told to stand on one foot, while your friend is allowed to stand on both feet. Who do you suppose will win this pulling match? Obviously, your friend has a clear advantage because they have a more solid foundation to pull from. This is a simple example, but it is very applicable to the way our muscles operate depending on how they are being used. When proper mechanics are taking place and muscles have a solid foundation to pull from, they can generate a lot of force very efficiently and do their job well. If these muscles do not have a solid base to pull from, it will be like trying to win a tug-of-war match on one foot. The muscles will be unable to generate the force they need to create the movement efficiently and thus will have to work much harder. For example, when you lift your arm up, the deltoid muscle is pulling your humerus bone (the bone to which the deltoid is attached, or the bone the muscle is pulling on) up, as your scapula and clavicle bones (other attachment of the deltoid, or the bone/s the muscle is pulling from) are, or should be, held fixed. [378, 379, 380, 381]

The second consideration when talking about how muscles pull on bones is the angle from which they are pulling. In biomechanics, this is called the torque angle and lever arm system. This system consists of an axis of rotation (in the body, this would be a joint), a point of resistance some distance away from the axis of rotation (the length and weight of the bones creating the joint), and the line vector of gravity or some other point of resistance. An easy example is to do a push-up. First, do a regular push-up from the ground. Then try to do the same push-up, but instead of having your hands on the ground, do it against your kitchen counter. Which one is easier? As I am sure you will discover when you try it, push-ups from the kitchen counter are much easier, but why? The answer is simple; the torque angle relative to gravity is different. This concept can also be applied to how muscles work inside our body. The position of bones relative to one another and the muscles pulling on them will create either a biomechanically advantageous or biomechanically disadvantageous torque angle, with efficient or inefficient movement mechanics, respectively. This can get quite complicated and fascinating if you really want to get into it, but for now, just simply understand the concepts. All muscles do is pull on bones. Two main factors affect how efficiently the muscles pull the bones. One factor is having a solid foundation, and the second is having a good position (torque angle) to pull from. [382, 383, 384, 385, 386, 387, 388, 389, 390, 391, 392, 393, 394, 395, 396, 397, 398]

Think about the importance of this for a minute. If your body does not or is not able to provide your muscles with the two things muscles need to do their job well: a good position and a solid foundation to pull from, then your muscles will not be able to do their job effectively. If muscles cannot do their job, we learned, by way of the Law of 100% motion, that job doesn't just disappear. Something must do it. So if the muscles don't or can't do the job, where do you suppose that workload goes? That's right; the only other place it can go is the passive tissue structures: joints, bones, tendons, ligaments, fascia, and cartilage. Your biomechanics will be faulty, tissue-wasting, and unsafe. In other words, if you don't understand how to create a good position and solid foundation for your muscles, you will most likely accelerate the wear and tear degeneration of your body.

THE **PREMIER** BODY METHOD WILL TEACH YOU HOW TO ACHIEVE BOTH OF THESE FACTORS SO YOUR MUSCLES CAN WORK EFFICIENTLY LIKE THEY ARE SUPPOSED TO.

BUILDING MOVEMENT:

Building Movement is the central concept of The PREMIER Body Method for human movement education. We are using The PREMIER Body Method to build a biomechanically correct, functional human being from the ground up. Whether you are an injury-free athlete training to improve performance, an average person wanting to live an active life, or someone with a debilitating chronic physical injury, learning and training more effective and efficient movement mechanics will make all the difference in the world [399, 400, 401, 402, 403, 404, 405, 406, 407, 408]. **Building movement is the idea of breaking the key aspects of large movements down into smaller component pieces. A larger movement is broken into its components, which are each then broken down into smaller pieces, and so on, until the most basic fundamental piece is met. By doing this for all the major biomechanical movements of the human body, we have created a road map for dissecting human movement down to the most foundational level. If we take this road map of human movement and train it in reverse, we have a clear training program to teach human biomechanics from the most basic fundamental level all the way back to the largest, most complex movements the human body is capable of.**

Here is a practical example. Suppose we have an athlete with shoulder pain caused by impingement [409]. There is nothing weird or tricky, just primary shoulder impingement syndrome caused by dysfunctional scapular mechanics that create a protracted and elevated scapular position [410, 411, 412, 413, 414, 415]. A common approach to rehabilitation involves strengthening the mid and lower trapezius, or muscles along the mid and upper portion of the back [416, 417]. A bent-over row is one of the most effective exercises to train the mid and lower trapezius [418, 419, 420].

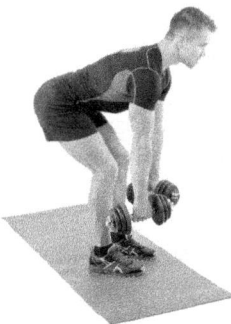

Can I just assign my patient a bent-over row as a treatment protocol? I can, but only if I want to narrow-mindedly address this aspect of the patient's condition without acknowledging that there are likely other holes in the system. To be more complete, we must recognize that the exercise of a bent-over row, while a fantastic exercise to train the mid and lower trapezius, is a high-level, complex movement pattern for the human body to perform. In addition, if this person has a scapular dysfunction causing his or her shoulder impingement, I would bet money that this is not the only hole in his or her system that needs to be corrected.

Now, as a specialist, I can try my best to look for and identify all the holes and faults individually when people come to me with pain, or I can train each movement pattern by breaking it down into its individual component pieces all the way back to the fundamental level, and then build this movement from the ground up. This approach lets me find and fill in all of the holes.

Let's continue our example by dissecting the bent-over row, breaking it down into its component pieces of movement mechanics. To begin with, you need to be able to row AND hold the correct bent-over position, which requires you to execute an RDL or Romanian deadlift position [421, 422]. So, we have already broken the bent-over row exercise into two components, the row and the RDL pattern. Next, to perform an effective RDL pattern, you need to have Full Spinal Control (discussed in detail in later chapters), which consists of three main parts: lumbopelvic control in the low back region, scapulothoracic control in the upper back and shoulder area, and cervical spine neutral control in the neck and head area.

Proper lumbopelvic rhythm for performing a correct RDL requires you to first be able to effectively perform a Hip Hinge movement pattern. To perform an effective Hip Hinge, you must be able to achieve correct lumbopelvic hip mechanics by segregating hip movement from lumbar spine movement. This is most effectively learned through a bridge movement pattern involving hip extension with proper core stability, as the trainee must learn how to use the hips to generate the power needed to create the major motion while maintaining lumbar spine and pelvic neutral. [423, 424, 425, 426, 427, 428, 429, 430, 431, 432, 433, 434]

We can continue to break down core stability into its individual component pieces. We have also not even begun to talk about the other two spinal control pieces, scapulothoracic control and cervical spine neutral control, or the row portion of the full bent-over row exercise. I have also omitted other steps in this example for simplicity's sake. What we are concerned with here is the concept of building movement. I think you get the idea. The upshot of the above description is that if you do not understand core stability, you cannot perform a bridge; if you cannot perform a bridge, you cannot perform a Hip Hinge; if you cannot perform a Hip Hinge, you cannot perform an RDL; and if you cannot perform an RDL, then you cannot effectively execute a bent-over row.

If you cannot effectively perform a bent-over row, then there is no reason to have this exercise be a part of a rehabilitation program to correct shoulder impingement. Also, keep in mind that when I say 'effectively perform,' I mean every single detail of every single aspect of the movement. I am not just talking about the key piece of the exercise intended to correct the injury. For example, if the scapulothoracic and row portions of the bent-over row are mechanically correct and thus effective in training the mid and lower traps to help the impingement syndrome, but faulty lumbopelvic mechanics are also present, you could be compromising lumbar spine health, leading to low back pain. If this is the case, this movement pattern or exercise should not be performed for two reasons. The first is obvious: the exercise or movement pattern is helping one area but possibly putting another at risk. This is an unacceptable cost-to-benefit ratio.

Never fix one area of the body at the expense of another.

The second reason for not performing a movement or exercise this way is less apparent but possibly even more critical. An imperfect movement pattern should be a big clue that more deep-seated biomechanical dysfunctions are present. In other words, there are holes in the system you are missing, so you are not succeeding in correcting the dysfunction as a whole. I hope we can all agree by now that the purpose is to correct dysfunction as a whole!

CATEGORIES OF MOVEMENT:

We just learned about the concept of building movement. So the next logical question is, what are we building towards? Yes, we have said the goal is to build a fully functional human being from the ground up, but what does that functional human consist of? The way I see it, there are three main categories of movement. The three major motions of the human body that encompass all of the mechanics necessary for the functional life the world demands of us **are hip-hinging motions, pulling motions, and pressing motions.** Hip hinging motions can be classified as any movements involving the hips and legs used to move the body's center of mass up and down or around the earth [437, 438, 439, 440, 441, 442, 443, 444, 445]. Pulling motions involve the back, shoulders, and arms where weight or resistance is away from the body's center of mass and must be pulled towards the body's center of mass [446, 447, 448, 449, 450]. Pressing motions involve the chest, shoulders, and arms where weight or resistance is close to the body's center of mass and needs to be driven away from the body's center of mass [451, 452, 453, 454, 455]. The mechanics of each of these motions will be discussed in detail later. For now, we'll look at their practical aspects.

These three motions account for all major muscles in the body and, when performed with correct mechanics, account for all smaller stabilizing muscles as well. All of the functional movements that life requires of us can be placed into one or more of these three categories. In fact, many of the most functional movements are a combination of all three major motions at the same time. An elementary example of this is the gait cycle when walking or running. The gait cycle involves hip-hinging mechanics, as the leg is moved back and forth mainly through hip flexion (bringing the leg up and forward) and extension (bringing the leg back). The gait cycle also involves both pulling and pressing mechanics, as the arm is moved back and forth in a rhythmic manner, mainly by shoulder flexion to bring the arm up and extension to bring the arm down and back [456, 457, 458]. These movement mechanics are most prominent in the gait cycle during sprinting, but they even happen during walking.

Nearly all basic human tasks can be categorized into these three major motions. Every time you sit down on or get up from a chair, bed, or toilet, you bend over to pick up or put down something, you climb up or down stairs, you lift or carry something, or you run, jump, or walk, you use a Hip Hinge type movement pattern. You employ pulling mechanics whenever you pick something up, carry something in your arms, or even open your car door. You use pressing mechanics to reach over your head, push a shopping cart, or wash a dish.

In exercise, you can work every major muscle in the body using these three major motions. Every compound exercise movement or lift requires at least one of these three major motions. Many, such as our example of sprinting, combine all three motions. Motions requiring movement of the hips and legs, such as running, jumping, squatting, deadlifting, lunging, throwing, the clean, and the snatch, are all based on hip-hinging mechanics. Motions using the shoulders, arms, and back, such as pull-ups, lat-pulls, countless variations of the row, the clean, the snatch, climbing a rope, rock wall, or ladder, and throwing a baseball or football, all involve pulling mechanics. Motions using the chest, shoulders, and arms, including push-ups, dips, all variations of the bench press, overhead press, and punching, all involve pressing mechanics. The end stages of The PREMIER Body Method progress to these three major motions, which are then applied to an exercise-training program.

A CONTROLLED FORM OF TRAUMA

One aspect of training and conditioning the human body the right way that I find particularly fascinating is the anabolic effect (anabolism) and the healing response it creates. Anabolism refers to the metabolic process of building up tissue structure in the body. You can easily remember that anabolism refers to building up when you think about anabolic steroids – the performance-enhancing drugs that body-builders, baseball players, and others have used to gain bulk. [459, 460, 461, 462, 463, 464, 465, 466, 467, 468]. However, we are not talking about artificial anabolism through taking anabolic steroids here; we are talking about the body's natural and healthy anabolism. Many times, this anabolic effect gets discussed among athletes and strength coaches in terms of getting bigger, faster, and stronger, or amongst fitness enthusiasts in terms of shedding fat, looking lean and ripped, and feeling great. [469, 470, 471, 472, 473, 474]

However, when we think about anabolic response from an injury standpoint, one of the best parts of an elevated anabolic effect is the tissue growth and healing response it stimulates. [475, 476, 477, 478, 479, 480, 481, 482, 483, 484, 485, 486, 487, 488, 489, 490, 491, 492, 493, 494, 495, 496]

To further discuss anabolism in the body, we must understand that metabolic processes are controlled by our body's hormones. Hormones regulate many of the significant physiologic processes in our bodies. These processes include metabolism, appetite, strength, lean muscle mass, body fat percentage, body composition, tissue integrity, heart rate, blood pressure, energy and fatigue, mood, sex drive, emotions, and stress. Many factors affect hormone levels, including genetics, various environmental factors, nutrition, sleep, physical activity, and physical, emotional, and mental stress. We cannot control all of these factors, but we can control some. [497, 498, 499, 500, 501, 502, 503, 504]

One major factor influencing hormone regulation that we can control (mostly) is physical activity, aka exercise. The type of exercise is important. Intensity and duration are the two main factors that influence hormones during exercise. Training the body the "right way" will produce an anabolic effect. We will discuss how to regulate hormones the "right way" in the next section. For now, let's finish discussing how these hormones promote a healing effect in the body. [505, 506, 507, 508, 509, 510, 511, 512, 513]

Basically, the way I see it, exercise is really a form of trauma to the body. Correct exercise training is a controlled, mild form of trauma performed in a precise way to produce a specific result. Something cool and amazing happens when you consistently train your body the right way: you teach it how to recover from damage. You train your body to recover from trauma. Your body learns how to heal more efficiently. The way I see it, **healing is a skill.** You can train yourself to be better at that skill! [514, 515, 516, 517, 518, 519, 520, 521, 522, 592, 593, 634, 635]

Imagine yourself in really good shape versus yourself really out of shape. Now imagine that each version of you is casually walking down the street. You accidentally step off the curb wrong, mildly twisting your ankle. Compared to the out-of-shape version of you, the in-shape version will recover much faster and possibly more completely from that sprained ankle. That's because your body is accustomed to recovering quickly and efficiently from damage when you train consistently. When you step off the curb wrong, your body says, "Oh, some more damage, no problem. You damage me all the time; I know exactly what to do with this!" Because you consistently "exercise," your body consistently produces all of the enzymes, hormones, immune factors, and everything else responsible for tissue damage repair, and thus can get to work healing right away. This is opposed to the really out-of-shape version of you that does NOT produce these enzymes, hormones, immune factors, etc, on a regular, consistent basis (not to nearly the same extent, anyway).

Think about an NFL football player. Some studies suggest that playing in just one NFL game is the equivalent of five to six 30-mile-per-hour car accidents over the course of 3 hours. [523, 524, 525, 526, 527, 528, 529, 530] Imagine yourself getting in five consecutive 30 mph car accidents within three hours! Do you think you would recover quickly enough to go through it again one week later? Now imagine doing this 18 weeks straight! How do these football players do it? How is it that they can take so much abuse, bounce back, and recover so quickly, then be ready to go one week later? How are they able to do this 17 weeks in a row, or for 22 weeks if they make the Super Bowl?

I will tell you how. These athletes have literally taught their bodies how to recover at this extreme rate by being in such great physical shape and condition. It is almost unbelievable when you think about it. Of course, there are also many other factors involved here that we are not discussing for the simplicity of staying on topic, such as nutrition, genetic ability, rest, sleep, therapy, and medical treatments. However, superior conditioning is one of the primary factors. It is fascinating!

This is also a very extreme example, which, in the long run, usually does not end well for most of these players. This extremely high level of training and abuse does take its toll over the long haul, and the vast majority of these players end up with long-term permanent structural damage and severe injury. At this extreme level, damage to the passive structures of the body surpasses the physical limits because the workload is so great that both the active and passive tissues are typically maxed to the extreme. Even if the mechanics are correct, and the active tissue muscles are doing as much work as they can, there is still more work to be done. This can cause permanent structural damage, as explained in the Active and Passive Tissues section earlier in this book.

Still, this example demonstrates just how incredible the human body is and what it is capable of. Scale back this same phenomenon to a better-balanced level, and we can use the anabolic effect to our advantage in terms of healing from injury and taking control over our body. Consistency in training is critical for this, and we will further discuss training consistency in later sections. **You must be consistent!**

TRAINING THE ANABOLIC EFFECT

So, what is the best strategy, in terms of training, to stimulate a healing anabolic effect for the body? This is not a physiology or endocrinology text, so I will summarize this effect as simply as possible. For this discussion, the two main groups of hormones in the body are anabolic hormones and catabolic hormones. The anabolic category contains hormones such as human growth hormone (hGH), growth hormone-releasing hormone (GH-RH), testosterone, insulin-type growth factor (IGF), thyroxin, and insulin, as well as others. These hormones promote tissue growth and repair. The majority of the hormones on the anabolic side are responsible for the "good" effects that we want. Examples include promoting good metabolism and muscle tone, building lean muscle mass, burning body fat, increasing energy and vitality, and accelerating tissue healing and recovery. [469, 470, 471, 472, 473, 474, 475, 476, 477, 478, 479, 480, 481, 482, 483, 484, 485, 486, 487, 488, 489, 490, 491, 492, 493, 494, 495, 496, 533]

The catabolic category includes hormones such as cortisol, glucagon, and epinephrine. These hormones promote body tissue breakdown and are produced in response to stress. When their levels are too high, catabolic hormones can cause "bad" effects that we don't want, such as lean muscle breakdown, body fat storage, low energy, and depressed mood. [531, 532, 534, 535, 536, 537, 538, 539, 540, 541, 542]

Don't take me too literally when I call these two categories "good" and "bad". In reality, neither is all good or all bad. Both groups of hormones are essential and are in constant balance and fluctuation with each other. All hormones, including these two groups, are extremely important and vital to human physiology and health. Just like everything else in the body, their balance is critical. By labeling anabolic hormones as "good" and catabolic hormones as "bad," I am just giving you an easy way to think about them in terms of exercise and healthy tissue effects. [543, 544, 545, 546, 547, 548, 549, 550, 551, 552]

Exercise influences these hormone groups. We can influence higher production of either the anabolic side or the catabolic side, depending on the type of exercise we do. Really, we are influencing both sides simultaneously when we exercise, but the type of exercise can increase the production of one compared to the other. The two factors that need to be considered when discussing how exercise influences hormone regulation are the duration of training and the intensity. Duration is simply how long your workout, training session, or competition lasts. [543, 544, 545, 546, 547, 548, 549, 553, 554, 555, 556, 557, 558, 559, 560]

The intensity of training is determined by the exercise physiology definition, not the general definition of how hard it is overall. In exercise physiology, the term intensity is defined as single max effort [561]. This means the most you can do in one moment. For example, a max-out lift, or as much weight as you can lift just once without being able to lift it twice, is just about the highest intensity you can get. The way I think of it is, how many times in a row can I do this, or how long could I keep this up? If my answer is not that many times, or not that long before I absolutely have to stop, then the activity is high intensity. Take sprinting the 100-meter dash versus running a marathon. Both are hard physical things to do, but the 100-meter dash is at a higher intensity. If I begin to sprint the 100 meters as fast as possible, I can only keep my pace up for about 10 or 15 seconds before I must slow down or stop. On the other hand, I can keep my pace up for hours to run that slower-paced marathon. So, in terms of exercise physiology, sprinting is high-intensity, while running a marathon is low-intensity, even though running a marathon is a very hard thing to do.

So, how do exercise and exercise intensity relate to anabolic and catabolic hormones? First, consider what happens to our hormones during an exercise training session. Catabolic "bad" hormones will increase in relation to duration or time of activity, and they continue to rise until the activity stops [562, 563, 564, 565, 567, 568, 569, 570, 571, 572, 573, 574]. It doesn't matter what the activity is; however, certain types of activity or exercise will cause faster catabolic rise than others. On the other hand, the anabolic "good" side will spike like a bell curve, with the height of the spike determined by the intensity of training. The higher the intensity of training, the higher the anabolic spike. [575, 576, 577, 578, 579, 580, 581, 582, 583, 584, 585, 586, 587, 588, 589, 590, 591, 594]

Marathon running, therefore, will actually produce a minimal anabolic spike. It is also a long-duration activity, so the catabolic hormones will rise for a long time over the course of the running. In contrast, high-intensity sprinting intervals over a short duration cause a high anabolic spike, while the catabolic side will remain relatively low. This is why a hundred-meter sprinter is much more muscular and defined than a skinny marathon runner. When the anabolic side outweighs the catabolic side, the body will become stronger, have more energy, better muscle tone, and promote better tissue recovery and healing. [469, 470, 471, 472, 473, 474, 475, 476, 477, 478, 479, 480, 481, 482, 483, 484, 485, 486, 487, 488, 489, 490, 491, 492, 493, 494, 495, 496, 533, 595]

When you're training the "right way," the anabolic side outweighs the catabolic side. That way, you are continually supporting the healing and growth of lean muscle and other body tissue, burning fat, promoting increased energy, and feeling great. The key is to train with higher-intensity activities for short durations. This is why high-intensity interval training methods like P90X, T25, CrossFit, and circuit training work when done correctly. An easy example is running a mile. A mile is four laps around a track. If you want to boost hormone regulation in favor of the anabolic side, you would be better off sprinting the straightaways as fast as you can and walking the curves of the track for four laps, as opposed to just running the four laps at one continuous slower pace.

Now, if you are an endurance athlete or someone who loves to run, jog, bike, or do other endurance "cardio" based activities, do not fear. I am not saying these endurance activities are bad or that they shouldn't be done. I am saying that these longer and slower activities are low intensity, so they will not produce a large anabolic output. We will discuss in a later section what you can do if your ultimate goals are based on endurance. As you will see below, you can easily modify your cardio program to make it more anabolic.

An important concept is that exercise's effect on the balance between anabolic and catabolic hormones is on a spectrum. If you are an endurance athlete or a person who only partakes in endurance "cardio" based activities, your activities are skewed toward the catabolic end of the spectrum. This can literally and figuratively create problems in the long run, with such issues as decreased healing and recovery ability of the body, overtraining syndrome, and possible accelerated degenerative processes (wear and tear) on certain body tissues and structures. [596, 597, 598, 599, 600, 601, 602, 603, 604, 605, 606, 636]

The fix here isn't to stop the endurance activity but to understand this process and add some form of higher-intensity training to the routine to balance this hormone-regulatory effect. You can add some sprints to your run, swim, or bike ride once you're good and warmed up, hit the track for some interval training, or go to the gym for some resistance training.

The other key when performing higher-intensity training is to end it in a relatively short period of time. This way, you will be spiking up the anabolic side while keeping the catabolic side low. Most decently in-shape people should limit their time from 20 to 40 minutes of high-intensity training. This time frame can be pushed further in very well-trained individuals. [582, 607, 608, 609, 610, 611, 612]

Once, I was in Guadalajara as a team doctor during the Pan American Olympic games. I was on a shuttle traveling from the Olympic Village to the sporting venue I was covering that day and was fortunate to sit next to one of our Olympic distance runners. I was just making simple conversation with her, and being the nerd I am, I began talking to her about her training and preparation for the Games. Throughout the conversation, I kept thinking, "Wow! I wish all the injured distance athlete-patients I am treating back home could hear this conversation." Even I, with as much as I thought I knew about exercise physiology, was amazed at how little distance running this US Olympic distance runner was actually doing to get herself in shape. Don't get me wrong. At this level of competition, she was running a lot, but not nearly as much as you would think. Her training was actually pretty well-rounded. She utilized resistance training, interval training, and many other modes of cardio training, such as biking and swimming throughout her exercise programs. She understood the principles discussed in the previous paragraphs and pages. She knew that by saving and preparing her body the "right way," she would perform better at her overall main goal of putting up a great distance time at the Pan American Games.

STRETCHING, FLEXIBILITY, AND MOBILITY

Stretching is always a big topic of conversation. Everyone wants to know about stretching. How important is it? How much should I do? When should I do it? Some people swear by it, while others hate it. In my opinion, the body does not need flexibility through stretching as much as it needs mobility through proper movement. **Flexibility** and **mobility** are similar but not the same.

Flexibility refers to the elasticity of soft tissue structures in the body, mainly in musculature and connective tissue. While many people are not flexible enough, others are actually too flexible. Extreme flexibility is not necessary for correct human functional movement and can be detrimental to physical body health and performance. A common example is gymnasts and dancers who end up with musculoskeletal problems later in life. While their extreme flexibility serves them well during competition when they are young, it also creates excessive motion in the joints, which, in turn, creates increased loading stress on those joints and, sooner or later, increases structural and degenerative changes. [613, 614, 615, 616, 617, 618, 619]

Mobility, however, refers more specifically to the functional range of motion within the body, particularly the joints. A person can have too little mobility, termed hypomobile, or too much mobility, termed hypermobile. Having correct mobility is extremely important for correct human functional movement, but, curiously, the best way to gain and achieve correct mobility is through correct movement, not through stretching. People often try to increase flexibility by stretching beyond normal ranges of motion, thus sacrificing proper

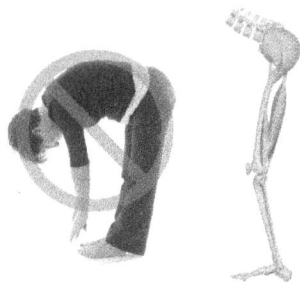

mechanics. These people think they are stretching and gaining flexibility, while in reality, they may be putting passive tissue structures in harm's way. This doesn't work well and may jeopardize physical body health by going past normal physical capability limits, causing structural damage. A typical example is when people attempt to stretch their hamstrings by bending their spines. Bending all the way over from the back will not add any extra stretch to the hamstrings; it will just put more strain on the spine [620, 621, 622, 623, 624, 625, 626, 627, 628, 629, 630, 631, 632, 633]

So, back to stretching in general, I am about to throw out a radical idea here. **If you have perfect human functional biomechanics, there is actually zero need for static stretching.** Before all you flexibility addicts go crazy on me and throw this book away, let me explain. I am not saying that one should never stretch or that stretching has no value. I myself do utilize stretching at times. However, think about it from a movement and mobility standpoint. If you are consistently moving through correct full ranges of motion with perfect mechanics, all day, every day, one hundred percent of the time, then there is absolutely no need to stretch anything. You are already perfectly mobile for everything you need to do because you are doing it and living it every day. [637, 638, 639, 640, 641, 642, 643, 644, 645, 646, 647, 648]

Stretching and the need to stretch are really just other ways for your body to compensate. Something is or feels tight because it is not in balance with the rest of the body. It is tight because it is not moving correctly, and that's because *you* are not moving it correctly, or in other words, your mechanics are faulty. So, the need to stretch is really just your attempt to compensate for a movement dysfunction your body is already compensating for. You are compensating for a compensation!

Here is a common example among athletes and the general population alike. I have had countless patients and athletes come to me because of tight hamstrings. They all tell me that they stretch their hamstrings over and over, but they still feel tight. The first thing I ask them is how often they stretch their hip flexors. Most of the time, these tight-hamstring people don't even know what the hip flexors are, let alone how to stretch them effectively.

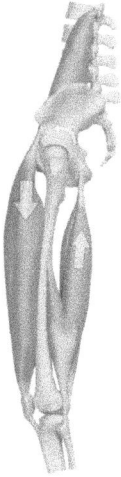

Tight hip flexors will rotate the pelvis forward into an anterior pelvic tilt, which lifts the back of the pelvis where the hamstrings attach (the ischial tuberosity). This pulls apart the bones where the hamstrings attach, creating tension through the hamstrings. The muscles are not even really tight; they just feel tight because of the way the body is being improperly controlled. These people can continue to stretch and stretch the hamstrings without relief. It is not until they understand what is causing the tension and learn to stretch out the hip flexors that they can relieve the tension in their hamstrings. [649, 650, 651, 868, 869]

Now, if you are following along, you might wonder why the hip flexors are tight and whether they should really be stretched. You are right to wonder. There is a reason the hip flexors are tight, and it goes back to movement again. The hip flexors are tight because of improper control of the pelvis, spinal, and core mechanics. If you were to consistently control the movement of your pelvis, hips, and spine through correct core stability mechanics on a day-to-day basis, your hip flexors would not have to compensate and become tight. Therefore, the pelvis will not be pulled into an anterior tilt, and the hamstrings will not feel as though they are tight; neither the hip flexor nor the hamstrings will need to be stretched. [652]

There are countless examples like this all over the body. Here is one for all the runners out there who are continually suffering from tight iliotibial bands, or "IT Band Syndrome." These poor people continue to roll out those tight IT bands on that foam roller until they are ready to cry! This helps a little bit for a short time but usually does not take the tightness away for any length of time. This is because, as you are starting to realize, it is not tightness that is the real problem. It is a movement dysfunction problem. Why did those IT Bands get tight in the first place?

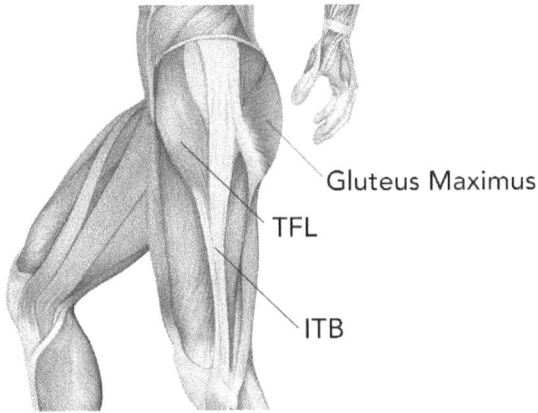

We know that the IT Bands originate from a muscle called the tensor fasciae latae (TFL). There is also a large attachment to the powerful gluteus maximus muscle into the IT Bands. This muscle and fascial complex is mainly responsible for lateral stability of the core, hips, and the whole lower extremity from side to side. So, if you are not correctly controlling the movement in the lateral, side-to-side plane, the lateral plane's musculature becomes unbalanced. This can cause tight IT Bands. To be a bit more specific, faulty lateral plane mechanics usually stem from a dysfunction of the gluteal muscle group, which is being under-utilized, thus forcing the other main lateral hip stabilizer, the TFL (which is directly connected to the IT Bands, remember) to compensate and pick up the slack for the glutes. This, in turn, overworks the TFL and thus creates tension in the IT Bands. [653, 654, 655, 656, 657, 658, 659, 660, 661]

By now you are thinking one of two things. You could be thinking, "Okay, I get it, but why then are the glutes underperforming?" Or you are thinking, "This is way too complicated and is a load of crap." The good news is that I have a good answer for each of you. If you're wondering why the glutes are underperforming, which we would call inhibited, it is because they are not being used properly. This assumes that there is no underlying pathology, such as a nerve lesion or structural abnormality, and we are dealing with a true mechanical dysfunction. It goes back to what muscles really do: pull on bones. Remember the two considerations regarding how well muscles pull on bones: they need a stable base and a good angle from which to pull. Returning to the anatomy of the glutes and TFL, we see that both muscle groups are anchored to the pelvis. So weak glutes, like tight hamstrings, result from poor pelvic control and core stability mechanics. If your core cannot control and hold the correct position for the pelvis, especially during higher-level athletic movements like running, then the glutes will not have a good angle or a stable base to pull from. Over time, this will create an inhibition in the glutes as they learn to underperform, thus forcing the TFL to take over and become overworked, eventually leading to tight IT Bands. [662, 663, 664, 665, 666, 667, 668, 669, 670, 671, 672, 673, 674, 675, 676]

This complex biomechanical stuff actually does have a practical side. If you do not care about the details of biomechanics and just want to know how to move without pain, you're not alone. And you're in the right place! We will soon switch gears from discussing the physiological theories and facts to describing how you can learn to move correctly. The exercises in later pages have the sole purpose of teaching you how to train your body to move correctly. In reality, all these complicated biomechanics don't matter if you just understand how to move and use your body correctly. Moving correctly is really not that hard to learn.

First, though, let's get back to talking about whether we should be stretching. In a perfect world with perfect movement, where the goal is to have normal functional human physical capabilities, you would not need to stretch. In the real world, however, perfect biomechanics are not possible 100 percent of the time. Also, normal functional human physical capability is not always the goal, especially if you're an athlete who pushes your body beyond normal limits. So, in the real world, there are three main reasons a person should stretch: therapeutic purposes, intelligent compensatory purposes, and alternative goal purposes. We will cover the "how-to's" of stretching later in the book and just introduce the "whys" here.

Stretching has many different types of **therapeutic purposes**. One primary purpose is to assist during and following recovery from an injury. When injured, the body is in an unbalanced state. Stretching, along with other forms of therapy, such as joint mobilization, soft tissue procedures, massage, chiropractic adjustments, foam rolling, ice, heat, cold baths, hot baths, therapeutic ultrasound, electric stimulation (E-stem or TENS), athletic taping, kinesio taping, and bracing and casting, can all help to promote the recovery and tissue healing process after an injury. [677, 678, 679, 680, 681, 682, 683, 684, 685, 686, 687, 688, 689, 690, 691, 692, 693, 694, 695, 696, 697, 698, 699]

Stretching can also be a very useful tool in accelerating the rehabilitation and retraining of biomechanics, especially if, like most people, you have had faulty biomechanics for a long time. The worse your mechanics are, the more unbalanced your body is or will become. When done correctly, stretching can be a fantastic way to supplement the biomechanical retraining process.

Return to that example of tight hamstrings caused by tight hip flexors caused by faulty pelvic-spine-core mechanics. The correct way to address this case is to learn and retrain the pelvic core mechanics. But, if the hip flexors have become tight in the process of compensation for this dysfunction, stretching the hip flexors along with the pelvic core training can also help. It's true that the hip flexors will naturally loosen up over time on their own if the movement is retrained well enough, but you can speed up this process by helping the body loosen up the hip flexors through careful stretching. We do this all the time in my clinic.

Another example is when we retrain correct squatting mechanics and notice that the patient has trouble getting the form correct due to ankle tightness on one side. In this situation, we take a time-out from the squat training to mobilize the tight ankle so it can function properly and allow the squat mechanical training to proceed correctly. Mobilizing and stretching the ankle just makes the whole process faster and easier. Keep in mind these are just examples. We are really interested in the concepts here and being able to apply them to the entire body whenever an imbalance is noted and the situation is appropriate. [700, 701, 7-2, 7-3, 704, 705, 706, 707]

The second main reason someone should stretch is for **intelligent compensatory purposes**. This occurs when you want to consciously "compensate for the compensation" due to real-world circumstances.

Once you have achieved a level of correct mechanics and your body has all the mobility and flexibility it needs for healthy, functional human movement capabilities, you will understand that real-life situations can and will often force you to break the rules of perfect mechanics. An easy example of this is a long car ride or plane flight. The simple act of sitting in that seat for an extended period forces the body into a terrible biomechanical position for too long, leading to an imbalance in your well-trained body. Once you get out of that seat and go back to moving correctly, your body will slowly conform back to its ideal balance. However, if you can help your body deal with this situation faster and safer, then you are an **intelligent mover**. The first thing I do when I get off a plane is stretch my hip flexors, thoracic spine, pecs, and lats. [708, 709, 710, 711, 712, 713, 714, 715]

The third main reason someone should stretch is for **alternative goal purposes**. However, before we discuss this directly, we must first discuss another key concept. This is the concept of ultimate goals.

ULTIMATE GOALS:

This entire book focuses on the goal of achieving the highest quality level of <u>perfect</u> human movement. We've talked about this goal but have not yet asked, "<u>Perfect</u> for what, exactly?" We have mentioned the application of movement education for purposes such as decreasing the probability of injury, rehabilitation from injuries or chronic pain, increased ability to exercise, and improved sports training and performance. Learning and applying this knowledge can dramatically improve each of these.

I believe that the main goal is to protect and preserve the physical structures of the human body.

PERFECT HUMAN MOVEMENT INVOLVES MAKING THE MUSCLES DO AS MUCH OF THE WORK AS POSSIBLE BY PLACING AS LITTLE OF THE WORK-LOAD AS POSSIBLE ON THE JOINTS, CARTILAGE, LIGAMENTS, AND TENDONS.

This preserves your body's structures and produces high levels of strength, power, and athletic ability. This is the primary goal of functional human mechanics.

However, there is an interesting concept here: extreme performance may not be consistent with ideal movement and proper musculoskeletal balance. At first, it would seem that ideal human mechanics should be ideal for everything, from protecting the body to achieving maximum athletic performance. This **IS** true most of the time; however, many extreme peak-level performance examples are inconsistent with the ideal functional human biomechanics described here.

Take major-league pitchers as an example. Studies show that many pitchers have altered rotational ranges of motion in their throwing shoulder [716, 717, 718, 719, 720, 721]. These changes in the shoulder allow for a greater range of motion and more of a whip-like action while throwing, allowing for faster speeds. From a health standpoint, you certainly don't want an excessive range of motion in your shoulder. However, if you happen to be standing on the mound in Game Seven of the World Series, and you're not thinking about your health over the next fifty years, or your overall baseball career, or the pain you're in now, and you're only thinking about striking out the batter, you might actually welcome this excessive shoulder motion! So, eventually, you need to decide what your ultimate goal is. Is it long-term health, fitness, and function, or is it to achieve the highest level of extreme peak performance possible in the moment? For most of us, it's the former.

There are many examples of sacrificing perfect functional mechanics for better performance at the highest levels of sport. This occurs because these highest peak-level performance maneuvers go beyond normal and sustainable human capabilities. This realization was a breakthrough for me.

I REALIZED THAT IDEAL FUNCTIONAL MECHANICS ARE WITHIN THE STRUCTURAL LIMITS OF THE HUMAN BODY. STILL, IT IS POSSIBLE, AND, IN SOME CASES, DESIRABLE, TO GO BEYOND THE STRUCTURAL LIMITS DEPENDING ON ONE'S ULTIMATE GOALS.

The fact is that people can force themselves beyond their normal limits to achieve exceptional performance in some instances. However, this has its consequences. Continually passing structural limits will eventually wear down the body's structures, causing pain and/or injury. Performance beyond normal human capabilities is possible but will lead to the same structural damage as improper normal mechanics in daily life.

Another instance of this can be seen during the Olympic snatch lift [722, 723, 724, 725, 726]. A perfectly executed snatch places the shoulder and elbow in a significantly compromised position. In fact, it is one of the worst positions I can think of to place these two joints in with an extremely weighted load on top of them. However, suppose your ultimate goal is not to preserve the shoulder and elbow joints but to put hundreds of kilograms over your head in a fraction of a second. In that case, you need to use proper Olympic snatch form, not proper tissue-sparing biomechanics, for tissue preservation. Again, it comes down to your ultimate goals.

BACK TO STRETCHING FOR ALTERNATIVE GOAL PURPOSES

If your ultimate goal is to achieve a certain level of human performance beyond normal function and physical capability limits, then stretching, among other techniques, may be necessary. Take the martial artist, for example, who requires extreme hip flexibility, such as doing the splits, to perform certain kicks and other maneuvers [727, 728, 729, 730]. This hip range of motion is beyond what is necessary for normal human functional ability, but it is necessary if your goal is to progress as a high-level martial artist. Stretching is an essential tool that can help the martial artist achieve these goals. The same applies to gymnasts, dancers, cheerleaders, and those who excel at yoga and pilates [731, 732, 733, 734, 735, 736, 737, 738, 739, 740]. Again, these are all just examples. The real value here is to understand the concept and be able to apply it accordingly.

When athletes and others force themselves beyond capacity for an alternative goal, they require further intelligent compensation to counteract structural damage. Think again about the pitcher forcing his shoulder beyond normal functional range of motion to achieve the alternative ultimate goal of increased velocity while throwing. Hopefully, this person is doing so in an informed way.

The pitcher should recognize the consequences of this action, which pushes normal structural limits and increases and accelerates the degeneration of body structure. This, in the worst-case scenario, will lead to structural damage of the shoulder (GHJ) joint and possibly a labral and/or rotator cuff tear [716, 717, 718, 719, 720, 721, 741, 742, 743, 744]. In my opinion, as long as we understand the consequences of our actions and are willing to accept them, then it is all good. If the pitcher agrees that the increased wear and tear and possible lifelong structural damage to the shoulder is worth the shorter-term sports success, then that is his decision, and I support it one hundred percent. I love sports and the athletes that play them! They are capable of extraordinary feats, showing us just how incredible the human body is.

The pitcher should intelligently "compensate for the compensation." This happens in two ways.

First, suppose the pitcher knows he is forcing his shoulder beyond normal functional capacity, and the consequence (the body's compensation) is an altered range of motion and excess hypermobility. In that case, he must "compensate for the compensation" by doing some corrective training to counteract this effect. In this example, the pitcher can increase his shoulder training. He would go beyond routine maintenance training and perform higher volumes and varieties of rotator cuff, scapular, and shoulder girdle exercises, among others. [745, 746, 747, 748, 749, 750, 751, 752]

The second and even more critical way this person must "compensate for the compensation" is by achieving a higher level of perfection in terms of overall <u>perfect</u> body mechanics at all other times, aside from the time he knowingly forces his body out of the normal ideal range. I like to think of it as a gas tank. If I know there are certain times that I will need to burn up a lot of gas, then I want to conserve as much gas as possible at all other times. This is another critical reason for athletes to understand <u>perfect</u> human movement mechanics. As athletes, we are constantly pushing our bodies to the limits and, many times, past the limits. If you do not understand how to conserve the gas in the tank between those times that push your body's limits, then you will run out of gas at one point or another! Just in case you are not following completely, the gas in the tank represents the finite physical integrity of your body. So, we are talking about reducing the risk of injury, faster recovery between training and competition, and prolonging careers! You tell me if this is important or not! [753, 754, 755]

MAKING A CHOICE

The real key here is understanding the concept of ultimate goals and knowing the difference between maintaining correct functional mechanics to preserve your body and consciously sacrificing correct mechanics for an alternative ultimate goal. If you understand the difference, then you can make a choice. The sad part is most people don't make that choice because they don't know the difference. It's sad because the reason why it happens is that they were simply never taught. It is due to blind ignorance, and in this case, ignorance is not bliss; it is chronic pain, poor health, and a poor quality of life.

This choice, by the way, is not limited to these extreme athletic efforts like our last several examples. The choice to move better goes down to the most basic and simple movements. You can choose to do something as simple as getting out of a chair properly or improperly. If you understand the difference, then you have the power to make a choice between the two. If you don't know how to properly move your body, you don't get to make that choice. [756, 757, 758, 759, 760, 761]

This book opens with a story about a former patient of mine suffering from chronic back and sacroiliac pain due to repetitive stress in these areas caused by having poor mechanics throughout most of her life. It was improper hip-hinging mechanics throughout this patient's life that led her to destroy her back. Other doctors told her not to perform Hip Hinge motions anymore, and in an ideal world, I would agree. In the real world, however, we don't always get to just completely avoid anything we want. Sure, this patient can avoid doing the exercise of a Hip Hinge or squat in a gym, but what happens when this person has to sit down on and stand up from a chair, get into and out of her car, get on and off her bed, and even get up from the toilet? You can't go through daily life without hip-hinging mechanics. **Life**

demands certain physical requirements of us. In the real world, this woman needs to improve her hip-hinging mechanics, even if it will cost her a little bit in the process. She is better off knowing how to do it the best way possible rather than continuing with the same horrible mechanics that brought her to our clinic in the first place.

Again, it goes back to making a choice, but this woman never had the luxury of that choice since she was not taught how to use her body correctly until the damage had been done. Her mechanics were so poor for so long that she used up her physical body structures by constantly going beyond her physical capability limits. The gas tank for her lower back was completely empty. Because of this, she destroyed her physical structure beyond the body's ability to recover and repair the damage.

This woman, like so many people out there, will most likely be in continued pain for the rest of her life. At the age of 40, that is a long way to go with debilitating pain. The continued pain will limit her ability to play with and care for her two small children. It will limit her work and financial contribution to her family. It most likely will put stress on her relationship with her husband. It will, on some level, create feelings of resentment and sadness. She will miss out on activities with her friends. She will miss out on so many of the joys we all take for granted until it is too late. She will most likely turn to chronic pain, sleep, and anti-depressant medications. She will become more and more sedentary, which will cause her overall health to decline rapidly. She will develop depression and have a poor quality of life for almost half of her life, maybe more than half.

My goal is not to force everyone to exercise, be healthy, and train like an Olympic champion. My ultimate goal is to give the world a choice. A choice between knowing and understanding how your physical body works and not. In my mind, the choice is obvious.

NUTRITION

This is not a nutrition book, but you cannot have a healthy physical body and train well without good nutrition, so I need to at least mention nutrition. Good nutrition is essential for everyone. The subject of nutrition can seem a bit overwhelming at times. Countless diet plans, vitamins, supplements, and changing information can be confusing and frustrating, making you feel like you don't even want to deal with it. In the past few years or even months, you've probably heard that fat is bad, fat is good, eat more protein, go vegetarian, and carbs are bad, but if you're an athlete, you need to carb load. It is hard to make sense of the conflicting information, and as soon as you think you have it all figured out, you get hit with a new idea that completely changes things. It doesn't need to be this difficult.

Good nutrition is actually quite simple. The problem is that people often will ask what constitutes good nutrition, but they don't like the answer. People are always looking for the magic trick or secret to good nutrition, allowing them to eat bad food while still being healthy. Well, the biggest secret of all, and one that you'll hear from any credible authority in nutrition, is that there are no shortcuts. Good nutrition is good nutrition, no matter how you slice it! In my mind, it is pretty simple; eat plants and meat, in that order, as close as possible to the way they come from nature. Plants include vegetables, fruits, nuts, legumes, and seeds. Meats include animal-source foods like fish, chicken, eggs, beef, deer, buffalo, and even insects. That's it! You just cannot get any healthier than that. If it is not on the list, you probably don't need it. [762, 763, 764, 765, 766, 767, 768, 769, 770, 771]

Another easy way to think about it is that if it doesn't grow from the ground, walk, fly, or swim, it is not good for you. I have never seen a cookie or a candy bar growing out of the ground. If you're ever unsure, think about how processed it is or how much it has been changed from how nature gave it to us. More processed foods are generally worse for you. An easy example of this is a baked potato versus French fries. Both are made from the same potato plant growing out of the earth, but the only change to the baked potato is that it has been heated. The French fries have been cut up, fried in oil at extreme temperatures, and salted, making them very different from how they came out of the ground. Therefore, the fries are worse for you. This simple rule holds true for just about everything, so think about it the next time you are deciding what you are going to feed your human body. [772, 773, 774, 775, 776, 777, 778, 779, 780, 781, 782, 783, 784, 785, 786, 787, 788, 789]

These principles are true due to human evolution over hundreds of thousands of years. For about 99% of those years, humans have been eating unprocessed foods, not far removed from how the earth gave them to us. A caveman ate plants right out of the ground. He killed animals, caught fish when he could, and occasionally found fruit growing from a tree or vine. Everything was fresh, and most was eaten raw. (In today's world, it is not safe to eat raw meat and other animal products for the most part, so don't try!) This is how our species, and all of our direct ancestor species' survived for hundreds of thousands, even millions of years. It was not until quite recently that our human species decided to artificially and radically change our food. Our nutritional physiology cannot evolve fast enough to keep up with these changes. I believe this changed diet is behind the vast majority of today's health problems. (790, 791, 792, 793, 794)

For more in-depth knowledge on this subject, I would recommend reading "The Paleo Diet" by Loren Cordain. This style of eating is purportedly the closest to the diet of early humans, before the influx of heavily processed foods, and, in my opinion, the healthiest.

Good nutrition stems from understanding what you are putting in your body. It's not that you can never have anything "bad." No one is entirely perfect 100% of the time. It's wonderful to enjoy food. However, most people need to start using food as fuel. As your base, learn to eat for purpose, not pleasure. That way, when you do eat for pleasure, it is actually pleasurable, not guilt-ridden. That is not to say that eating healthy is not pleasurable either! With a better understanding of the things you are putting in your body, you can make better choices.

Nutrition is vital for everyone, including athletes, people pursuing physical fitness, and those healing from injury. We must remember that when we exercise, we break down body tissue and use up energy stores. If you are injured, you already have broken down tissue. This body tissue must be rebuilt, and the energy stores must be replaced. Our diets, the foods we eat, and the liquids we drink become these building blocks and the energy needed to recover from physical activity and/or injury. What you eat and when you eat it throughout

the day, especially in the morning and pre- and post-workouts, is criti-
cal. (795, 796, 797, 798, 799, 800, 801, 802, 803, 804, 805, 806, 807, 808, 809, 810, 811, 812)

Finally, there is one more nutrient to mention: physical challenge. Challenging our bodies physically is a vital source of nutrition, just like any other. Physical fitness (exercise) is nourishment. Physical stimulation and challenge are essential for proper human health. Just like your body can't live without vitamins and minerals, your body can't achieve proper health without exercise. The goal of good health and nutrition is to have a healthy body, balanced metabolism, and strong cellular function. Your body needs the proper nutrients from the foods you eat to build it from the inside out. We must also challenge our bodies from the outside in through exercise and physical fitness training.

Physical activity helps to regulate the same physiologic processes in our bodies that good nutrition does. Countless research shows that physical activity influences hormone balance and regulation, metabolism, mood, energy, and many other physiological processes. Our bodies need to be physically challenged. It is a necessary component of life. All the hard work and dedication you are putting into your diet to improve your health will fall short of reaching its full potential without a good fitness training program alongside it (and vice-versa). Challenging your body physically is a vital nutrient. Make sure you give your body all the nutrients it needs. (813, 814, 815, 816, 817, 818, 819)

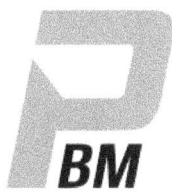

PREMIER BODY METHOD
PBM

PERFORMANCE
READY
EDUCATIONAL
MOVEMENT
INTEGRATION
ENHANCEMENT
REHABILITATION

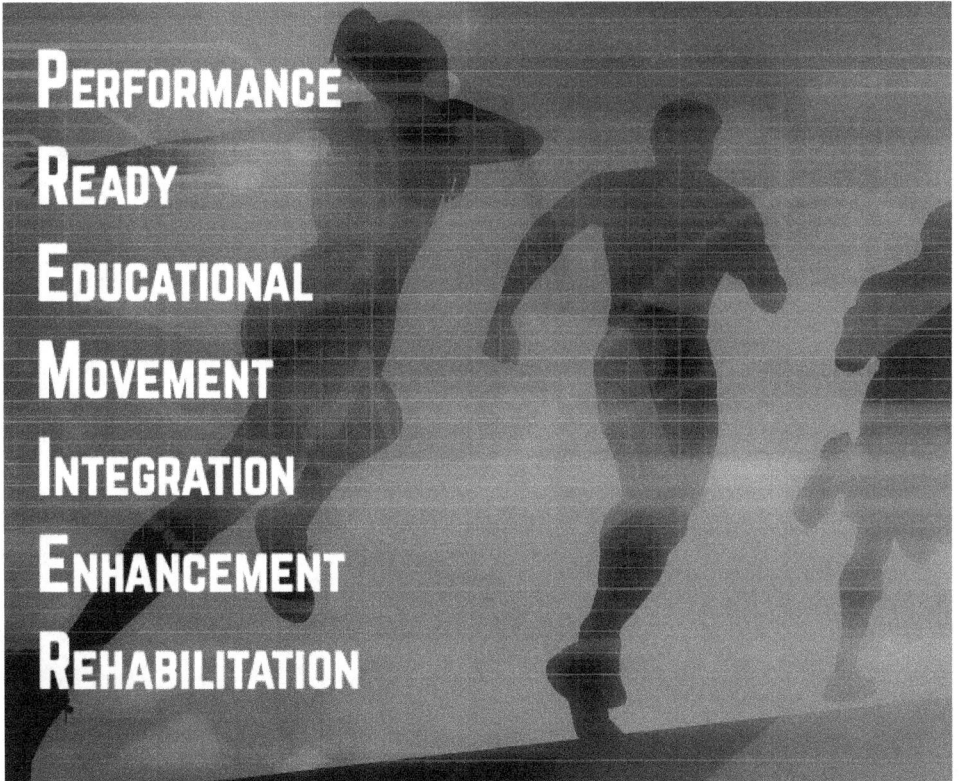

PART TWO
THE PREMIER BODY METHOD

Now that we have learned our key concepts, it is time to get to work and put them to use. The rest of this book will outline The PREMIER Body Method, the specific step-by-step program for building human mechanics through human movement education. Since this is an educational process, mastering it will take time, consistency, effort, and dedication. Consistency in training and application to everyday life are the biggest keys to success.

THE PREMIER BODY METHOD OVERVIEW

THE LANGUAGE OF MOVEMENT

Through this program, we will attempt to retrain control of body mechanics. In many ways, it will be like learning a new language, not a new spoken language but, rather, a new language of movement. Just like learning a new foreign language, learning this new language of movement is challenging; however, once you are fluent, you can continue to use it easily and automatically. Remember this analogy throughout your training. The program can be overwhelming or even tedious, especially in the beginning, but if you stick with it, you can achieve your physical goals before you know it. I've worked with hundreds of patients who felt overwhelmed when they started and were surprised when proper movement became second nature to them. So, I encourage you to stick with it.

THE "CORE" OF HUMAN BIOMECHANICS

SETTING THE STAGE FOR THE SYSTEM BY CREATING A SOLID FOUNDATION

There are a lot of mistaken beliefs about what "core strength" is and how to achieve it. Many people think having a strong "core" means having rock-hard abs. They believe sit-ups, crunches, and trunk rotations will strengthen your core. Neither of these beliefs is true. Some people think that "core strength" means protecting the lower back. This isn't wrong, but it is still only a small piece of the puzzle. As you will learn throughout The PREMIER Body Method, proper core stability involves much more than strong abs and a straight low back. True core stability involves what we classify as **Full Spinal Control** or control of the entire length of the spine from the pelvis to the top of the head.

The first primary goal for proper human movement is to achieve Full Spinal Control. The spine is the centerpiece of the human body. It is the foundation of the musculoskeletal system. No body movement will be completely correct without proper spinal control and alignment. The spinal column provides the working foundation for all movement mechanics. Remember that muscles pull on bones, and the pulling is more effective when they pull from a stable base. When controlled correctly, the spine provides that stable base for many of our large muscles. When positioned in the correct spinal alignment, the spine will also provide good torque angles from which muscles can pull. [820, 821, 822, 823, 824, 825, 826, 827, 828]

To learn how to achieve Full Spinal Control, we will break it down into three components. This goes back to the key concept of building movement. The three main components of Full Spinal Control are **Lumbopelvic Control, Scapulothoracic Control, and Cervical Spine Neutral Control.** The training will begin with lumbopelvic control, as the pelvis is the foundation of the spine. Once pelvic control is achieved through proper core stability, training can begin to branch up and down the biomechanical chain, first to the lower back position and hips. The training then continues to scapulothoracic control, building the upper back and shoulder girdle positions, and cervical spine neutral control centering on the neck and head positions. Once Full Spinal Control is understood, we can continue to build off the hip to the rest of the lower extremity and off the shoulder girdle to the rest of the upper extremity. This progression will allow us to completely rebuild a biomechanically correct, functional human body.

LUMBOPELVIC CORE CONTROL

We begin with pelvic control because the pelvis is the cornerstone of the body. Connected to the pelvic bone are the human body's largest and most powerful muscles, including the glutes, hamstrings, hip flexors, quads (partial), and hip adductors. Even the latissimus dorsi, one of the most powerful upper extremity muscles, is anchored to the pelvic bone by the thoracolumbar fascia.

The position and stability of the pelvis are critical for the proper function and force production of all of these and also many smaller muscles, making pelvic position and stability crucial for the control of hip mechanics. The spinal column sits directly above the pelvis, and so pelvic position and stability also dictate spinal mechanics all the way up to the skull. The lower extremity is built off the hip, and the upper extremity is built off the spine through the scapulo-thoracic articulation. Because of its cornerstone role, the pelvis is the best place to start. [829, 830, 831, 832, 833, 834, 835, 836, 837, 838, 839]

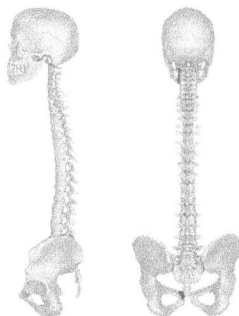

Here, we will learn how the pelvis moves and how to control this movement to prevent excessive motion of the pelvic position away from pelvic neutral. This is done through the proper control and coordination of core stability.

THE CORE'S JOB IS NOT TO CREATE MOTION BUT TO PREVENT IT.

Its job is to prevent the pelvic bone from moving relative to the rest of the torso (the thorax). Visualize a runway model walking down the runway. This is an excellent example of poor pelvic control! Now, the model has an alternative ultimate goal of looking beautiful and sexy, which she is accomplishing. Still, this walk is ugly in terms of correct mechanics and structural body health. [840, 841, 842, 843, 844, 845, 846, 847, 848]

When the pelvis and torso are locked together as one unit, the core is doing its job. If the core is not doing its job, the pelvis and torso move independently, leading to excessive motion in the spine and poor hip mechanics. Many of the traditional "core" and "ab" exercises like crunches, sit-ups, and rotation machines at the gym defeat the purpose of core stability and, in my opinion, can cause many spinal and other mechanical problems. Yes, these traditional exercises can strengthen the abdominal muscles, but at what cost? There are much more effective ways to strengthen the core and abdominal muscles that don't defy the true purpose of core stability. We want to train the core, not necessarily just to be stronger; we want to train core stability to do its job better and more efficiently. Always remember that the job of core stability is not to create motion but to prevent it. [849, 850]

The pelvis and thorax are like two independent parts, with the spine serving as a connecting rope between them. If these two pieces are allowed to move independently of one another without control, the spine, like the rope in the middle, will be tugged, pulled, and torqued around haphazardly. This can create bad biomechanical positions and excessive spinal stress, which causes repetitive damage, degeneration, and injury to the spine. An uncontrolled pelvis relative to the thorax and lower extremity will also create bad torque angles and non-solid foundations to pull from for all of the muscles attached to it, therefore creating non-ideal mechanical positions, faulty hip mechanics, and compromised body regions, such as hip, thigh, knee, foot/ankle, and even shoulder, upper extremity, and neck problems. [851, 852, 853, 854, 855, 856, 857, 858, 859, 860]

To truly understand lumbopelvic core control and stability, we must first be aware of the pelvic position in relation to the tri-planar axis of our center of mass. We must always think in three dimensions because we live in a three-dimensional world. We use the tri-planar system to think in three dimensions when discussing biomechanics. [861]

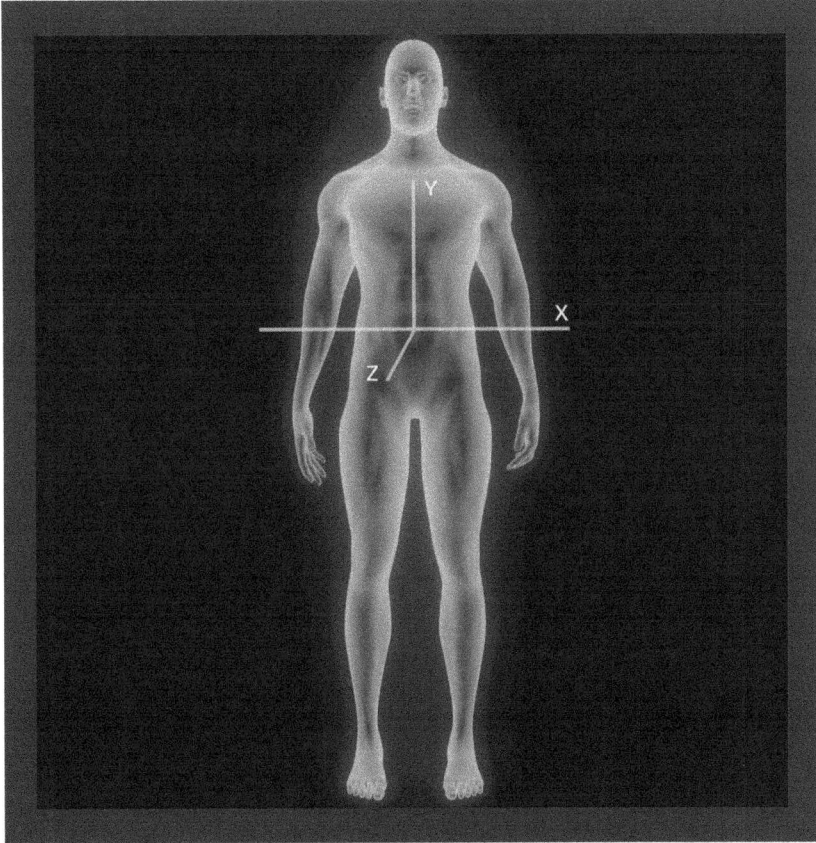

We can think of our center of mass as the center of this tri-axial system. If we imagine the human body, as seen from the front, super-imposed on this tri-axis, we have a basis for body orientation in three-dimensional space. The X-axis runs horizontally across the body from side to side. The Y-axis runs vertically up and down. The Z-axis runs horizontally from front to back. The X-axis and Y-axis form the XY plane, or **frontal/coronal plane**. It is a vertical plane that divides the front and back of your body. The XZ plane is the **transverse plane**, which divides the body into upper and lower halves, and the YZ plane is the **sagittal plane** of the body, which divides your body into right and left halves. All movement occurs in combinations of these planes. Therefore, when thinking about motion, we must always visualize what happens in all three planes.

Returning to pelvic control, we must learn to achieve a **pelvic neutral position (pelvic neutral)** to achieve a truly stable lumbopelvic core. Achieving pelvic neutral occurs in all three planes. In the XY or frontal/coronal plane, neutrality is achieved by the leveling of the iliac crests ('ASIS'), in which the tops of the pelvic bone on the sides of your waist are aligned and level. A dysfunction in the XY plane manifests as a hip hiking motion or Trendelenburg's sign, in which one side drops and/or the other rises or hikes up.

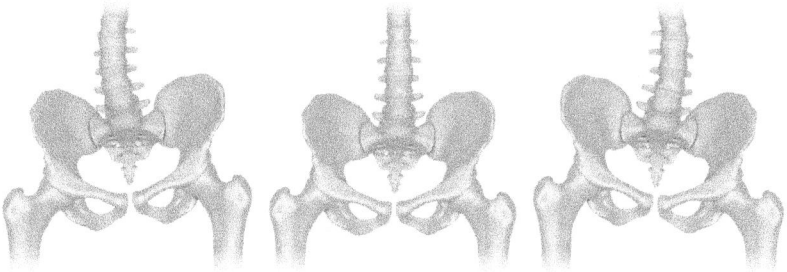

In the YZ or sagittal plane, the pelvic neutral position is at the center point in the anterior and posterior (front to back) pelvic tilt range. A dysfunction here is seen as an increase in posterior pelvic tilt or, more commonly, an increase in anterior pelvic tilt (due to a lower cross-type syndrome). You might see an anterior pelvic tilt in someone who walks and stands with a large curve in the lower back, commonly called sway back. This is perhaps the biggest mechanical fault (hole in the system) that we see all the time. It causes an unbelievable number of problems, such as back pain, facet syndrome, facet arthropathy, hip

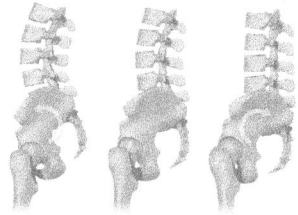

dysfunctions, ITB syndrome, bursitis, knee pain, patellar tendinitis, patellar femoral pain syndrome, lower cross syndrome, upper cross syndrome, even upper back, shoulder, and neck issues, and many more. (862, 863, 864, 865, 866, 867, 870, 871, 872, 873, 874, 875, 876, 877, 878, 879, 880, 881)

Finally, in the XZ or transverse plane, the pelvic neutral position is seen as neutral rotation of the pelvis in regards to the thorax of the body. When the pelvis is not XZ neutral, it is rotated relative to the torso (shoulders and thorax), and the spine becomes rotated. This looks like a baseball batter that has just swung too hard and missed the ball. This dysfunction can cause many issues, usually leading to excessive rotational stress on the joints and discs of the spine. Research shows that excessive rotational force on the spine's discs is the number one way to cause damage and injury to them. (882, 883, 884, 885, 886, 887, 888, 889)

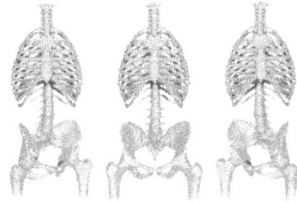

All three axial planes must be held in a comfortable neutral position to achieve pelvic neutral position. In other words, if you can hold all three planes of pelvic motion in a pain-free neutral position, then you have lumbopelvic core stability. Pelvic neutral is individual-specific; it must be learned specifically for each person based on individual anatomy, structural limits, and any pertinent pathology or injury. (865, 873)

Once pelvic neutral is achieved, the next step will be to learn how to maintain it. This will be the job of core stability, which we will discuss in detail in a later section. For now, let's finish discussing the other two fundamental pieces of Full Spinal Control: Scapulothoracic Control and Cervical Spine Neutral Control.

SCAPULOTHORACIC CONTROL

Once the pelvic position and lumbar spine are neutral, we can build the rest of the spine on top of it. The next piece to add is Scapulothoracic Control. Now that we have the lower portion of the spinal column tied down with proper pelvic position, it is time to tie the other end of the spine down with the correct scapular and thoracic spine position. The correct position for the scapula and thoracic spine is the **set scapular position**. This is the equivalent of pelvic neutral for the upper back and shoulder girdle.

Just like the pelvis does, the scapula, your shoulder blade, also moves in three dimensions in our tri-planar system. In the XY or frontal/coronal plane, the movement is reflected in the proper height of the scapula relative to the thorax/rib cage. In movement terms, it's the correct balance between elevation and depression of the scapula. If you shrug your shoulder blades up, you are elevating your scapulae. When you do the opposite and pull your shoulder blades down on your back, you are depressing your scapulae. The most common dysfunction here is excessive elevation as the shoulders become hiked up over the rib cage. Learning to depress the shoulder blades to the right level is critical for most individuals.

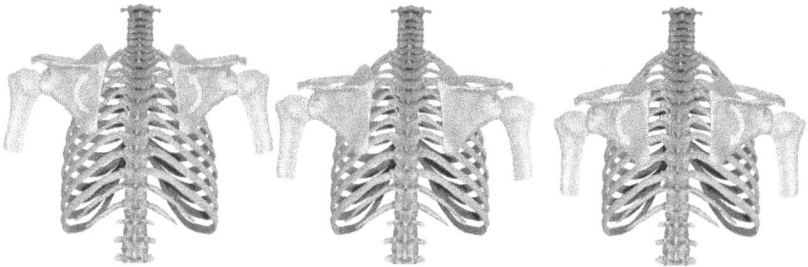

Scapular Movement in the XY or Frontal/Coronal Plane

In the YZ or sagittal plane, the set scapular position is the center in the range of anterior and posterior (front to back) scapular tilt. If you slump your shoulder blades forward, you create an anterior tilt for the scapulae. Doing the opposite causes a posterior tilting of the scapulae. A dysfunction here appears as an increase in anterior tilting as the scapula rounds up over the top of the rib cage. This is most often coupled with excessive elevation of the scapula, as discussed above.

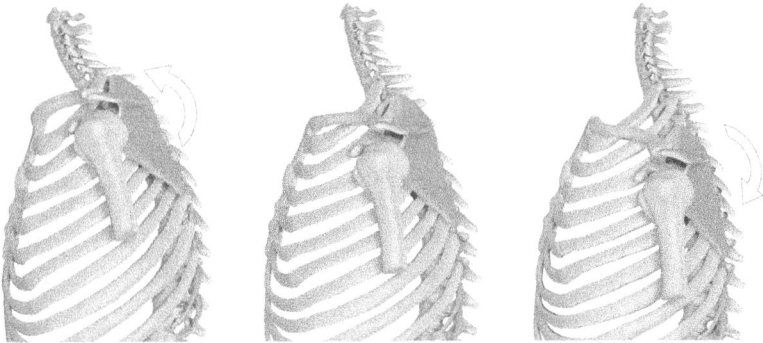

Scapular movement in the YZ or Saggital Plane

Finally, in the XZ or transverse plane, the set scapular position is the balance between the retraction and protraction of the scapula. If you pinch your shoulder blades together on your back, you are performing retraction of the scapulae. If you do the opposite and move your shoulder blades apart, you are protracting the scapulae.

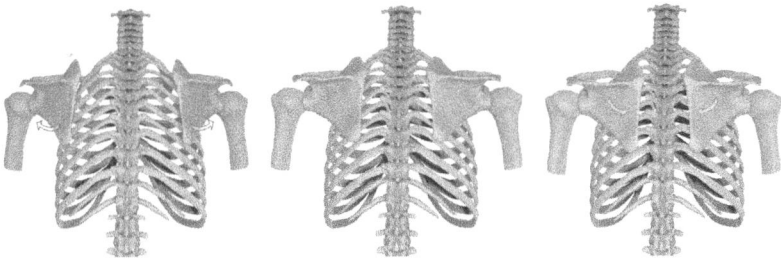

Scapular movement in the XZ or Transverse Plane

The most common dysfunction here is excessive protraction, again as the shoulder blade is rounded up and over the top and side of the rib cage. All three of these dysfunctions, excessive elevation, anterior tilting, and excessive protraction, commonly occur together in what's known as upper cross syndrome or scapular dyskinesis. Most people just call it bad posture!

The goal is to achieve a set scapular position, aka scapular neutral, for the thoracic spine and shoulder girdle, just as we want to attain pelvic neutral for the pelvis and lumbar spine. The set scapular position is the neutral position for all three planes of motion for the scapula, thoracic spine, and shoulder girdle. For most people, pulling the shoulder blades back and down while extending the thoracic spine will reverse the most common faults and help to achieve this set scapular position. Again, however, the set scapular position is individual-specific. (890, 891, 892, 893, 894, 895, 896, 897, 898, 899, 900, 901, 902, 903, 904, 905, 906)

Once the set scapular position is achieved, the next step is to learn how to maintain it. This will provide us with the correct position (good torque angles to pull from), a solid foundation from which to pull for much of the upper extremity, and the foundation to build the final piece of Full Spinal Control: Cervical Spine Neutral Control.

CERVICAL SPINE NEUTRAL CONTROL

The final piece to creating Full Spinal Control is Cervical Spine Neutral Control. With the pelvis, lumbar spine, thoracic spine, and shoulder girdle all in place, we need to top it off with the correct head and neck position. The spinal column works as a single unit, like a row of dominos. It will be much easier to put the neck into proper alignment once the pelvis, lower back, and upper back are in line. Learning and achieving this final piece of Full Spinal Control is critical because if the neck is out of position, it may pull the rest of the spine with it. Thus, Full Spinal Control will be lost. I bring this up because some people, especially those with issues/injuries in the lower back or lower extremities, sometimes have trouble understanding why they need to be concerned with the neck, as it doesn't seem to have anything to do with their condition. It does. The human body works as one machine. One faulty part can jeopardize the whole thing. It is like executing an offensive play in football. Ten out of eleven players may do exactly what they are supposed to, but if the right guard misses his block and the quarterback is sacked, then the whole play is unsuccessful.

A recent patient of mine was a collegiate baseball player. He was a pitcher who came to me in his off-season complaining of pain in his lower back while pitching. We assessed his mechanics and found he was overloading too much weight onto the front half of his body during hip-hinging mechanics (hip-hinging mechanics will be discussed later). This was overworking his lower back and also decreasing the velocity of his fastball. He went through the PREMIER body method program, and once completed, not only was his back pain gone, but his fastball velocity was up 3 miles an hour on average. He went from being a good collegiate player to being a great collegiate player, with scouts approaching him. Needless to say, he was thrilled – and shocked!

Would you like to know what one of the faultiest parts of his mechanics was? Since we are in the neck section of this text right now, yes, it was indeed his neck. The problem happened mainly during his hip-hinging motions, especially his squats. The faulty neck position threw off his whole spinal position, leading to hyperextension in his lower back and causing his injury. The faulty neck position, which was causing him to lose Full Spinal Control, was also creating a faulty pelvic position that, in turn, decreased his force and power production in the hips and thus decreased velocity while throwing. Once corrected, his spinal control improved, his hip mechanics improved, his squat max went up by 30+ pounds, the velocity while throwing went up, and his back pain was gone. Dramatic results, and they were primarily due to correcting the neck!

The cervical spine (neck) and head also move in three dimensions on our tri-planar system, like the pelvis and the scapula do. Movement in the XY or frontal/coronal plane is lateral side-to-side bending, such as when you lean your head to one side. In the XZ or transverse plane, it is seen as rotation, like shaking your head no. In the YZ or sagittal plane, it appears as flexion and extension, like nodding your head. Most neck dysfunction occurs in the front-to-back flexion and extension position. It appears as an excessive extension of the cervical spine in what is known as an anterior head carriage. You commonly see this when someone sits in front of the computer. I call this turtle man syndrome because the head

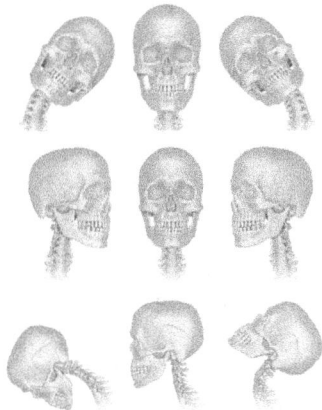

protrudes outward from the body. This is usually caused by poor spinal control below the neck, in the upper and lower back, and even down to the pelvic position. Remember that it works both ways, as in our baseball example above. It does not matter if the problem comes from the bottom up or the top down (chicken or egg). The whole thing needs to be fixed!

Once the cervical spine neutral position is achieved, it is held by a group of muscles called the deep neck flexors. The specifics on how to position the head and neck correctly, as well as how to activate the deep neck flexors, will be discussed in detail in a later section. For now just understand the importance of achieving cervical spine neutral, as it completes Full Spinal Control and thus helps provide the solid foundation and correct torque angles for our human body to work from. (907, 908, 909, 910, 911, 912, 913, 914, 915, 916, 917, 918, 919, 920, 921, 922, 923, 924)

PUTTING IT ALL TOGETHER – FULL SPINAL CONTROL

Full Spinal Control is the biggest key to the mechanics of the entire body. It does not matter if you are talking about simple everyday movements and tasks for the sport of life, elite-level athletic movements for a specific sport, or anything in between. The major motion in human movement comes or should come from the hips, legs, shoulders, and arms. The spine is designed to work in a neutral, stable position during movement, meaning there should be no major motion in the spine. Our large, powerful, strong muscles in the extremities, or hips and shoulders, are designed to produce the force necessary for movement and major motion. These muscles are the glutes, hamstrings, quads, iliopsoas, hip adductors, pectorals, latissimus, deltoids, biceps, and triceps. These are powerful prime movers. Now think about the spinal column and core musculature, the erectors, quadratus laborum or QL, transverse abdominus, internal and external obliques, rectus abdominus, pelvic floor muscles, the mid and lower trapezius, the rhomboids, the serratus anterior, the deep neck flexors, the multifidi, and all of the other smaller spinal stabilizers. These are not prime movers! These are designed to be postural stabilizing muscles. They are designed to help hold our pelvis, spine, thorax, shoulder girdle, neck, and head stable, thus creating a solid foundation for the big boys (extremity musculature) to pull from, and if held in the correct position, will also provide the proper torque angles for the big boys to pull from. With the spinal column, pelvis, torso, head, and neck held solid, the prime movers of the extremities can produce powerful force and proper movement. Achieving and maintaining Full Spinal Control is the foundation.

I cannot stress enough the importance of understanding this point. Full Spinal Control must be the number one priority of movement. Whether you are deadlifting, squatting, sprinting, climbing stairs, getting up from a chair, or just walking around, Full Spinal Control should be involved. In my opinion, this differentiates the people who understand how to train their body well from the amateurs who don't.

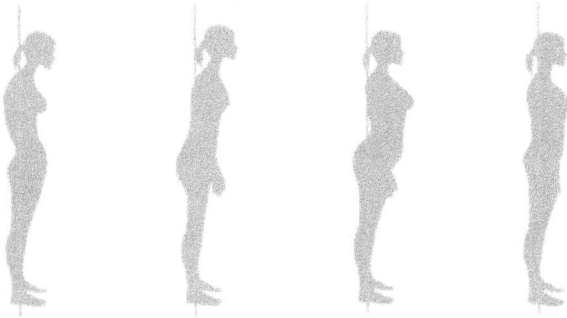

Most amateurs think only about the parts that are moving. For example, if an amateur is doing a bench press exercise, he thinks about moving the weight up and down with his arms. The pro who really understands how to train his body well does not think about arm movement; that is just what is happening. The guy who knows what he is doing is thinking about all the parts that aren't moving, like his pelvic position, set scapular position, neck position, and so on, while the actual movement is occurring. He is focusing on Full Spinal Control and creating a good position and solid foundation for his moving parts to work from. Make Full Spinal Control your number one priority and focus no matter what you are doing. You will be amazed at the results!

RETRAINING THE NEURO-MUSCULOSKELETAL SYSTEM FROM THE GROUND UP

Proper movement starts with the lumbopelvic core. This is the foundation of our house. Starting with lumbopelvic core stability is like building a house using solid concrete rather than unstable mud. If we do not lay this groundwork, we cannot get good results, regardless of which body part or skill we focus on. If the foundation's concrete has not been laid, there is no point in hammering boards and nails together to build a building. If you begin to rehabilitate or train at any level other than the very beginning, you will leave the potential for holes in the system to persist. Compensation patterns form or persist, and re-injury and predisposition to new injury are possible. However, if you build from the ground up, just as in building a new house, you can fill in the holes along the way and have a fully functioning system at the end. **Do not put up boards and nails before concrete.**

We have already discussed biomechanics as occurring in the three-dimensional tri-planar system. Basic posture also appears in this tri-planar system. In fact, biomechanics and posture are really the same thing. **Biomechanics is just posture in motion, and posture is biomechanics held in a static position.** If you cannot achieve correct basic static posture, you cannot achieve correct posture in motion, which is correct biomechanics.

Core stability is essential for correct posture and biomechanics. A comfortable pelvic neutral position is necessary for core stability. Therefore, the trainee must be able to maintain a pelvic neutral position to achieve proper posture and biomechanics. The trainee must first learn to achieve a pelvic neutral position statically before learning to hold pelvic neutral through motion. Again, this must be achieved in all three planes, as explained above, to be correct. There must be no hip hiking in the coronal plane (ASIS' must be level), no rotation in the transverse plane (the pelvis must be in alignment with the shoulders bilaterally), and no excessive anterior or posterior pelvic tilt in the sagittal plane (a neutral tilt must be held). Your body should be in a pelvic neutral position no matter what position your body is in, whether standing, seated, lying supine, prone, on your side, or even hanging upside down. Trainees must understand this position and how to tell whether or not they are in it before beginning the first exercise. This may take as little as a couple of minutes for some, or much, much longer, such as days or even weeks, for others to learn. [829, 830, 831, 832, 833, 834, 835, 836, 837, 838, 839, 851, 852, 853, 854, 855, 856, 857, 858, 859, 860]

Another characteristic of a true pelvic neutral position is that it is pain-free (or as close as possible given certain pathology). If the trainee is trying to put the pelvis into pelvic neutral and teach the core to keep it there, it needs to be a pain-free, comfortable, and healthy position. Otherwise, what is the point? This is why we must be specific to the individual, based on individual anatomy. You can see this by going back to the example of facet syndrome and facet arthropathy. Suppose you have facet arthropathy and degenerative structural changes to the joints in your lower back from repetitive long-term stress. In that case, your anatomy is different, and you may have a neutral position different from someone without this condition. Also, you may and most likely will have a different neutral now than you did ten years ago because your body has acquired a different structure. Remember, like rocks in a river, our body's structures will change over time. [296, 297, 298, 299, 300, 301, 254, 255, 256, 257, 258, 259, 260, 261, 262, 263, 264, 265, 266, 267, 268, 269, 270, 271, 272, 273, 274, 275]

By now, you may realize that pelvic neutral is not a single position that you should be in all the time. It is more of a concept and an awareness. Pelvic neutral, like all mechanics of the body, is a living thing, constantly changing and evolving over time as your body changes over time, like rocks in a river. Once you fully understand pelvic neutral, you will realize it is more of an awareness than anything else. With this awareness, you will constantly work to tweak, fine-tune it, and improve pelvic neutral. We are getting a bit ahead of ourselves now, though.

The easiest way to find the pelvic neutral position is to find anatomical neutral, which is the same for everyone, and then find your pelvic neutral, which is specific to the individual. To find anatomical neutral, we roll and shift the pelvis through the full range of motion for each of the three planes, one at a time. You can determine the center, middle, or neutral of each plane of motion once its end ranges have been established.

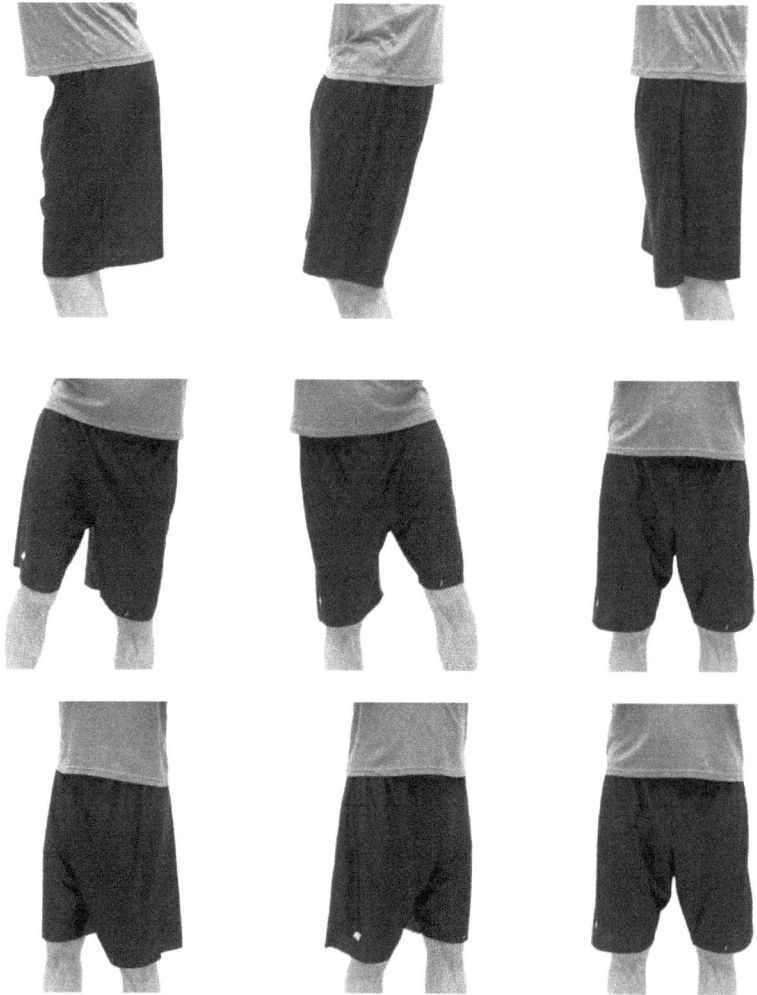

The next step is to fine-tune this position specific to the individual to find your pelvic neutral. You may need to deviate slightly from anatomical neutral to find the ideal neutral position for a particular individual. This is because, as explained in the physical capability limits key concept at the beginning of the book, we are all individual-ized in terms of anatomical structure. This is especially true when the trainee attempts to correct injury due to dysfunction.

ANOTHER EASY WAY TO DISCOVER THE IDEAL NEUTRAL POSITION FOR THE INDIVIDUAL IS TO FIND THE MOST COMFORTABLE POSITION CLOSEST TO THE MIDDLE OF ALL THREE PLANES OF MOTION.

Perfecting this can take some time and fine-tuning over several days, weeks, or even months. Nonetheless, once the ideal neutral posi-tion for the individual is found, the mechanics of the rest of the body can begin to fall in line.

It is worth noting that achieving pelvic neutral is a continual work in progress. You can never stop working at it or any of the funda-mental basics. Continual practice, reinforcement, and awareness are the keys to success.

Once you achieve a pelvic neutral position, the next step will be to teach the core how to keep it there. Remember that the core's job is to prevent, not create, major motion. The core is preventing the pelvis from moving relative to the thorax. If these two pieces, the pelvis and thorax, are held together as a single unit, then the spine will be held stable. If the pelvis and thorax are held together in comfortable pelvic neutral, the spine will be held stable in a pain-free, healthy, and safe position. [849, 850, 865, 873]

Now we are finally ready to begin **Core Bracing Stage I**, which is the first exercise to train the lumbopelvic core component of Full Spinal Control. The first step is to lie on a stable but comfortable surface in the supine (face-up) position in an unloaded spinal position without gravity weighing down the spine. The hips and knees should be flexed (bent) so that the soles of the feet are flat on the ground, spaced about hip-width apart. The knees must be held slightly wider than foot width and never caving inward. Caving inward is a common dysfunctional pattern and a sign of gluteal, especially gluteus medius, inhibition or weakness, and is a hole in the system. It must not be allowed, for it may be a part of the larger underlying dysfunction. The pelvis must be in the individual's specific neutral position.

In the supine position, special attention must be paid to the anterior to posterior, or front to back, sagittal plane pelvic tilt. The lumbar spine (lower back) should not be arched up off the floor (indicating anterior pelvic tilt), nor should it be smashed down into the ground (indicating posterior pelvic tilt). The shoulders should be back and down with the scapula flat on the floor, not rounded and caved in up off the floor. The cervical spine (neck) should also be in a neutral position. We do not want to see chin jutting or excessive lordosis in the C/S. This is all before we even begin the exercise. This much attention to detail is necessary.

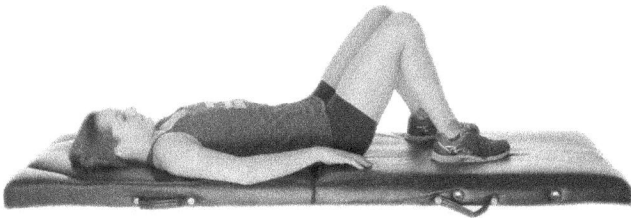

Now that we are in the correct starting position, we can start the core bracing exercise. It involves a series of steps that must be performed in the proper order, as each step builds upon itself to create movement. You should not progress to a subsequent step until the previous step(s) have been mastered—remember, don't hammer boards and nails before laying concrete! Staying patient can be tedious since some people will require a tremendous amount of focus and concentration.

The following chapters outline the specific step-by-step progressions of the PREMIER Body Method's human movement education.

PART THREE
HUMAN MOVEMENT EDUCATION

The PREMIER Body Method's Human Movement Education program has three separate levels of learning. Each level builds off the previous one as functional movement is built from the ground up.

Level I consists of individual fundamental pieces of movement. These foundational pieces are first learned individually with high focus given to every detail.

Level II then takes the individual foundational pieces learned in Level I and puts them together to create basic functional human mechanics.

Level III continues to build more advanced and complex human movement and takes the functional full-body mechanics learned in Level II and applies strength and endurance to them. This is an important step because it is not only necessary to understand how to move, but you must also have a certain level of fitness to be able to move that way and physically apply this knowledge in the real world and/or sports world. With this final step, these mechanics will not only be able to be performed, but they will also be able to be performed consistently throughout the day or throughout whatever activity, sport, or event the individual needs to accomplish. Level III ends by progressing the trainee to a full body strength and conditioning program for basic fitness and human function. The end result is a fully functioning human, ready to continue a basic fitness exercise program for health or return to higher-level sports performance training without pain and knowing how to reduce the risk of injury.

LEVEL I: FULL SPINAL CONTROL

Level I of Human Movement Education begins with learning Full Spinal Control, which is pivotal for proper human biomechanics in healthy and injured individuals alike. Full Spinal Control consists of three components: Lumbopelvic Core Control, Scapulothoracic Control, and Cervical Spine Neutral Control. Each piece will be learned thoroughly and separately before moving to the next. Once all three pieces of spinal control are learned, they will be added back together to achieve Full Spinal Control.

CORE BRACING SERIES:

The Core Bracing Series is designed to teach the basics of core stability and to train the first key component of spinal control, Lumbopelvic Core Control. This series consists of five basic exercise progressions as follows:

STAGE I CORE BRACING (THREE DETAILS OF CORE STABILITY/10-SECOND HOLDS)

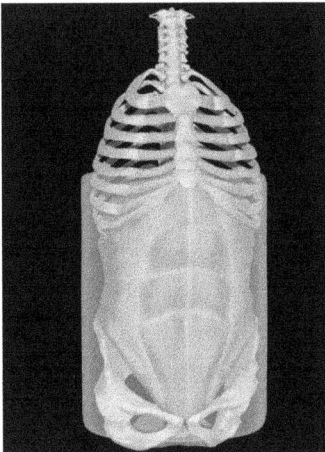

The goal of core bracing is to create stability in the pelvic and lumbar spine region of the body. Remember, the job of core stability is to lock the pelvis to the thorax, thus preventing pelvic and lower spinal movement. Learning to core brace involves an understanding of the core. Think of the core as a big vertical cylinder, like a can of soda, all the way from the pelvis to the shoulders. It has a floor, walls, and a roof. The floor consists of three muscles: Puborectalis, Pubococcygeus, and Iliococcygeus. These are known collectively as the pelvic floor muscles. The walls consist of the Transverse, Oblique, and Rectus Abdominus, as well as the QL, Erector Spinae, and other deeper spinal stabilizers, along with all associated fascia and connective tissue. We may, to a more or lesser extent, include the thoracolumbar fascia and possibly the Latissimus Dorsi here as well, but this will come later. The roof is the Thoracic cage and its associated intercostal musculature and fascia, which is already a fairly solid structure. The diaphragm is a free-floating structure inside the center of this core cylinder. [925, 926, 927, 928]

Essentially, we want to create a solid cylinder while keeping the diaphragm free-flowing. In other words, you must hold tight to the pelvic floor and abdominal muscles while breathing naturally. The abdominal musculature must be solid all the way around, not just in front. The pelvic floor is a commonly overlooked part of core stability. The pelvic floor must be kept tight. This completes the three-dimensional core cylinder, which creates tensegrity and, thus, structural stability. If the pelvic floor is not solid, energy will be lost through the bottom of the core structure, disrupting core stability. [929, 930, 931]

Think of the core as a can of soda. Before you pop the can lid, all three walls are intact and solid. The can is very stable this way. You can't crush or bend it or do anything else to destroy its integrity with your bare hand. Now pop the lid. You have disrupted the integrity of one of the walls, and now you can bend and crush the can easily. Core stability works very similarly to this. One must have a solid core in all three dimensions, not just the pretty six-pack abs in front. Hence, three main components are needed to achieve core stability. The three components of core stability are: solid kegel, solid abdominal wall, and natural breathing.

This exercise begins in the supine position. The trainee lies supine with knees bent, feet flat, and shoulders, neck, and face relaxed.

1. Performing a kegel to tighten the pelvic floor is the first key component of core stability. It's not an exercise just for women after childbirth. The easiest way to do this exercise is to imagine you are urinating and then cutting it off midstream to hold it in. Performing

this action will activate all three main muscles of the pelvic floor. This is because the same nerve that innervates the sphincter muscle that controls urination also innervates the pelvic floor muscles. When you activate one, you activate them all.

2. The second component of core stability is abdominal bracing. The entire abdominal wall must be held rigid all the way around. This includes your six-pack abs, your obliques, your transverse abdominis, and other spinal stabilizing muscles in your back. Press your thumbs into your sides just above the iliac crests (the top sides of your pelvis). If you activate your core properly, you will resist this jabbing of the thumbs. You can also imagine that you are bracing for impact as if you are about to be punched in the stomach. Remember that the walls need to be solid all the way around, not just the "six-pack" in front. This should not be done by sucking in, as with hollowing, nor by pressing the abdominal muscles out. Just create rigidity in the abdominal wall.

3. The third component of core stability is free, normal breathing. Breathing is the most difficult part of the initial stage for most people. The first two steps of creating rigidity in the pelvic floor and the abdominal wall will create the stability needed to sufficiently lock the pelvis in the neutral position. However, if you cannot achieve this solid stability while breathing at the same time, your system will not be able to move with proper biomechanics. If your brain has to choose between core stability and breathing, it will choose breathing. If you cannot achieve core stability and breathe normally at the same time, your brain will drop its focus on core activation and choose breathing to keep you alive. In other words, your brain will continuously tell your body to inhibit and shut down core stability in favor of breathing. This is an unbelievably fundamental and rudimentary component of basic human neuro-musculoskeletal function. Incorrect core activation is a major dysfunction and a huge hole at the most fundamental level of the system.

So, the Stage I Core Bracing exercise is simply to practice and train these three main details of core stability to work together as they should. The exercise is to hold the proper brace activation in the pelvic neutral position for ten seconds while focusing on normal, relaxed breathing. Hold a kegel, keep the abdominal wall solid, and breathe normally all at the same time for around ten seconds. The goal is to train your body to be able to activate the core while breathing normally. This should be practiced as a series of ten-second holds, and trainees should not progress to stage two until they can do all this perfectly.

It is extremely important to keep in mind the true goal of core stability, which is to lock the pelvis in place in the pelvic neutral position. There are a lot of details to think about here, especially for someone with a dysfunction. Some may be able to coordinate all this within just a few tries, while others may require more time.

DO NOT MOVE ON UNTIL THIS STAGE IS MASTERED - EVERY DETAIL!

One tip that helps in learning and retraining this level of control over all these details is to create a running checklist in your mind. As you are performing the exercise, continuously review and repeat your checklist over and over the same way. For this Stage I Core Bracing exercise, you have four basic checkboxes: pelvic neutral, check; kegel, check; abdominal wall, check; and normal relaxed breathing, check. Repeat and review this checklist repeatedly as you perform the ten-second Core Bracing hold. This can be a bit monotonous, but the monotony helps train the neurology, which is the point.

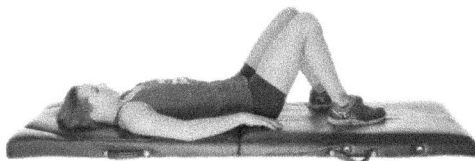

Core Bracing Position

Core Bracing Stage I

Goal/Purpose:

- Focus the mind and reinforce the details of core stability fundamentals.

Beginning Position:

- Supine (face up) on an exercise mat or foam roller.
- Pelvic neutral.
- Lower extremity flexed, hip-width apart.
- Attention to upper body posture, Scapular position, and C/S neutral.

Movement/Action:

- Turn on core stability by activating and holding solid the kegel muscles of the pelvic floor (holding urination) and the abdominal wall (bracing for a punch) while breathing normally all at the same time for 10 seconds, then relax, then repeat.

Key Notes/Common Faults:

- Pain/discomfort/straining of any kind.
- Faulty breathing pattern.
- Loss of pelvic neutral position and/or excessive lumbar

Remember that this stage, like all stages, ideally should be pain-free. Since no movement occurs in this exercise, pain can be positional or the result of pressure. Positional pain can occur if the pelvic position is faulty, meaning the pelvis is not in the ideal neutral position for the individual. A faulty position can put extra pressure or tension on various structures such as joints, cartilage, ligaments, tendons, and/or nerves. If this is the case, adjust the pelvic position to the most relieving position possible, thus creating a better neutral position for the individual.

If the position is optimized and does not cause discomfort, but you are still experiencing pain, then the pain is most likely due to pressure, probably because normal, relaxed breathing is not occurring. This results in increased intra-abdominal pressure, as if one is bearing down. This is also known as the Valsalva maneuver. Increases in intra-abdominal pressure cause a rise in intra-thecal pressure, which represents the pressure within the spinal canal. Depending on the pathology involved, increases in intra-thecal pressure can cause increased pain, possibly severe. These conditions would be along the lines of Myelopathy, Radiculopathy, discogenic pain, disc bulges or herniation, or other spinal conditions. Normal breathing must be maintained. [932, 940, 941, 942, 943, 944, 945, 946, 947]

STAGE II CORE BRACING WITH LIMB INITIATION (HEEL LIFTS)

Once you have successfully learned stage one core bracing and can hold your core solid in the correct position while breathing normally, you are ready to begin stage two of these progressions. The starting position here will also be supine. Remember, everything you do from here will build on itself, so the first step of progression two should always be 'see progression one'. Lay supine; achieve pelvic neutral in all three planes; core brace while breathing normally; and check off all other items on your checklist. Now, we build from here. You are now ready to learn how to initiate limb movement while maintaining core stability.

So far, we have learned what core stability is. Now, we have to learn how to use it. You are not walking around all day squeezing and contracting a constant kegel and the abdominal wall while trying to breathe. Stage one simply teaches the body how to coordinate the three key details of core stability so that they function together correctly. This is so you can turn core stability "on" correctly when necessary.

The next task is to integrate this into a true motor firing pattern, which means putting core stability activation together with movement.

As we move throughout the world, there is (or should be) a continual series of turning "on" and "off" core stability, which occurs in accordance with our movements. It is kind of like a light switch. When I need to use it, I turn it on; when I don't need it anymore, I turn it off to conserve energy. [933, 934]

For example, if someone needs to bend down and pick something up, just before the movement to bend down and lift begins, the core should come "on" to lock everything in place and ensure the body mechanics work efficiently. Now, with the core stable, the movement can take place. Once the movement of picking up the object is complete, the core can then be shut "off." This "on/off" system should occur with all movements, such as lifting, getting up and down from chairs, in and out of the car, climbing stairs, and even getting on and off the toilet! Everything! Eventually, with enough practice, this will become automatic.

This is a good time to mention the true meaning of "on" and "off" core stability. When we say "on," that does not necessarily mean complete 100% contractile tension is on. When we say "off," that does not necessarily mean that 0% of contractile tension is completely flaccid off. We are talking about a continuum of relative muscular tension given the body position and the body movement to take place. So don't think of that light switch as a black-and-white on/off switch. Think of it as a dimmer switch, like in a dining room. You can ramp up "on" for more light (stability) when you need it, and ramp down "off" for less light (stability) when you don't need it as much.

For example, if I were to do a free squat, the starting position would be for me to stand in place, then perform the movement of a squat pattern, and then return to the starting standing position. The correct core activation sequence is core stability "off" at the starting standing position; then just before the squat movement takes place, the core should come "on" to maintain proper pelvic/spinal control while the hip creates the major motion of the squat. Once the squat movement pattern is complete and I am back in the starting standing position, my core will relax "off" again, only to come right back "on" so another squat rep can proceed.

Now, just to hold and maintain the correct standing posture for my starting position, my core must be activated to a certain extent. That means that the "off " here is really on to, let's say, 10% contractile tension above resting muscle tone. In order to maintain my proper pelvic/body position through the squat movement, I must ramp "on" my core stability to, let's say, around 35% contractile tension. ^{(Percent} numbers are just examples and not necessarily accurate, as the exact percentages depend on several factors.)

Now, suppose I am going to perform another squat, but this time, I put 225 pounds on my back. Holding the starting "off" position here may take 40% contractile tension throughout my core musculature with this amount of extra load. Just before I initiate the squat movement, my core must now ramp "on" all the way to 80% contractile tension to maintain stability with this amount of load. Once the movement is complete, my core can ramp back down to the 40% tension "off". So the "off" and "on" of core stability is relative depending on the body position and the movement/activity taking place. Remember, the main purpose of core stability is to maintain pelvic neutral. So, really, you are ramping core stability up and down to whatever level is necessary to maintain pelvic neutrality no matter what you are doing. (Percent numbers are just examples and not necessarily accurate, as the exact percentages are dependent on several factors.)

Core Bracing Stage II (aka heel lifts) is designed to teach and train the ability to utilize this "on/off" system of core stability in accordance with movement. The sequence (firing order) goes like this:

- From the supine starting position, first turn "on" core bracing (which involves everything learned in Core Bracing Stage I)
- Then lift one foot off the ground (just a few inches is all that is needed; we just want to initiate limb movement)
- Then, put the foot back down
- Then, turn "off" the core (relaxing everything).

This teaches you the actual firing pattern that takes place as you move throughout the world. Walking, running, jumping, reaching to get a glass out of the cupboard, and all other movement patterns are all an eloquent and rapid series of on > off > on > off by different muscle groups (really, it is more like ramp up > ramp down > ramp up > ramp down). This beginning Stage II progression is teaching you this motor pattern. So it is on > lift > down > off > on > lift > down > off.

After learning the order, which shouldn't take long, the key is to perfect the movement. You need to be conscious of any changes in pelvic position in all three planes when you lift your foot. If you have perfect lumbopelvic core stability, there will be no difference in pelvic position when your foot is relaxed on the ground and lifted in the air. Correct core stability at this stage locks the pelvic bone to the thorax to make one single unit. If you are strict with yourself, as you need to be, you will most likely find achieving this core stability extremely diffi-cult. Even the slightest bit of pelvic movement, tilting, rocking, rotat-ing, whatever, in this simple low-load exercise can and will translate into much larger problems when you are up on your feet moving throughout the world or performing higher-level exercises. [935]

You can practice on a foam roller to provide more of a challenge and greater feedback in terms of keeping the pelvis stable. We desig-nate the use of a foam roller for this and all the other progressions in this series as the advanced versions of these basic technique exercises.

Practice this exercise in sets of 10 to 20, back-and-forth between sides (right and left leg, on and off between each repetition).

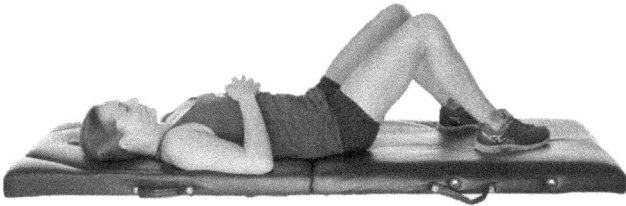

Core Bracing Stage II - Heel Lifts - Beginning Position

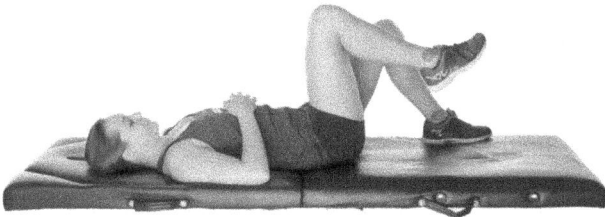

Core Bracing Stage II - Heel Lifts - Movement Position

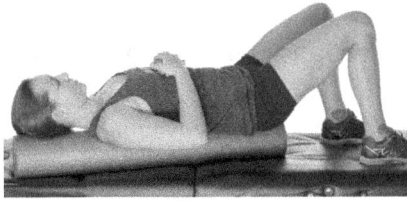

Advanced Core Bracing Stage II - Heel Lifts - Beginning Position
on Foam Roller

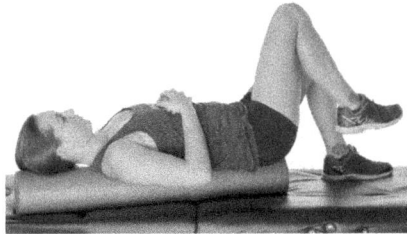

Advanced Core Bracing Stage II - Heel Lifts - Movement Position
on Foam Roller

Core Bracing Stage II

Goal/Purpose:

- Continued reinforcement of the core stability "on/off"
  system with increased stability control and integration with
  a hip flexion mechanism.

Beginning Position:

- Supine (face up) (note: for advanced - on a foam roller.)
- Pelvic neutral.
- Lower extremity flexed, hip-width apart.
- Attention to Scapular and C/S neutral.

Movement/Action:

- Turn the core "on" and "off" in accordance with extremity movement.
- Activate core stability "on" by way of Core Bracing I, lift one heel off the ground by way of hip flexion, then relax heel lift back to the starting position, and then relax core stability "off."
- Repeat with the opposite side.

Key Notes/Common Faults:

- Pain/discomfort/straining of any kind.
- Faulty breathing pattern.
- Loss of pelvic neutral position, seen as rotational disconnect and/or tilting and/or hiking and/or low back arching.
- Instability on the foam roller (falling off the foam roller).
- Other body region compromise.

When designing rehabilitation and exercise programs, remember that beginning-stage motor learning (i.e., training neurology) is more effectively done through higher frequency, not volume. This means you would be better off doing two sets in the morning, two at midday, and two at night, for a total of six sets in a day, rather than six sets together at one point in the day, then not again until the next day. This goes for basic neurological training only! Once you progress to more difficult exercises that place more physical and neurological demands on the body, you need more recovery time and longer rest periods. [936, 937, 938]

Also, keep in mind that as volume increases, recovery time must also increase. First, neurology needs repetition in order to become ingrained, and second, you need to avoid the fatigue factor. Once fatigue sets in, movement patterns will likely revert to the old, ingrained, faulty patterns. If this occurs, you will not be accomplishing the goal but reinforcing the problem. **Perfect practice makes perfect!**

Ideally, this exercise also should be done free of pain, so minor adjustments may be required depending on whether certain pathologies are involved. Common pathologies that may cause pain here can be specific to the hip joint, such as hip degenerative joint disease, arthritis, labral tears, femoral acetabular impingement, hip tendinitis, especially the hip flexor tendon/s, and other joint lesions. If the exercise is causing pain, the first attempt is to change the pelvic position, as it may not be in the correct neutral position. If this does not work, attempt to change the angle of motion at the hip joint by adjusting foot placement to allow for increased or decreased hip flexion, rotation, abduction, and/or adduction at the starting position. Moving the feet further out, closer in, wider, or narrower while in the starting position can change this angle of motion at the hip. Also, as the heel is raised, you can adjust the lift angle by bringing the knee wider or narrower.

If this does not work, next, attempt to limit the range of motion to a pain-free range. Remember that the heel lift mainly utilizes the hip flexor muscle group: Iliopsoas, Rectus Femoris, and Sartorius. If there is tendinitis or other injury present in any of these muscles, pain may occur.

If the pain does not originate from the hip joint, it may come from the sacroiliac joints or the lumbar spine in the lower back. The SI joints can be aggravated by unbalanced torque from side to side or any unilateral movement involving one side at a time. If this is the case, try paying more attention to maintaining pelvic neutral. Also, one of the main hip flexor muscles, the psoas muscle, originates on the lumbar spine and may cause torque, rotation, extension, or compression of the lumbar spine. This can cause pressure to the Facet joints in the spine, mechanical stenosis to the IVF spaces or the spinal central canal, causing radicular or myelopathic complications, and/or increased pressure on the spine's discs. [932, 940, 941, 942, 943, 944, 945, 946, 947]

Any of these scenarios can cause pain. If none of these attempts successfully eliminate the pain, then this exercise may be beyond your current limit capacity and, thus, should not be done. If this is the case, it may indicate that you have trouble with other hip flexion movement patterns. If you cannot perform this exercise now, don't give up. There are ways to handle this situation. First, I recommend seeking proper medical and mechanical evaluation for your pain and injury. The main idea here is to determine the true source of your pain. Either the pain you are experiencing is an injury that will heal with time, or it is a true structural issue that may never truly heal 100%.

If the injury will heal with time, you only need to temporarily pause your training progression and continue to practice and train all previous exercise progressions up to this point. Continue to do this until your injury heals and you can perform this exercise pain-free. Then, you can proceed through the rest of the training program.

If the source of your pain is a true structural issue that may never heal to 100%, then you must accept this fact and continue to move through the training progressions while leaving this particular exercise out of the routine. This may sound harsh or cruel, but it's not meant to be. This is where seeking correct medical advice from a trained professional comes into play.

STAGE III CORE BRACING WITH CONTINUED LIMB INITIATION (HEEL DRIVES)

Now that Core Bracing Stage I has helped us understand core stability and how to achieve it, and Core Bracing Stage II has helped us understand how to use core stability correctly as an "on/off" continuum according to movement, we have learned and installed the main value of this entire training and rehabilitation system.

The basic firing pattern of core stability "on/off" applies to all fundamental movement patterns.

Each fundamental movement pattern sets the stage for bigger, more complex movement patterns. Each movement builds on previous movements. This continues throughout the entire program, with constant reinforcement. Trainees must first be able to perform large human movements with correct mechanics. Then they gain the strength and endurance of these movements and can repeat these mechanics continuously throughout daily life, fitness and exercise programs, and athletic training at a level necessary to achieve their specific goals. At that time, we have built a functional human being.

Core Bracing Stage III (heel drives) is the same fundamental pattern applied to a new movement. During the movement, core stability should be turned "on" and "off" to meet the demands of the movement activation, just as in Core Bracing Stage II. The movement activation, this time, introduces a hip extension pattern. The trainee begins in the same supine starting position, and the motion is a heel drive. The trainee drives one heel at a time into the ground to activate hip extension by way of glute contraction. The heel should be pushed slightly out and away from the body (like pressing a gas pedal) as the drive down occurs, not pulled back towards the buttock. The heel itself does not move along the ground.

This down-and-away line of drive helps to create greater activation of the glutes and less activation of the hamstring. If this movement causes hamstring cramping, it may be because the trainee is pulling the heel down and back towards the buttock instead of the correct down-and-out pattern. Also, as in the heel lift from Core Bracing Stage II, high, forceful contraction is unnecessary here. We simply need to initiate the movement. Do not be concerned with range of motion and strength of contraction at this point. The pelvic position, as always, must be held neutral by superior core stability. Overexertion of the heel drive could cause the pelvis to rotate.

So the pattern is as follows:

- Core stability "on" (as learned in Core Bracing Stage I).
- Heel drive (one side at a time).
- Relax the heel drive.
- Core stability "off."

This is then repeated for the subsequent leg. This exercise can be done on the foam roller for a more advanced challenge.

This should be done in sets of 10-20 back and forth between sides (right and left leg), on and off between each repetition.

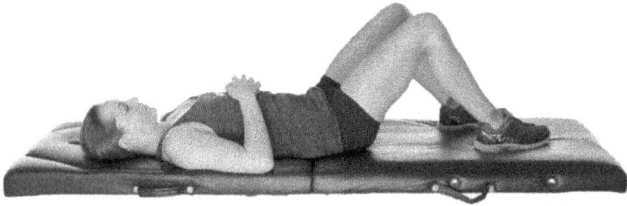

Core Bracing Stage III - Heel Drives - Beginning Position (use Foam Roller for Advanced)

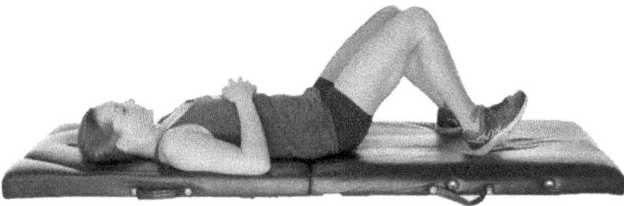

Core Bracing Stage III - Heel Drives - Movement Position (use Foam Roller for Advanced)

Core Bracing Stage III
Goal/Purpose:

- Continued reinforcement of the core stability "on / off" system with increased stability control and integration with a hip extension mechanism.

Beginning Position:

- Supine (face up) on a foam roller.
- Pelvic neutral.
- Lower extremity flexed, hip-width apart.
- Attention to Scapular and C/S neutral.

Movement/Action:

- Turn the core "on" and "off" in accordance with extremity movement.
- Activate core stability "on" by way of Core Bracing I, drive one heel into the ground in a down and away direction by way of hip extension, then relax heel drive, and then relax core stability "off."
- Repeat with the opposite side.

Key Notes/Common Faults:

- Pain/discomfort/straining of any kind.
- Faulty breathing pattern.
- Loss of pelvic neutral position, seen as rotational disconnect and/or tilting and/or hiking and/or lower back arching.
- Instability on the foam roller (falling off the foam roller).
- Other body region compromise.

This exercise ideally should be done pain-free, so minor adjustments may be necessary based on specific pathologies. Common pathologies that may cause pain here can be those specific to the hip joint, such as hip degenerative joint disease, arthritis, labral tears, hip tendinitis (especially glutes or hamstrings), and other joint lesions. If pain is due to hip pathologies, first attempt to change the pelvic position, as it may not be in the correct neutral position. If this does not work, attempt to change the angle of motion at the hip joint by adjusting foot placement to allow for increased or decreased hip flexion, rotation, abduction, or adduction at the starting position. Moving the feet further out, closer in, wider, or narrower in the starting position can do this.

Range of motion is not of concern since this is an isometric exercise in which the heel does not move, but overdoing it by driving the heel down too hard is possible. Do not try to put a hole in the ground!

If the pain does not originate from the hip joint, it may be coming from the sacroiliac joints, hip area, or the lumbar spine in the lower back. Remember, the SI joints can be aggravated by unbalanced torque from side to side. If this is the case, try paying more attention to maintaining pelvic neutral. Since the heel drive mainly uses the hip extensor muscle group of the glutes and hamstrings, with slight activation of the hip rotators, pain may occur if tendinitis is present in any of these muscles.

One of the hip rotator muscles, the piriformis, originates on the sacrum and may cause torque, rotation, or compression of the Sacroiliac joints. This can cause pain to the SI joints or change the position of the lumbar spine, putting pressure on the Facet joints in the spine or causing mechanical stenosis to the IVF space/s or the spinal central canal, causing radicular or myelopathic complications, or increased pressure on the discs of the spine.

Each of these scenarios may cause pain. If no attempts are successful at eliminating the pain, then this particular exercise may be beyond the trainee's current limit capacity and thus should not be done. If this is the case, it may also be a sign that this particular person may have trouble with other hip extension movement patterns. [932, 940, 941, 942, 943, 944, 945, 946, 947]

After successful mastery of Stage III, the trainee can progress to Stage IV Core Bracing.

STAGE IV CORE BRACING WITH CONTINUED LIMB INITIATION (FALLOUTS)

Continued reinforcement of the core "on/off" system will occur throughout the rest of this program as we progress to more complicated movements. For now, we will continue to apply our "on/off" system to several smaller pieces of movement until we have enough individual pieces built to add together to create larger body mechanics. The rest of the Core Bracing Series will complete all the major motions of the hip in accordance with our core stability system. We have already done hip flexion with the heel lifts and hip extension with the heel drives. Stage IV Core Bracing continues with the fallout exercise to train hip abduction. The exercise is similar to Stage II and Stage III Core Bracing, except instead of lifting or driving the heel, it involves abducting the hip as the knee falls out to the side of the body. This exercise should be done with a TheraBand secured around the knees to provide the resistance needed to activate the hip abduction.

The starting position is the same, with the trainee supine with knees bent, feet flat, shoulders, neck, and face relaxed, and in pelvic neutral. The movement pattern is to abduct the hip by moving the knee out to the side, one side at a time. This must be done in accordance with our core stability "on/off" system, so the pattern is:

- Core stability "on" (as learned in Core Bracing Stage I).
- Hip abduction knee fall out.
- Return hip/knee to the starting position.
- Core stability "off."

This is then repeated for the subsequent leg. This exercise can be done on the foam roller for a more advanced challenge.

This should be done in sets of 10-20 back and forth between sides (right and left leg), on and off between each repetition.

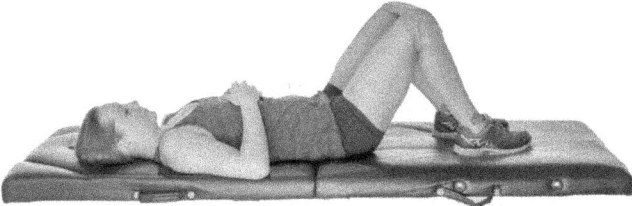

Core Bracing IV - Fallouts - Beginning Position

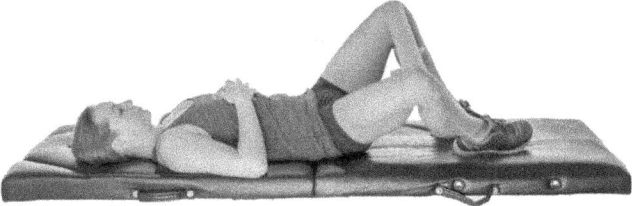

Core Bracing IV - Fallouts - Movement Position

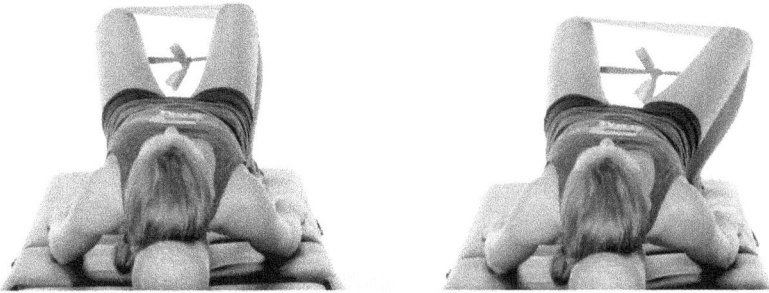

Core Bracing IV - Fallouts - Advanced with Foam Roller (Top View)

Core Bracing Stage IV
Goal/Purpose:

- The integration of core stability, as learned in Core Bracing Stage I, into a basic and fundamental motor firing pattern involving hip abduction, i.e., learning to turn the core "off" and "on" in accordance with movement.

Beginning Position:

- Supine (face up).
- Pelvic neutral.
- Lower extremities flexed, hip-width apart, with a TheraBand secured around the knees.
- Attention to Scapular and C/S neutral.

Movement/Action:

- Turn the core "on and off" in accordance with extremity movement.
- Activate core stability "on" by way of Core Bracing I, move one knee (leg) out to the side laterally by way of hip abduction, then return the leg to the starting position, and then relax core stability "off."
- Repeat with the opposite side.

Key Notes/Common Faults:

- Pain/discomfort/straining of any kind.
- Faulty breathing pattern.
- Loss of pelvic neutral position, seen as rotational disconnect and/or tilting and/or hiking and/or lower back arching
- Other body region compromise.

Remember, as with everything, pelvic neutral must be maintained. The most common fault with fallouts is pelvic rotation. It can happen in one of two ways. One is that pelvic neutral is simply not maintained as the hip abduction movement occurs, and the pelvis is allowed to rotate with the movement. The trainee must separate pelvic movement from hip movement, or, in other words, create movement at the hip without the pelvis moving at the same time.

The second way pelvic rotation can occur is at the end range. If the movement of hip abduction is performed as it should without pelvic movement, but the trainee overdoes the motion by going too far, the range of motion of the fallout moves beyond the hip's range of motion. The movement will then be transferred to the pelvis and spine. So, the goal here is to get as much pain-free motion out of the hip without the pelvis moving and without going beyond the end of the hip's range of motion. This sounds simple, but I cannot stress enough the importance of this concept. This is a huge dysfunction for many people. Understanding how your body moves is the whole point of this program. Not understanding when the hip is moving and when the spine is moving is a premier (*no pun intended*) example of the need for this program.

Again, depending on the presence of certain pathologies, minor adjustments may be necessary to avoid pain. Usual suspects here can be specific to the hip joint, such as hip degenerative joint disease, arthritis, labral tears, hip tendinitis, or other joint lesions. If this is the case and the exercise is causing pain, you should first attempt to change the pelvic position, as it may not be in the correct neutral position. If this does not work, try to change the angle of motion at the hip joint by adjusting foot placement to allow for increased or decreased

hip flexion, rotation, abduction, and/or adduction at the starting position. Moving the feet further out, closer in, wider, or narrower in the
starting position can do this.

If this does not work, next attempt to limit the range of motion to a
pain-free range. This range may be as small as zero, as this exercise
may be done isometrically if necessary. For zero-range movement,
secure a non-elastic belt or strap around the knees to provide resistance
so the hip abduction can be activated by pressing the knees out against
the belt without actual movement.

If the pain does not originate in the hip joint, it may come from the
sacroiliac joints or the lumbar spine in the back. The lumbar spine and
SI joints can be aggravated by unbalanced torque from side to side. If
this is the case and torque is unbalanced, then try paying more attention to maintaining pelvic neutral. If this does not work, the trainee
may perform the abduction movement bilaterally instead of unilaterally. This is done by moving both knees out together simultaneously
instead of one side at a time. This will create more of an equal pull
across the spine and SI joints and minimize any lumbar spine rotation
and SI joint torque.

If none of these attempts successfully eliminate the pain, then this
particular exercise may be beyond the trainee's current limit capacity
and thus should not be done. If this is the case, it may also indicate that
this particular person has trouble with other hip abduction movement
patterns. [932, 940, 941, 942, 943, 944, 945, 946, 947]

STAGE V CORE BRACING WITH CONTINUED LIMB INITIATION (BALL SQUEEZE)

We will complete the four major hip motions with Core Bracing Stage
V, the ball-squeeze for hip adduction. Yes, for all you sticklers out
there, there are indeed six major hip motions. We have left out hip
internal rotation and hip external rotation. This is because, in real-life
movement, these motions are rarely, if ever, isolated and are instead
coupled with the other four hip motions. For example, you see hip
external and internal rotation when the hip flexes and extends during a
correct squatting pattern movement. Even above with our fallout exer-

cise, labeled as hip abduction, the hip is actually externally rotating as well as abducting during that movement. Also, keep in mind that other specific exercises can be applied if specific internal and external rotations of the hip want to be trained individually.

The ball squeeze exercise is just as it sounds. It requires a ball like a large (basketball size) rubber handball. Begin in the supine starting position with knees bent, feet flat, and shoulders, neck, and face relaxed. Place the ball between the knees. The movement pattern is to adduct the hip by squeezing a ball or padded object that is placed between the knees. This must be done in accordance with our core stability "on/off" system. So the pattern is:

- Core stability "on" (as learned in Core Bracing Stage I).
- Hip adduction by squeezing the knees together.
- Relax the squeeze and return to the starting position.
- Core stability "off."

This exercise can be done on the foam roller for a more advanced challenge.

The trainee should perform 3-5 sets of 10-20 reps.

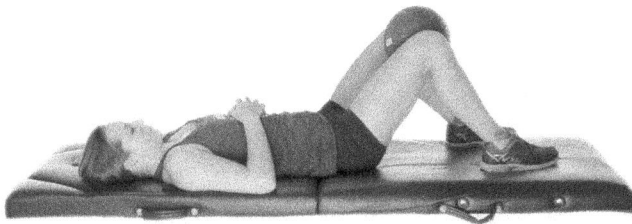

Core Bracing Stage V - Ball Squeeze - Beginning Position

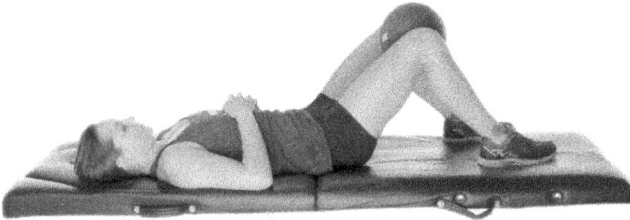

Core Bracing Stage V - Ball Squeeze - Movement Position

Core Bracing Stage V - Ball Squeeze - Advanced with Foam Roller (Top View)

Core Bracing Stage V
Goal/Purpose:

- The integration of core stability, as learned in Core Bracing Stage I, into a basic and fundamental motor firing pattern involving hip adduction, i.e., learning to turn the core "off" and "on" in accordance with movement.

Beginning Position:

- Supine (face up).
- Pelvic neutral.
- Lower extremities flexed, hip-width apart, with a ball between knees.
- Attention to Scapular and C/S neutral.

Movement/Action:

- Turn the core "on" and" off" in accordance with extremity movement.
- Activate core stability "on" by way of Core Bracing I, squeeze both legs into the ball between the knees by way of hip adduction, then relax the squeeze, and then relax core stability "off."
- Repeat.

Key Notes/Common Faults:

- Pain/discomfort/straining of any kind.
- Faulty breathing pattern.
- Loss of pelvic neutral position, seen as rotational disconnect and/or tilting and/or hiking and/or lower back arching.
- Other body region compromise.

As with everything, ideally, this should be done pain-free. The firmness of the ball affects the movement range. A soft, flexible ball will allow for a greater range, while a firm, non-flexible ball makes this exercise nearly isometric and can be used to attempt to reduce pain if it is present with a more squeeze-able ball. It is a bilateral movement, so we shouldn't worry too much about unequal torque or rotation on the spine or SI joints. If there is pain, one may attempt to change the angle of movement at the hip again by changing foot placement at the start position.

The hip joint adductor and hip flexor tendons can be sources of pain here, so ensure the pelvic position is neutral, limit the range of motion, and ensure the trainee is not overdoing it by squeezing too hard.

If none of these attempts successfully eliminate the pain, then this particular exercise may be beyond the current limit capacity and thus should not be done. If this is the case, it may also be a sign that this particular person may have trouble with other hip adduction movement patterns.

IMPORTANCE OF THESE BEGINNING EXERCISES AND DETAILS

By now, you may be questioning the importance of all these little tedious technique exercises. How are these really going to help you? Do you really need to do this stuff? I know you just want to get to the good stuff, but the level of detail in the beginning Level I exercises is what lets you get to the fun stuff and excel at it. It's like math. If your goal is to pass calculus, you will not be able to meet your goal unless you first learn how to count, add and subtract correctly, and do algebra. If you can't add and subtract, you will have a hell of a time trying to pass calculus. In this program, you can't excel at Level III unless you first master Levels I and II. Skipping right to the higher-level movements can lead to problems such as pain, injuries, and/or poor results and performance gains.

Now that we have completed the Core Bracing Series and learned the initial aspects of core stability and pelvic control, the first component of Full Spinal control, we are ready to progress to the second major component, thoracic spine and scapulothoracic control, taught by the Scapular Setting Series.

SCAPULAR SETTING SERIES:

The scapular setting series is designed to teach and train the second major piece of Full Spinal Control, thoracic spine and scapulothoracic control. This creates a solid foundation from which the shoulder and upper extremities can work.

STAGE I-A SUPINE SCAPULAR SETTING (SCAPULA ONLY)

We will now branch up the mechanical chain to the thoracic spine and shoulder girdle by learning the proper thoracic spine and scapular position. This is known as the set scapular position, or scapular neutral, and is achieved through a scapular setting motion. We will first learn this movement position in an unloaded supine position. Begin in the supine starting position with knees bent, feet flat, and shoulders, neck, and face relaxed. As with all movements in this program, we will use pelvic neutral and our core stability "on/off" system in accordance with the movement.

The scapular setting motion is best understood as the combination of depression and retraction of the scapulae, or pulling the shoulder blade back and down. Think of your shoulder blades as two big triangles on your back, with their points facing downward. The goal of this movement is to tuck the bottom points of these triangles into your back pockets.

The exercise (firing pattern) is as follows:

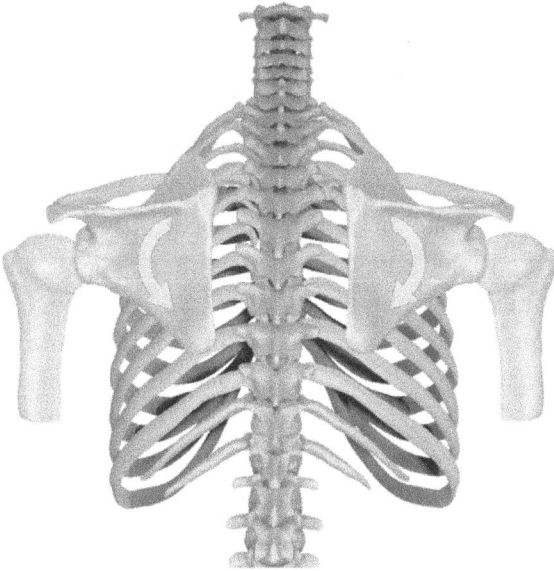

- In the supine starting position, first turn core stability "on" (as learned in Core Bracing Stage I).
- Then, achieve the set scapular position by using the scapular setting motion (pull shoulder blades back and down).
- Relax the scapular setting motion
- Turn core stability "off."
- Repeat the sequence.

This exercise can be done on the foam roller for a more advanced challenge. It should be done in sets of 10-20 (core on and off between each repetition).

There are two main things to remember as the scapular setting motion is taking place. Number one, we do not want excessive movement in the spine, particularly the lumbar spine, to occur along with the scapular movement. This is commonly seen as hyperextension of the lower back up off the ground and is a major faulty pattern here. This is another example of why proper pelvic Core Control is so important. If proper core activation ("on") is achieved prior to the scapular movement, then the pelvis and, thus, the spine should already be locked in a stable position. If this is maintained correctly, the scapular setting motion should occur without spinal movement, thus avoiding hyperextension.

The second main thing to remember is the set scapular position itself. It is similar to the neutral pelvic position, as the scapula can be moved up (elevation), down (depression), forward (protraction), and back (retraction), none of which are neutral. The anatomical set scapular position is classified as the middle position in all planes of motion, and you can identify it just as you did pelvic neutral. Move the scapulae to the end range for all positions and planes of motion, and then settle into the center middle spot. Once this neutral spot is found, you can fine-tune it specifically for the individual based on their unique anatomical structure and physical capability limits.

Most people grossly err towards the protracted and elevated position of the scapula, as the shoulders round and slump forward to create what we call "bad posture." The goal is to train your shoulders to be back and down, but not necessarily smashed back and down excessively to the point of straining. The human body likes balance and neutrality, not extremes.

Remember that with all positions and movements, certain structural pathology can change physical capability limits and an individual's ideal neutral. Once the individual ideal set scapular position is learned, it should be the position of movement achieved in this Stage I scapular setting exercise and all other progressions in this series.

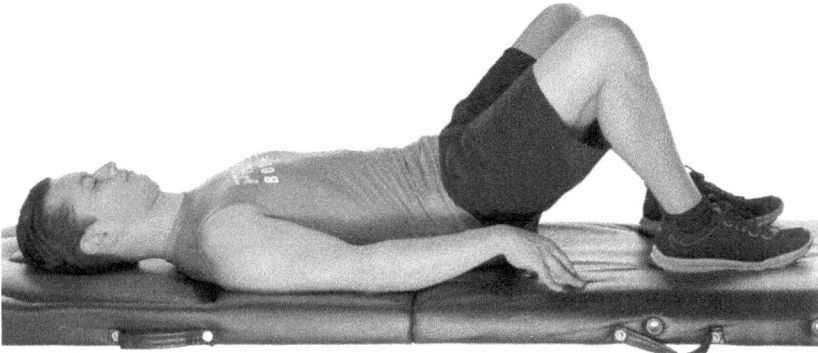

Scapular Setting I-A - Supine Scap Setting - Beginning Position

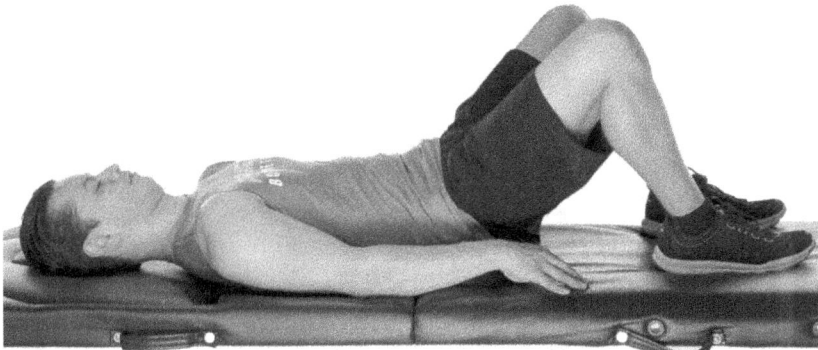

Scapular Setting I-A - Supine Scap Setting - Movement Position

Supine Scapular Setting Stage I
Goal/Purpose:

- The integration of core stability, as learned in Core Bracing
  Stage I, with the second fundamental component of Full
  Spinal Control, a set scapular position.

Beginning Position:

- Supine (face up).
- Pelvic neutral.
- Lower extremity flexed, hip-width apart, with a ball between the knees.
- Attention to Scapular and C/S neutral.

Movement/Action:

- Turn the core "on" and "off" in accordance with extremity movement.
- Activate core stability "on" by way of Core Bracing I, depress and retract the scapulae bilaterally by pulling the shoulder blades back and down, with the upper extremity and C/S relaxed, then relax the scapulae, then relax core stability "off."
- Repeat.

Key Notes/Common Faults:

- Pain/discomfort/straining of any kind.
- Faulty breathing pattern.
- Loss of pelvic neutral position, seen mainly as lower back arching.
- Overactivation/straining at the neck.
- Other body region compromise.

Since this exercise ideally should be performed pain-free, minor adjustments may be necessary if certain pathologies are involved. Common pathologies which may cause pain here can be specific to the shoulder joint. Possibilities include degenerative joint disease, arthritis, labral tears, tendinitis, and other joint lesions. The thoracic spine and cervical spine are also involved because several muscles of the scapula and shoulder are connected to the mid back and neck. Pathology such as nerve compression or neuropathy, thoracic outlet syndrome, myelopathy, radiculopathy, discogenic pain, disc bulges or herniation, and other spinal conditions may be aggravated and cause pain. In addition, several muscular, facial, and bursa layers between the scapula and thoracic (rib) cage can be a source of injury or pain. If pelvic neutral is lost, the lumbar spine and thus all the various pathologies discussed already for the low back and hip may also be involved here.

This is the case as we progress and continue to build movement. As we build movement, we are adding each piece to the next. Nothing ever goes away, so as we progress, all previous pieces are still involved to a certain extent. Therefore, we need to keep in mind all pathologies that may be involved and that more pathology may be involved as we continue to build more movement.

Whenever an exercise causes pain, we must alter the position or movement to achieve pain-free posture or motion. As before, checking and adjusting the pelvic neutral position is a good place to start since everything is built on this.

Pain in the upper back or underneath the shoulder blade (retro-scapular pain) may be a problem with a rib or sub-scapular bursitis. The fix here is to limit the amount of scapular setting motion. Too much retraction and depression of the scapula may create compression, friction, and increased pressure on the thoracic spine, posterior costovertebral joints (ribs), and the bursas underneath the scapula. Limit the setting range of motion to a pain-free range, and learn to fine-tune the set scapular position so it is as comfortable as possible.

The shoulder joint itself is not moving in this Stage I exercise and should not cause pain. If this exercise is causing pain specific to the shoulder joint (GHJ), the cause may be positional. Try to change the arm position to alleviate this. Try moving it, turning the arms out (palms up) or down (palms down), or neutral (thumbs up), or perhaps moving the arms further out away from the body, or closer in, and so on.

Pain can also originate from the cervical spine, such as C6 or C7 discogenic referral pain, which can mimic pain in the scapular area (retroscapular or intrascapular pain). It feels like upper back or shoulder pain but is not pain from the thoracic spine, ribs, or the bursa at all. Neck, mid-back, shoulder blade, or arm pain may also be referred neurological pain from radiculopathy, myelopathy, or other peripheral neuropathy. If this is the case, special attention must be given to the neck position and the range of motion for the scapular setting movement, as many of the muscles attached to the scapula are also anchored to the cervical spine.

If none of these attempts successfully eliminate the pain, then this particular exercise may be beyond the trainee's current limit capacity and thus should not be done. If this is the case, it may also be a sign that this particular person may have trouble with other shoulder and/or upper extremity movement patterns. [932, 940, 941, 942, 943, 944, 945, 946, 947]

STAGE I-B PRONE SCAPULAR SETTING (SCAPULA ONLY)

The next progression in the scapular setting series is to move to the prone (face down) position. This increases the difficulty for two main reasons. First, you will now be moving the scapula and shoulder girdle against gravity without the luxury of having the ground to guide you, so the movement is slightly harder to control.

Second, the pelvic neutral position is more difficult to achieve and maintain when face down. This is the first time in the program we will not be in the supine starting position, and achieving the correct position while face down may take some getting used to. Depending on individual body type, gravity will usually pull the pelvis out of the neutral position and into an anterior tilt position when lying face down, thus forcing the lower back into extension. Before proceeding, special attention and focus must go to rolling the pelvis back to the correct neutral position. A bolster or pillow underneath the abdomen may help while learning this new position.

Once the correct prone position is achieved, begin the exercise (firing pattern).

- Starting in the prone starting position, turn core stability "on" (as learned in Core Bracing Stage I).

- Achieve the set scapular position by way of scapular setting motion (pull shoulder blades back and down).
- Relax the scapular setting motion.
- Core stability "off."

This sequence is then repeated. This should be done in sets of 10-20 (core on and off between each repetition).

Please keep in mind that turning the core off and on does not mean rolling in and out of the neutral pelvic position. Remember to keep the continuum of contraction in mind. "On" does not mean 100% contractile tension on, and "off" does not mean 0% contractile tension off. The degree of contraction is on a sliding gray scale of relative muscular tension given the body position and the body movement to take place. When face down, the core will most likely have to have a greater activation level in the "off position." The purpose of turning the core "on" here is to provide increased stability to maintain the neutral position as the scapular setting movement occurs.

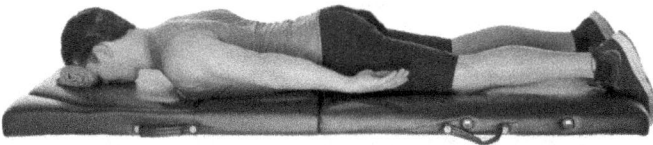

Stage 1-B Prone Scap Setting - Beginning Position

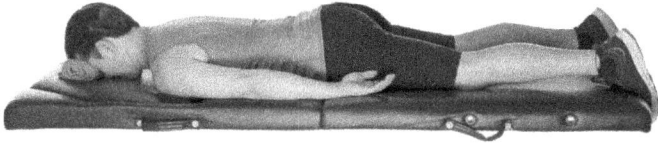

Stage 1-B Prone Scap Setting - Movement Position

Prone Scapular Setting Stage I
Goal/Purpose:

- The integration of core stability, as learned in Core Bracing Stage I, with the second fundamental component of Full Spinal Control, a set scapular position.

Beginning Position:

- Prone (face down).
- Pelvic neutral (use bolster assistant if necessary).
- Attention to C/S neutral.

Movement/Action:

- Turn the core "on" and "off" in accordance with extremity movement.
- Activate core stability "on" by way of Core Bracing I, depress and retract the scapulae bilaterally by pulling the shoulder blades back and down, with the upper extremity

and *C/S relaxed*, then relax the scapulae, then relax core stability "off."

Repeat.

Key Notes/Common Faults:

- Pain/discomfort/straining of any kind.
- Faulty breathing pattern.
- Loss of pelvic neutral position, seen mainly as lower back arching (use a bolster under the stomach to maintain neutral if necessary).
- Other body region compromise.

All the pathology discussed thus far can be possible here, so please refer to the above information if pain is present. In the prone position, one major adjustment that can be made to achieve and maintain proper pelvic neutral is to use a bolster lumbar type support under the abdomen. This can be useful if the trainee cannot achieve the proper position or if pain occurs with the exercise, especially pain originating at the spine.

If none of the attempts successfully eliminate the pain, then this particular exercise may be beyond the trainee's current limit capacity and thus should not be done. [932, 940, 941, 942, 943, 944, 945, 946, 947]

STAGE II PRONE SCAPULAR SETTING (SCAPULA + GHJ ROTATION)

The next progression in the scapular setting series is Stage II Prone Scapular Setting. This progression adds to the Stage I-b prone scapular setting exercise. Everything remains the same as in Stage I-b, but with the addition of upper extremity lift and external rotation of the GHJ (shoulder joint). The external rotation of the GHJ will help facilitate the scapular setting motion when done correctly.

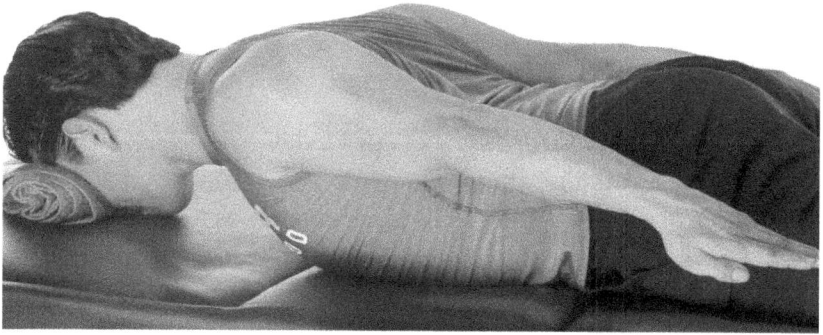

The sequence is as follows:

- Starting in the prone starting position, turn core stability "on" (as learned in Core Bracing Stage I).
- Achieve the set scapular position by way of scapular setting motion (pull shoulder blades back and down) while also externally rotating the GHJ.
- Relax the scapular setting and GHJ motion.
- Core stability "off."

This sequence is then repeated. This should be done in sets of 10-20 (core on and off between each repetition).

Just as in the stage I progression, turning the core off and on does not mean rolling in and out of neutral position. If necessary, a bolster or lumbar support can help control this.

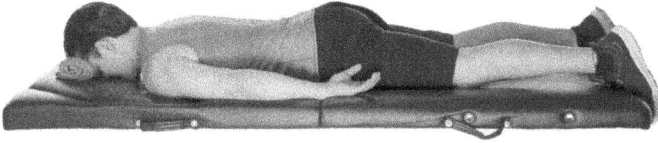

Stage II Prone Scap Setting - Beginning Position

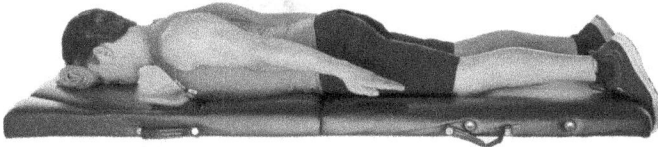

Stage II Prone Scap Setting - Movement Position

Prone Scapular Setting Stage II
Goal/Purpose:

- The integration of core stability, as learned in Core Bracing
  Stage I, with the second fundamental component of Full
  Spinal Control, a set scapular position.

Beginning Position:

- Prone (face down).
- Pelvic neutral (use bolster assistant if necessary).
- Attention to C/S neutral.

Movement/Action:

- Turn the core "on" and "off" in accordance with extremity movement.
- Activate core stability "on" by way of Core Bracing I, depress and retract the scapulae bilaterally by pulling the shoulder blades back and down, *with upper extremity external rotation (turn the arms out),* and C/S relaxed, then relax the scapular/arms, then relax core stability "off."
- Repeat.

Key Notes/Common Faults:

- Pain/discomfort/straining of any kind.
- Faulty breathing pattern.
- Loss of pelvic neutral position, seen mainly as lower back arching (use a bolster under the stomach to maintain neutral if necessary).
- Other body region compromise.

All the pathology discussed thus far can be possible. The addition of GHJ motion can aggravate additional shoulder pathology, such as GH degenerative joint disease, arthritis, labral tears, bursitis, rotator cuff or biceps tendinitis, and other joint lesions. These pathologies can be controlled by limiting the range of motion for external rotation at the GHJ.

If none of these attempts successfully eliminate the pain, then this particular exercise may be beyond the trainee's current limit capacity and thus should not be done. [932, 940, 941, 942, 943, 944, 945, 946, 947]

STAGE III PRONE SCAPULAR SETTING (SCAPULA + GHJ ROTATION + T/S EXTENSION WITH C/S DNF)

The next progression in the Scapular Setting Series is Stage III Prone Scapular Setting, which adds to the Stage II Prone Scapular Setting exercise. Everything remains the same as Stage II, but with the addition of upper thoracic spine extension and the achievement of a neutral cervical spine position by way of deep neck flexor muscle group (DNF) activation; please see the DNF progression for cervical spine control in later sections for the specifics on this movement control piece. In the exercise program progression, the Cervical Spine (C/S) DNF stages I and II should be taught and learned before this Stage III Prone Scapular Setting exercise is attempted. This is starting to get into the concept of building movement now, where multiple pieces must first be learned and then added together to create larger movements.

So, the sequence for this exercise is as follows:

- Starting in the prone starting position, turn core stability "on" (as learned in Core Bracing Stage I).
- Achieve the set scapular position by way of scapular setting motion (pull shoulder blades back and down) while also externally rotating the GHJ. and extending the upper thoracic spine while achieving a DNF-neutral neck position.
- Relax the scapular setting, GHJ, T/S, and C/S motion.
- Core stability "off."

This sequence is then repeated. This should be done in sets of 10-20 (core on and off between each repetition).

Please keep in mind, just as in the Stage I and II progressions, turning the core off and on does not mean rolling in and out of pelvic neutral position. A bolster/lumbar support can be used to help control this if necessary. Also, it is extremely important to create thoracic spine (upper back) extension only. The lumbar spine (lower back) should not extend (arch up) at all.

Prone Scapular Setting Stage III
Goal/Purpose:

- The integration of core stability, as learned in Core Bracing Stage I, with the second and third fundamental components of Full Spinal Control, a set scapular position, and C/S DNF neck position.

Beginning Position:

- Prone (face down).
- Pelvic neutral (use bolster assistant if necessary).
- Attention to C/S neutral.

Movement/Action:

- Turn the core "on" and "off" in accordance with extremity movement.
- Activate core stability "on" by way of Core Bracing I, depress and retract the scapulae bilaterally by pulling the shoulder blades back and down, with upper extremity external rotation (turn the arms out), with C/S DNF activation, then relax the scapular/arm/neck movement, then relax core stability "off."
- Repeat.

Key Notes/Common Faults:

- Pain/discomfort/straining of any kind.
- Faulty breathing pattern.
- Loss of pelvic neutral position, seen mainly as lower back arching (use a bolster under the stomach to aid in maintaining neutral if necessary).
- Other body region compromise.

All the pathology discussed thus far can be possible, so if pain is present, please see the above information. With the addition of thoracic spine extension, make sure the movement of spinal extension comes only from the thoracic spine and not from the lumbar spine! It is very common to overextend the lumbar spine and thus lose the neutral pelvic position. This is faulty and should not be allowed for anyone, especially persons with low back pain and lumbar spine pathology. Excessive lower back extension, especially on a repetitive basis, may cause damage to the interspinous and supraspinous ligaments of the spine and create or aggravate other pathology.

With the addition of cervical spine involvement, it is important to pay close attention to any neck or upper extremity pain, as well as cervical spine pathology. A neutral cervical spine is a must here, so proper activation and control of the DNF neutral position neck is crucial. As stated above, this should be learned by way of the C/S DNF Series and mastered before Stage III Prone Scapular Setting is attempted.

If these areas are of concern and pathology is present, pain can be controlled by limiting the range of motion for thoracic spine extension and cervical spine activation. If none of these attempts successfully eliminate the pain, then this particular exercise may be beyond the trainee's current limit capacity and thus should not be done. More practice at Stage I and II scapular setting, as well as Stage I and II C/S DNF, may be necessary before the trainee is ready to attempt this Stage III progression. [932, 940, 941, 942, 943, 944, 945, 946, 947]

CERVICAL SPINE DEEP NECK FLEXOR (DNF) SERIES:

T he cervical spine deep neck flexor series is designed to teach the third and final piece of Full Spinal Control, the cervical spine complex and cervical spine neutral. This helps complete the solid foundation for the shoulder and upper extremity to work from since many of the muscles that work to create upper extremity movement are also anchored to the neck.

STAGE I CERVICAL SPINE DEEP NECK FLEXOR MUSCLE ACTIVATION (SUPINE DNF)

We now continue to move up the biomechanical chain to the cervical spine. Building on lumbopelvic and scapulothoracic control, we will now learn to achieve a neutral cervical spine position. We do this by activating a small group of muscles, collectively known as the deep neck flexors, or DNF for short. This DNF group consists of two muscles known as longus capitis and longus colli. These muscles are located along the anterior (front) side of the cervical vertebrae. Together, their actions elongate the posterior (back) side of the neck, opening up the intervertebral foramina (IVF) nerve root spaces and the facet joints of the neck. This helps create the cervical spine neutral position and reduces tension and stress on the other larger neck muscles. You can think of the DNF muscles as the core stability of the neck. Just as we activated the core to lock the pelvis in place and create a neutral and stable lumbar spine, we will now learn to activate the DNF muscles to stabilize the neck to achieve the neutral cervical spine position.

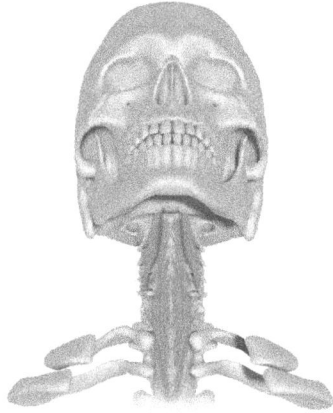

Begin in the supine starting position with knees bent, feet flat, and shoulders, neck, and face relaxed. Just as with everything else, DNF movement control activation is in accordance with core stability "on" and "off". The movement pattern or activation of the DNF is best accomplished by sliding the back of the trainee's head up on the ground. This can be a tricky activation to learn. I use the word activation because it is not a large movement but simply an activation of these muscles. While some small movement occurs as the neck is elongated and flattens out, the head should not lift from the ground in any way, nor should the trainee actively pull the chin back.

Pulling the chin back is a common mistake because the chin does come back slightly if the DNF activation is performed correctly, but the movement will likely be overdone if the trainee actively thinks of the movement as pulling the chin back. This can cause other larger muscles, such as the SCM and scalene muscles, to activate, creating compression and increased loading stress to the neck. So, the movement activation to create a neutral cervical spine by way of DNF activation is simply to slide the back of the head up on the ground. Do not overdo it! Another way to think about it is to imagine a string attached to the top back of the head is pulling upwards, causing the back of the neck to elongate, flatten, and stretch in a gentle, non-straining manner. This lengthens your spine long from the top.

The sequence for the exercise is as follows:

- Starting in the supine starting position, turn core stability "on" (as learned in Core Bracing Stage I)
- Achieve the neutral cervical spine position by way of DNF activation
- Relax the DNF activation
- Core stability "off". This sequence is then repeated.
- This should be done in sets of 10-20 (core on and off between each repetition).

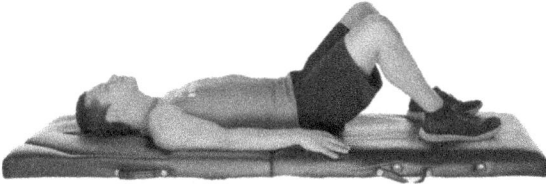

Stage I C/S DNF - Beginning Position

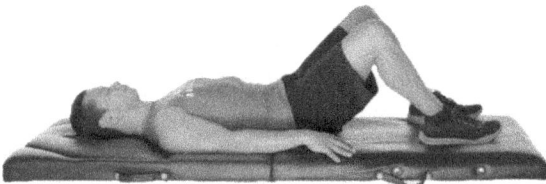

Stage I C/S DNF - Movement Position

CS/DNF Stage I
Goal/Purpose:

- The integration of core stability, as learned in Core Bracing Stage I, with the third fundamental component of Full Spinal Control, Cervical Spine DNF neutral.

Beginning Position:

- Supine (face up).
- Pelvic neutral.
- Lower extremity flexed, hip-width apart.
- Attention to Scapular and C/S neutral.

Movement/Action:

- Turn the core "on" and "off" in accordance with extremity movement.
- Activate core stability "on" by way of Core Bracing I, then activate the DNF muscles by sliding the back of the head up as if a string were pulling from the back top of the head (do not lift the head), then relax the DNF neck activation, then relax core stability "off."
- Repeat.

Key Notes/Common Faults:

- Pain/discomfort/straining of any kind.
- Faulty breathing pattern.
- Loss of pelvic neutral position.
- Activation of the superficial anterior neck musculature.
- Excessive chin retraction.
- Chin jutting.
- Other body region compromise.

All the pathology discussed thus far is possible, so if pain is present, please see the above information. The most common patholo-gies aggravated here are specific to the cervical spine. Watch out for neuropathy, thoracic outlet syndrome, myelopathy, radiculopathy, discogenic pain, disc bulges or herniation, facet pain, and other spinal conditions. If the larger muscles of the neck are tensed by over-acti-vating the motion, the cervical spine will most likely be compressed, and these conditions may be aggravated.

Also, remember that as the DNF muscles are activated, the poste-rior (back) of the neck will be elongated, opening the facet joints and the IVF nerve root space. This should take pressure off these structures, but it may stretch and tense the joint capsule of the facets, and pain may occur if the motion is taken too far. Once again, the goal is to find the best, most comfortable, neutral position specific for the individual based on each individual's structural and physical capability limits.

If no attempts are successful at eliminating the pain, this exercise may be beyond the trainee's current limit capacity and thus should not be done. This is an indication that seeking evaluation and proper guid-ance from a professional may be necessary. [932, 940, 941, 942, 943, 944, 945, 946, 947]

STAGE II CERVICAL SPINE DEEP NECK FLEXOR MUSCLE ACTIVATION (UPRIGHT DNF)

The stage II progression of DNF activation applies what we learned in the unloaded supine position to a loaded vertical standing position. The loaded spinal position increases the difficulty and may provoke pathology if present. The starting position is standing upright or sitting, with the back to a wall, depending on the trainee's comfort and ability based on physical capability limits due to pathology. The feet should be hip-width apart, with the heels placed about a foot from the wall with the pelvis and spine flush against the wall for support. Pelvic neutral, spinal position, and set scapular position should be main-tained. The head is also back against the wall for support and to allow the cue for DNF activation. We have basically just turned the supine position upright, with the wall taking the place of the ground. Keep in mind the concept of building movement here, as we are really beginning to add together the pieces of Full Spinal Control.

We are now ready to begin the sequence as follows:

- In the standing/seated starting position against the wall, turn core stability "on" (as learned in Core Bracing Stage I).
- Achieve the neutral cervical spine position by way of DNF activation (slide the back of the head up on the wall).
- Relax the DNF activation core stability "off."
- This sequence is then repeated.

This should be done in sets of 10-20 (core on and off between each repetition).

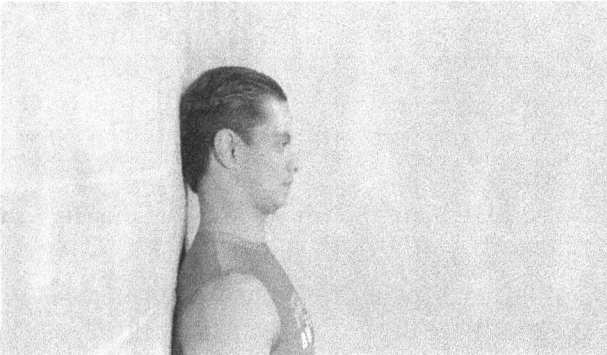

Stage II - CS/DNF - Beginning Position

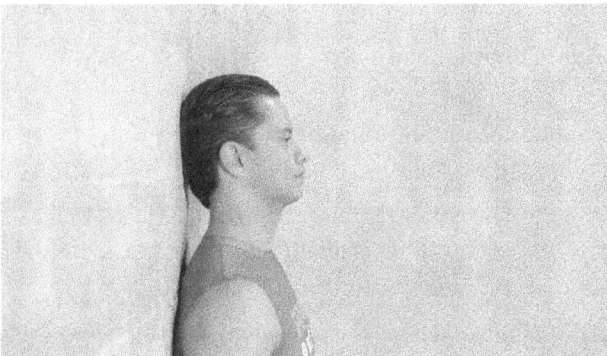

Stage II - CS/DNF - Movement Position

CS/DNF Stage II
Goal/Purpose:

- The integration of core stability as learned in Core Bracing Stage I, with the third fundamental component of Full Spinal Control, Cervical Spine DNF neutral.

Beginning Position:

- Standing or Seated with back against the wall.
- Pelvic neutral.
- Feet flat on the ground, hip-width apart, with knees slightly flexed.
- Attention to Scapular and C/S neutral.

Movement/Action:

- Turn the core "on" and "off" in accordance with extremity movement.
- Activate core stability "on" by way of Core Bracing I, then activate the DNF muscles by sliding the back of the head up as if a string were pulling from the back top of the head (do not allow the head to lift away from the wall), then relax the DNF neck activation, then relax core stability "off."
- Repeat.

Key Notes/Common Faults:

- Pain/discomfort/straining of any kind.
- Faulty breathing pattern.
- Loss of pelvic neutral.
- Activation of the superficial anterior neck musculature.
- Excessive chin retraction.
- Chin jutting.
- Other body region compromise.

All the pathology discussed thus far can be possible, so if pain is present, please see the above information. Remember, the trainee is now upright and, therefore, in a spinal (axial) loaded position. Spinal, rib, hip, lower, and even upper extremity pathology may be accentuated by gravity due to the upright loaded position. Special attention must be given to all neutral positions, or pelvic, spinal, scapular, and neck, along with leg and arm positions, especially if pain is experienced. All the adjustments discussed thus far can be made, especially to the three main spinal positions. Also, as said before, if pertinent pathology is present, such as lower extremity injury (like a sprained ankle that should not yet bear weight), this control exercise can be done seated instead of standing. The rest of the exercise remains the same.

If no attempts are successful at eliminating the pain, this exercise may be beyond the trainee's current limit capacity and thus should not be done. [932, 940, 941, 942, 943, 944, 945, 946, 947]

STAGE III CERVICAL SPINE DEEP NECK FLEXOR MUSCLE ACTIVATION (PRONE DNF)

The stage III progression of DNF activation applies the skills learned in the first and second stage progressions in the prone position. This increases the difficulty due to the loaded spinal musculature position and thus may increase the chance of pathology provocation. This exercise can be done in isolation, but I tend to do it in combination with Prone Scapular Setting Stage III. The starting position is lying prone, as in the Prone Scapular Setting Series. Remember that achieving and maintaining a pelvic neutral position is more difficult in the prone position, and a bolster may be used to assist the correct pelvic position if necessary.

When done in combination with stage III scapular setting, the sequence is as follows:

- Starting in the prone starting position, turn core stability "on" (as learned in Core Bracing Stage I).

- Achieve the set scapular position by way of scapular setting motion (pull shoulder blades back and down) while also externally rotating the GHJ. and extending the upper thoracic spine while achieving a DNF-neutral neck position.
- Relax the scapular setting, GHJ, T/S, and C/S motion.
- Core stability "off."

This sequence is then repeated. This should be done in sets of 10-20 (core on and off between each repetition).

Please keep in mind that, just as in the stage I progression, turning the core off and on does not mean rolling in and out of neutral position. If necessary, a bolster or lumbar support can help control this.

If you want to isolate this movement exercise from the scapular setting, simply remove the scapular and shoulder movement from the sequence. This may be necessary if certain shoulder pathology is present.

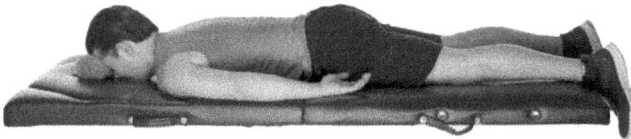

Stage III - CS/DNF Activation (Prone) - Beginning Position

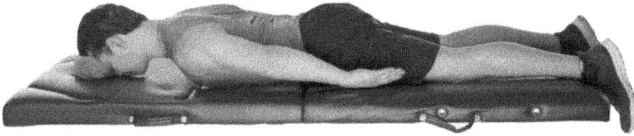

Stage III - CS/DNF Activation (Prone) - Movement Position

CS/DNF Stage III
Goal/Purpose:

- The integration of core stability, as learned in Core Bracing Stage I, with the third fundamental component of Full Spinal Control, Cervical Spine neutral.

Beginning Position:

- Prone (face down).
- Pelvic neutral (use bolster assistant if necessary).
- Attention to C/S neutral.

Movement/Action:

- Turn the core "on" and "off" in accordance with extremity movement.
- Activate core stability "on" by way of Core Bracing I, then activate the DNF muscles by lifting the head back with DNF activation, creating a long neck posture (do not extend the

head and neck by leaning the head back), then relax the DNF neck activation, then relax core stability "off."
- Repeat.
- This exercise is commonly done in combination with Prone Scapular Setting III.

Key Notes/Common Faults:

- Pain/discomfort/straining of any kind.
- Faulty breathing pattern.
- Loss of pelvic neutral.
- C/S extension.
- Activation of the superficial anterior neck musculature.
- Excessive chin retraction.
- Chin jutting.
- Other body region compromise.

This is an extremely difficult position and movement to control. There are many pieces and details to think about here. One of the best strategies for the trainee to develop and implement is to review a checklist in their mind. The checklist should begin here as follows: "pelvic neutral – check – core stability on – check - set scapula – check – neutral DNF neck – check," and so forth.

All the pathology discussed thus far can potentially cause pain, so if pain is present, please see the above information. Special attention must be given to all neutral positions, pelvic, spinal, scapular, and neck, as well as leg and arm positions, especially if pain is experienced. All the adjustments discussed thus far can be made, especially the three main spinal positions.

If no attempts are successful at eliminating the pain, then this particular exercise may be beyond the trainee's current limit capacity and thus should not be done. [932, 940, 941, 942, 943, 944, 945, 946, 947]

CONTINUED LEVEL I PROGRESS

Once the above basic progressions have been mastered, the trainee will have the ability to create Full Spinal Control, which consists of the three main pieces we have covered. The first is lumbopelvic control, which is learned via the Core Bracing Series progressions. As we have learned, this involves first learning and mastering basic core stability to lock pelvic neutral and then integrating core stability into an "on/off" system in accordance with movement. The Core Bracing Series applied this system to the major motions of the hip.

The second major piece of spinal control involves the thoracic spine and the scapulothoracic articulation. Control of this piece was learned by way of the Scapular Setting Series progressions. This series involved applying the "on/off" core stability system to thoracic spine and scapular movement control as the set scapular position is achieved.

The third and final piece of spinal control is for the cervical spine, and was learned in the Cervical Spine Deep Neck Flexor (DNF) Series progressions. This series involved once again applying the "on/off" core system to activate the deep neck flexor muscle group, which is utilized to create a long neutral neck position.

The next step of this human movement education course is to put these pieces together. You can achieve Full Spinal Control if you can achieve all three pieces of spinal control at the same time. Then, you can begin to learn how to move from the hips, the shoulders, the arms, and the legs while maintaining a stable spinal base. This is how the human body is designed to move. Certain muscle groups prevent motion, thus creating a stable base for other muscle groups to pull from and create the force necessary to move us throughout the world. So, from this point forward, we are no longer activating just the core; now, we are activating the core, shoulder, and neck simultaneously to achieve our Full Spinal Control Foundation.

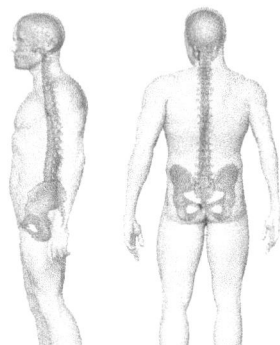

Think one more time about what muscles do and how they do it. They pull on bones, either pulling them together, as in the case of a pull-up, or pulling them apart, as in the case of a push-up. The positions of these bones are critical in determining how effective the muscles will be at pulling them. Returning to the tug-of-war example, imagine competing against a friend of equal size and strength, but your friend is standing on two feet, and you are standing on only one foot. You will lose the game every time because you do not have a solid support base to pull from. Similarly, if a muscle does not have a solid base to pull from, it cannot generate the force it should. Now, if you put your second foot on the ground while playing tug-of-war and create a stable base for yourself, you can pull more effectively. Similarly, when the muscles responsible for major movement have a solid, stable base of support from which to pull, they can create the force necessary for proper function.

The most powerful muscles in your body are the glutes, hamstrings, quadriceps, hip flexors, and hip adductors. These are the muscles of the hips, and since they are all attached to the pelvis, the position and control of the pelvis determines the functional ability of these powerful hip muscles. If the pelvis is held in a stable neutral position, locked in place by good core stability, these huge, powerful muscles will have a solid, stable base to pull from. Hip function, as well as the lower extremity as a whole, will be correct.

If your core stability is unable to lock the pelvis in the correct position, the hip muscles will not have a stable base to pull from. This will lead to decreases in force production and, thus, decreased functional ability and poor hip mechanics. We already know that decreased function in one area of the body will lead to increased demands in another area. Remember, total workload, or tissue stress, does not disappear when one area is underperforming but will have to be made up for by other areas of the body (Law of 100% Motion). Compensation patterns will ensue, eventually progressing to pain and/or injury.

The same can be said for the set scapular position and the cervical spine neutral neck position. These areas are (or should be) providing the solid base for the majority of the shoulder and upper extremity muscles. If these positions are not held stable in the correct position, the powerful muscles of the shoulders and arms will not be able to function correctly.

This is why it is so important to master the basics. As tedious as the basics may seem, it is what everything else is built on, all the way up to the highest levels of human performance. **Focus on the fundamentals of Full Spinal Control more than anything else, and apply Full Spinal Control to everything you do**. You will be amazed at the results.

Once these first basic progressions are learned perfectly, you will be ready to move on to more advanced movement patterns and exercises. The progressions continue as follows:

The first Level of The PREMIER Body Method is Movement Fundamentals. It is done mainly in an unloaded spinal position. The emphasis at this level is to learn fundamental control of the human body. It begins with learning the concept of Full Spinal Control and implementing the core stability on/off system. This fundamental pattern will be used throughout the entire progression series. That is, the pattern of core stability "on," then initiating the movement to be performed, completing that movement, and then core stability "off." However, from this point forward, it is not only core stability "on," it is core-shoulder-neck (Full Spinal Control) "on" as a whole unit. We will now begin to increase the range and difficulty of hip and shoulder movement while maintaining Full Spinal Control by combining all three spinal control pieces: pelvic/core, shoulder, and neck. These progressions are as follows:

GLUTEAL BRIDGE SERIES

The Gluteal Bridge Series Progressions are a continuation of Heel Drives and Fallouts, respectively, from the Stage II and III Core Bracing exercises, in that this series is designed to progress hip mechanics by way of glute activation. The gluteal muscle group is responsible for both hip extension and lateral hip stability. Thus, this series has two main parts: bridge exercise progressions to train glute/hip extension ability, and lateral movement exercise progressions to train lateral glute/hip stability. [939]

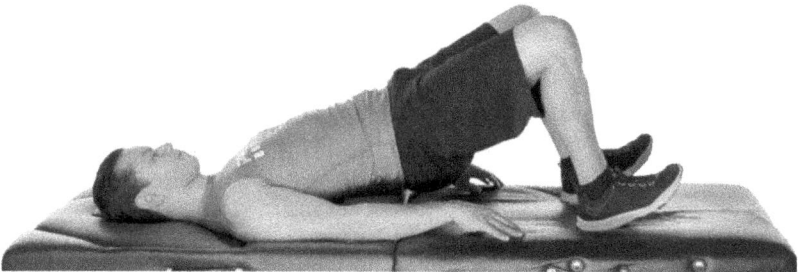

Performing the bridge movement pattern correctly reinforces the "on/off" sequence of core stability. The exercise begins in the supine starting position with Full Spinal Control. Begin the movement by first turning the core "on" to lock the pelvis and spine in neutral, and then begin to drive the heels down and out. In this exercise, both heels will be driven down at the same time and with enough force to lift the torso.

Focus here on correct hip and pelvic mechanics. The major motion should come from the hip and hip musculature, which include muscles designed to create motion. The pelvis and spine are held in the neutral position by the core stability musculature, whose muscles are designed to prevent motion. The movement can proceed as high as the hip's range of motion allows, but no further. Continuing the motion higher after hip extension has reached its end range of motion means the motion is coming from the spine and no longer from the hip.

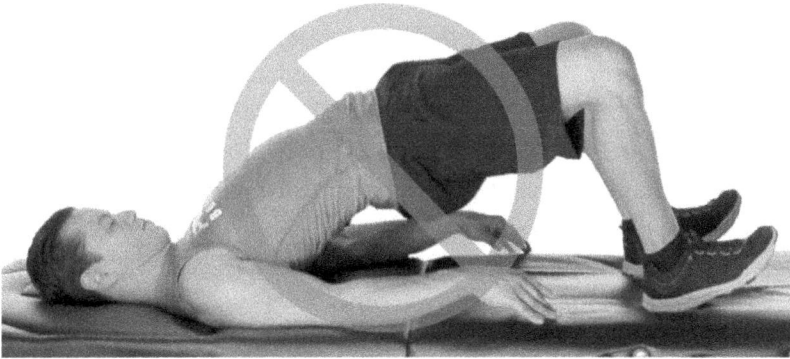

Any movement from the spine defeats the purpose of this and any other movement education exercise since the job of the pelvis and spine musculature is to prevent motion. The hip musculature should be doing the work to create motion, and the core should be doing the work to prevent motion at the spine and pelvis, thus allowing the hip to function with greater ease and efficiency. The real value and purpose of performing the bridge movement pattern is to train the body to use proper lumbopelvic hip mechanics to isolate extension motion at the hip joint from spinal movement.

For people with faulty hip and spinal mechanics, the actual fault is often to allow the spine and pelvis to move with the hip. This is not correct and can be seen with many real-life motions, even something as simple as walking with excessive extension in the lower back. Again, the hip should be doing the work to create motion, while the core and spinal musculature should do the work to prevent motion. Never go beyond the hip's range of motion during the bridge movement control exercise or any other movement/exercise involving hip extension.

The bridge movement series has three stages of progression. The Stage I Bridge is a basic bilateral bridge movement designed to train proper lumbopelvic core and hip extension movement mechanics. Stage II progression increases the difficulty of control by adding a unilateral component at the top of the bridge motion. This challenges not only the sagittal (front to back) plane of motion, but all three planes as the unilateral position takes place. In this Stage II progression, the unilateral position is held static, while the movement of the bridge motion is still bilateral with both legs. Stage III progression further increases the difficulty by applying the unilateral component to the entire bridge motion, thus making the movement a single-leg bridge exercise. The goal for all progressions is to maintain pelvic and spinal neutral through Full Spinal Control in all three planes of motion at all times during the exercises.

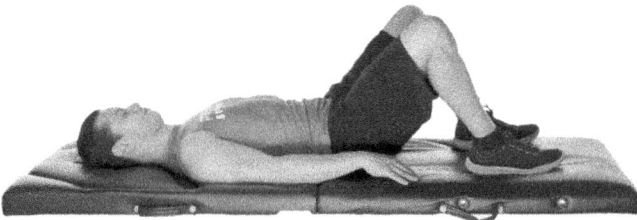

Glute Bridge - Beginning Position (For All 3 Stages)

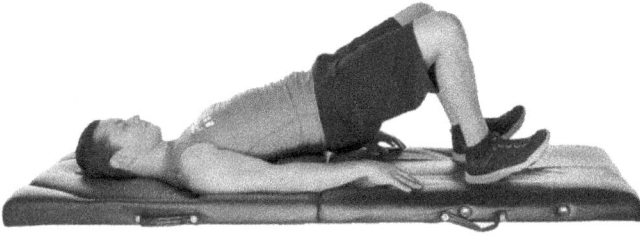

Glute Bridge Stage I - Movement Position

Glute Bridge Stage I - Goal/Purpose:

- Learn to distinguish and control hip extension without lumbar spine (lower back) extension (arching).

Beginning Position:

- Supine (face up).
- Achieve Full Spinal Control with Pelvic, Scapular, and C/S neutral.
- Lower extremity flexed, feet hip-width apart, knee width slightly wider than foot width.

Movement/Action:

- Activate core stability "on" by way of Core Bracing I. Then drive both heels into the ground by activating the gluteal muscles with enough force to create hip extension, thus lifting the pelvis and torso as one unit into a bridge position (do not permit low back extension), then relax the movement back to the starting position, then relax core stability "off."

- Repeat.

Key Notes/Common Faults:

- Pain/discomfort/straining of any kind.
- Faulty breathing pattern.
- Loss of Full Spinal Control.
- Loss of pelvic neutral position, seen as rotational disconnect and/or tilting and/or hiking and/or <u>lower back arching</u>.
- Other body region compromise.

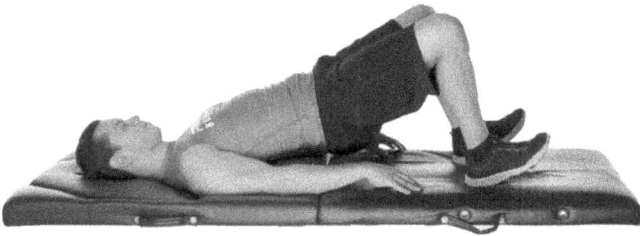

Glute Bridge Stage II - First Movement Position

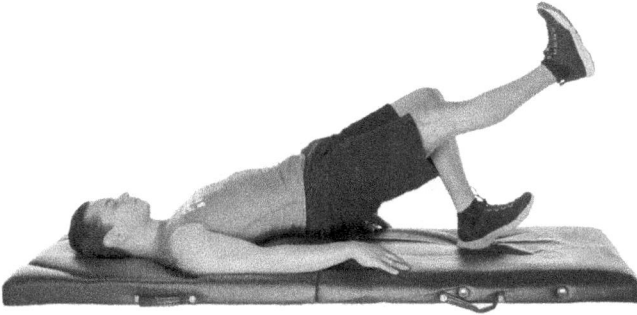

Glute Bridge Stage II - Second Movement Position

Glute Bridge Stage II Goal/Purpose:

- Learn to distinguish and control hip extension without lumbar spine (lower back) extension (arching).

Beginning Position:

- Supine (face up).
- Achieve Full Spinal Control with Pelvic, Scapular, and C/S neutral.
- Lower extremity flexed, feet hip-width apart, knee width slightly wider than foot width.

Movement/Action:

- Activate core stability "on" by way of Core Bracing I, then perform a bridge movement as described in Glute/Bridge Stage I, then hold the top bridge position while extending one leg out and back (kick-out by way of knee extension) while keeping the thighs parallel, then reverse the

movement back to the starting position, then relax core stability "off."
- Repeat with the opposite leg kick out at the top.

Key Notes/Common Faults:

- Pain / discomfort / straining of any kind.
- Faulty breathing pattern.
- Loss of Full Spinal Control.
- Loss of pelvic neutral position, seen as <u>rotational disconnect</u> and / or tilting and / or hiking and / or <u>lower back arching</u>.
- Other body region compromise.

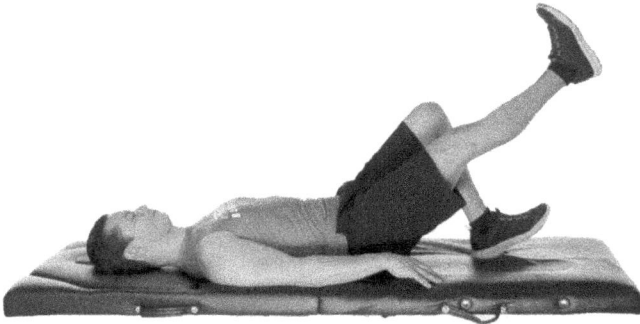

Glute Bridge Stage III - Movement Position 1 (Back Flat)

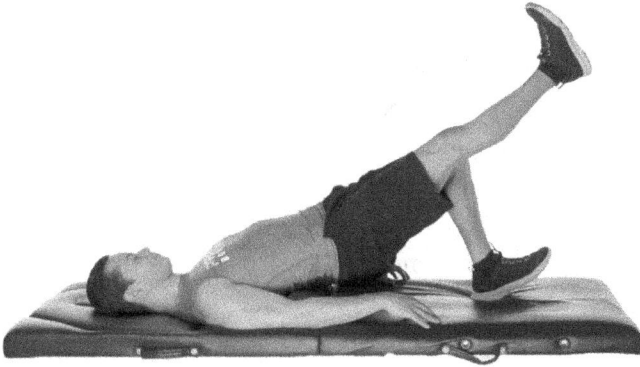

Glute Bridge Stage III - Movement Position 2

Glute Bridge Stage III Goal/Purpose:

- Learning to distinguish and control hip extension without lumbar spine (lower back) extension (arching).

Beginning Position:

- Supine (face up).
- Achieve Full Spinal Control with Pelvic, Scapular, and C/S neutral.
- Lower extremity flexed, feet hip-width apart, knee width slightly wider then foot width.

Movement/Action:

- Activate core stability "on" by way of Core Bracing I, then extend one leg out (kick-out by way of knee extension) while keeping the thighs parallel, then perform a single leg bridge movement (the same way as described in Glute/Bridge Stage I only with one leg), then reverse the movement back to the starting position, then relax core stability "off."

- Repeat with the opposite leg kick out at the start.

Key Notes/Common Faults:

- Pain / discomfort / straining of any kind.
- Faulty breathing pattern.
- Loss of Full Spinal Control.
- Loss of pelvic neutral position, seen as <u>rotational disconnect</u> and / or tilting and / or hiking and / or <u>lower back arching</u>.
- Other body region compromise.

The lateral hip stability portion of the Gluteal Bridge Series begins with the side-lying clam exercise, which is basically the Fallout exercise in a side-lying position. The goal is to achieve and maintain Full Spinal Control now in the side-lying position because, in the real world, our bodies are placed in many positions and must perform a wide variety of movements. The ability to maintain proper control of body mechanics is critical in all situations, so part of training includes learning to maintain correct posture and mechanics in various body positions. Doing so at this beginning Level I stage is an extremely important step leading to the ability to use these correct mechanics in larger movements, exercises, and real-world activities.

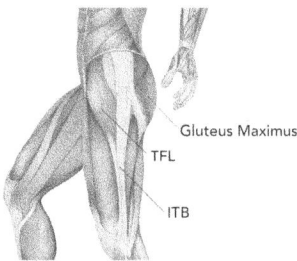

Gluteus Maximus

TFL

ITB

Lateral hip stability training continues with the side-lying hip abduction exercise. At this point in the training, it is important to note that two main muscles control the majority of lateral stability at the hip. These muscles are the gluteus medius (part of the overall glute complex) and the tensor fascia lata (TFL). These muscles work together to support and control lateral stability at the hip, but the glute should predominantly be in control. In many people with faulty mechanics, this often becomes reversed, with inhibition of the glute forcing the TFL to compensate and take over as the predominant lateral hip stabilizer. This root cause of dysfunction will branch out in different ways in different people. It can lead to various problems, such as ITB syndrome, trochanteric bursitis, MCL injuries, meniscus lesions, ACL injury, patellar tracking syndromes, and other forms of hip and knee pain/injury and/or ankle issues.

The root cause of this flip-flopping of lateral hip control is usually due to faulty anterior pelvic position that creates poor torque angles and a non-stable base for these muscles to pull from. Correct Full Spinal Control can allow the lateral hip stability to correct. Coupling slight hip extension with lateral motions can help ensure the glute, not the TFL, is doing the majority of the work in the lateral plane. For the side-lying hip abduction exercise, think of it as lifting the leg up and slightly back, leading with the heel.

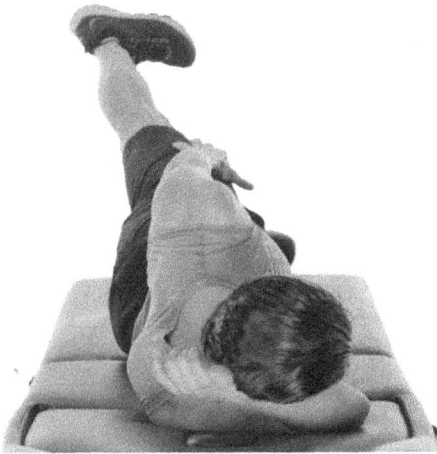

Getting this right is critical because lateral hip stability is involved in almost everything we do, such as any single leg effort like walking, running, sprinting, cutting, jumping, going up and down stairs, getting up and down from a chair, and squatting to pick something up. If you don't master these simple beginning technique exercises, you can't expect to get the movement right in daily life or the sporting world.

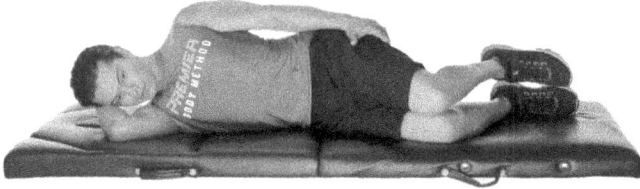

Side-Lying Clam - Beginning Position

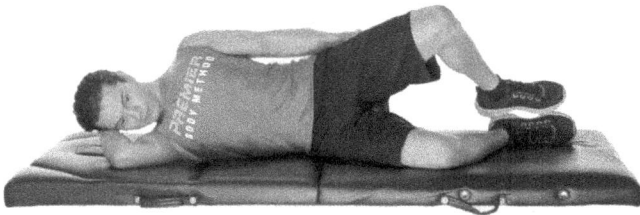

Side-Lying Clam - Movement Position

Side Lying Clam
Goal/Purpose:

- Learning to distinguish and control hip abduction without loss of pelvic neutral and / or Full Spinal Control.

Beginning Position:

- Side-lying position.
- Achieve Full Spinal Control with Pelvic, Scapular, and C/S neutral.
- Lower extremity flexed comfortably with hips and knees 60 degrees of flexion.
- Keep head, face, and neck relaxed.

Movement/Action:

- Activate core stability "on" by way of Core Bracing I, then lift the top side leg (knee) by way of hip abduction while keeping the feet together (as if the legs were a clamshell opening), then reverse the movement back to the starting position, then relax core stability "off."
- Repeat 10 reps, then switch to the other side.

Key Notes/Common Faults:

- Pain/discomfort/straining of any kind.
- Faulty breathing pattern.
- Loss of Full Spinal Control.
- Loss of pelvic neutral position, seen as <u>rotational disconnect</u> and/or tilting and/or hiking and/or <u>lower back arching</u>.
- Do not allow the body to roll back with the leg movement.
- Other body region compromise.

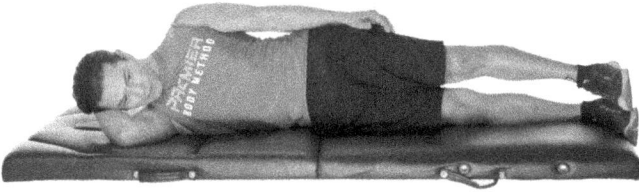

Side-Lying Hip Abduction - Beginning Position

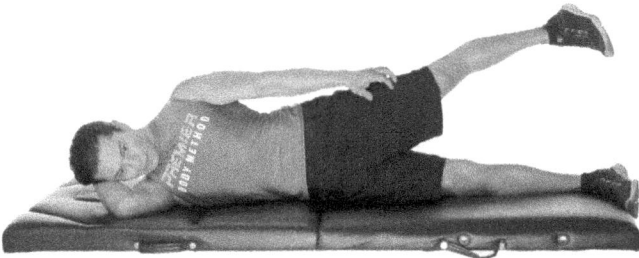

Side-Lying Hip Abduction - Movement Position

Side Lying Hip Abduction
Goal/Purpose:

- Learning to distinguish and control hip abduction without loss of pelvic neutral and/or Full Spinal Control.

Beginning Position:

- Side-lying position.
- Achieve Full Spinal Control with Pelvic, Scapular, and C/S neutral.
- The bottom leg is flexed for more stability, while the top leg is straight.
- Keep head, face, and neck relaxed

Movement/Action:

- Activate core stability "on" by way of Core Bracing I, then lift the top side leg by way of hip abduction (the leg should be lifted up and back utilizing the gluteus medius, not the TFL), then reverse the movement back to the starting position, then relax core stability "off."
- Repeat 10 times, and then switch to the other side.

Key Notes/Common Faults:

- Pain/discomfort/straining of any kind.
- Faulty breathing pattern.
- Loss of Full Spinal Control.
- Loss of pelvic neutral position, seen as <u>rotational disconnect</u> and/or tilting and/or <u>hiking</u> and/or <u>lower back arching</u>.
- Do not allow the body to roll back with the leg movement.
- Other body region compromise.

Remember, just as with all exercises and movements learned, no pain should be experienced. All the same pathologies and pain generators explained throughout the spinal control series may be accentuated here. Remember that lifting the pelvis and torso off the ground with the bridge exercises can make Full Spinal Control more difficult. For one, the spine will no longer have the support and tactile cue of the floor. Also, the position causes the posterior spinal musculature, especially the spinal erector group, to have increased activity and workload. These changes may increase the chance of pathology being aggravated.

The workload on the hip joint and hip musculature also increases. If the exercise is causing pain, first attempt to change the pelvic position, set scapular position, and/or DNF neck position, as these may not be in the correct neutral position. If this does not work, attempt to change the angle of motion at the hip joint to allow for increased or decreased flexion, rotation, abduction, or adduction during the movement. If this does not work, attempt to limit the range of motion to a pain-free range.

If the pain is not originating from the hip joint, it may be coming from the sacroiliac joints or the spine, including the neck. Again, an unbalancing from side to side can aggravate the spine and SI joints. If this is the case, try giving more attention to maintaining pelvic neutral and the set scapular position. As the hip extends during the movement, excessive movement in the spine often occurs. The result can be excessive torque, rotation, extension, or compression of the spine, thus causing pressure to the facet joints in the spine, mechanical stenosis to the IVF space/s or the spinal central canal, causing radicular or myelopathic complications, and/or increased pressure on the discs of the spine.

If cervical spine pathology causes pain, special attention must be given to the DNF position. Remember that cervical spine pathology can cause anything from local pain to upper and/or lower extremity pain.

Pain may occur in the side-lying position if Full Spinal Control is not maintained due to lateral bending in the spine. Pain may also occur in the down-side hip due to the pressure of lying on it. This usually happens with conditions such as trochanteric bursitis or deeper hip joint issues such as degenerative joint disease and/or labral injuries.

The addition of extremity movement may cause strain, tension, and/or over-activation, which may increase intra-abdominal and intrathecal pressure (Valsalva) and, thus, symptoms or pain. Also, pain can occur if an injury, such as tendinitis or tendinosis, occurs in any of the working muscles (e.g., the glutes and hamstrings).

Any of these scenarios may cause pain. If pain is present and no attempts are successful at eliminating the pain, then this particular exercise is beyond current limit capacity and thus should not be done. (932, 940, 941, 942, 943, 944, 945, 946, 947)

DEAD BUG SERIES

Core Bracing Stage II heel lifts continue to progress with the Dead Bug series. In this series, the time of activation and, thus, the strength and endurance of hip flexion increase, as does the range of motion of the hip flexion movement pattern. We also introduce shoulder and upper extremity movement in this series. Full Spinal Control must be maintained, and the main goal of this series is learning to move from the extremities while maintaining spinal control.

The Dead Bug series consists of three basic progressions, or stages I, II, and III. The starting position for each is supine. This series calls for the bilateral maintenance of the flexed hip position, but a unilateral version is possible if necessary, depending on core strength and control ability. In the supine position, the core is first activated "on," along with the rest of the Full Spinal Control foundation, i.e., core-shoulder-neck. Next, the hip/s and shoulders are flexed to 90 degrees. Dead Bug Stage I involves only arm movement, as the next step is to move the shoulder into further flexion one side at a time, back and forth. If shoulder or neck pathology is present, special attention may be needed regarding the shoulder movement. The goal is once again to maintain Full Spinal Control during the movement.

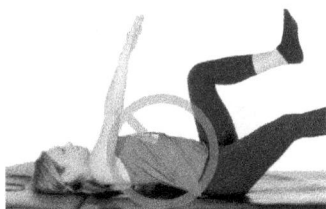

Do not arch the back!

Dead Bug Stage II involves only hip movement, as the hip is extended out past the 90-degree flexed position as far as Full Spinal Control will allow. Again, **the leg should be moved out only as far as neutral spinal alignment will allow.** It doesn't matter if you only move your leg out one inch and back as long as your spine is neutral. You are doing absolutely no good by moving the leg out through a big range of motion if the lower back is extending up off the ground and you are losing spinal control.

Stage III progresses the movement with the upper and lower extremities working together, as the arms and legs will flex and extend contralaterally (opposite arm and leg). As stated before, this is how the body is designed to work. Proper biomechanics require maintaining Full Spinal Control while creating movement with the hips, shoulders, legs, and arms. The contralateral movement of arms and legs during the Dead Bug Stage III exercise mimics many of the higher-level exercises and life movements the world requires of us and helps us gain the ability to perform these higher-level activities correctly.

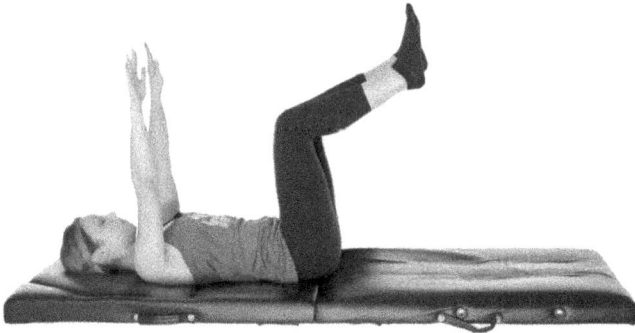

Dead Bug Beginning Position for Stages I, II, and III

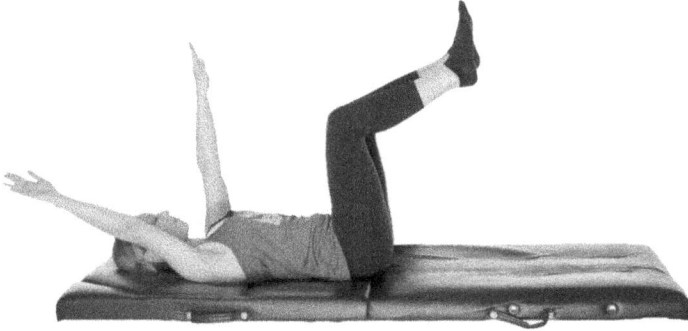

Dead Bug Stage I Movement Position

Dead Bug Stage I
Goal/Purpose:

- Integration of upper extremity movement with increased core activation to maintain pelvic neutral and / or Full Spinal Control.

Beginning Position:

- Supine (face up).
- Achieve Full Spinal Control with Pelvic, Scapular, and C/S neutral.
- Hips and knees flexed to 90 degrees bilaterally, shoulders at 90 degrees of flexion bilaterally.
- Keep head, face, and neck relaxed.

Movement/Action:

- Core stability is already on to a certain extent just to maintain the starting position. Begin the exercise movement by ramping up core stability "on" more to maintain pelvic neutral. Then, reach one arm out to further shoulder flexion, complete the arm movement back to the starting position, and ramp core stability down (not low enough to allow loss of pelvic neutral).

- Repeat 10 reps, alternating side to side.

Key Notes/Common Faults:

- Pain/discomfort/straining of any kind.
- Faulty breathing pattern.
- Loss of Full Spinal Control.

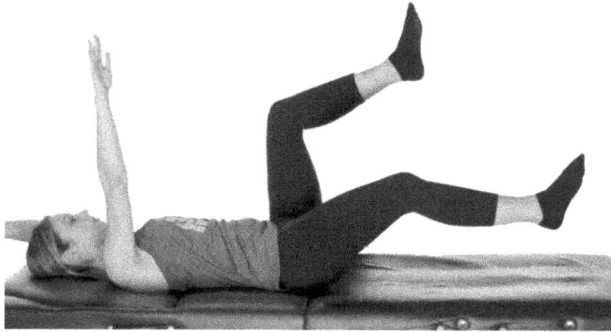

Dead Bug Stage II Movement Position

Dead Bug Stage II
Goal/Purpose:

- Integrate lower extremity movement with increased core activation to maintain pelvic neutral and/or Full Spinal Control.

Beginning Position:

- Supine (face up).
- Achieve Full Spinal Control with Pelvic, Scapular, and C/S neutral.

- Hips and knees flexed to 90 degrees bilaterally, shoulders at 90 degrees of flexion bilaterally.
- Keep head, face, and neck relaxed.

Movement/Action:

- Core stability is already on to a certain extent just to maintain the starting position. Begin the exercise movement by ramping up core stability "on" more to maintain pelvic neutral. Then, reach one leg out by way of hip extension, complete the leg movement back to the starting position, and ramp core stability down (not low enough to allow loss of pelvic neutral).
- Repeat 10 reps, alternating side to side.

Key Notes/Common Faults:

- Pain/discomfort/straining of any kind.
- Faulty breathing pattern.
- Loss of Full Spinal Control.

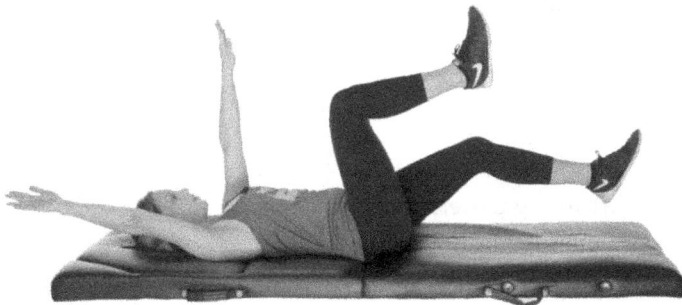

Dead Bug Stage III Movement Position

Dead Bug Stage III
Goal/Purpose:

- Integration of upper and lower extremity movement with increased core activation to maintain pelvic neutral and/or Full Spinal Control.

Beginning Position:

- Supine (face up).
- Achieve Full Spinal Control with Pelvic, Scapular, and C/S neutral.
- Hips and knees flexed to 90 degrees bilaterally, shoulders at 90 degrees of flexion bilaterally.
- Keep head, face, and neck relaxed.

Movement/Action:

- Core stability is already on to a certain extent just to maintain the starting position. Begin the exercise movement by ramping up core stability "on" more to maintain pelvic neutral. Then, reach one leg out while reaching the opposite side arm out. Complete the leg and arm movement back to the starting position, then ramp core stability down (not low enough to allow loss of pelvic neutral).
- Repeat 10 reps, alternating side to side.

Key Notes/Common Faults:

- Pain/discomfort/straining of any kind.
- Faulty breathing pattern.
- Loss of Full Spinal Control.
- Loss of pelvic neutral position, seen mainly as lower back arching. Do not allow the low back to arch up off the ground.
- Other body region compromise.

Remember, just as with all exercises and movements learned, no pain should be experienced. All the same pathologies and pain generators explained throughout the spinal control series may be accentuated here and must be kept in mind. Common pathologies that may cause pain here can be specific to the hip joint. They include hip degenerative joint disease, arthritis, labral tears, hip tendinitis, and other joint lesions. If this is the case and the exercise is causing pain, first attempt to change the pelvic position, as it may not be in the correct neutral position. If this does not work, attempt to change the angle of motion at the hip joint to allow for increased or decreased hip flexion, rotation, abduction, and/or adduction during the movement. Moving the knee further out, closer in, wider, or narrower can do this. If this does not work, next attempt to limit the range of motion to a pain-free range.

If the pain does not originate from the actual hip joint, it may be coming from the sacroiliac joints or the lumbar spine in the back. If this is the case, more attention should be given to maintaining pelvic neutral.

The Dead Bug mainly utilizes the hip flexor muscle group, including the iliopsoas, rectus femoris, and sartorius. If tendinitis is present in any of these muscles, pain may occur. Also, the psoas muscle originates on the lumbar spine and may cause torque, rotation, extension, or compression of the lumbar spine. This can place pressure on the facet joints in the spine, mechanical stenosis to the IVF space/s or the central spinal canal, causing radicular or myelopathic complications and increased pressure on the discs of the spine.

With the additional GH joint (shoulder) motion, consider shoulder pathologies such as GH degenerative joint disease, arthritis, labral tears, bursitis, rotator cuff or biceps tendinitis, and other joint lesions as possible sources of pain. Special attention to the set scapular position is necessary in these cases. Limiting the range of motion and/or altering the angle of motion at the GH joint can also control these pathologies.

If pain is caused by cervical spine pathology, special attention must be given to the DNF position. Remember that cervical spine pathology can cause anything from local pain to upper and even lower extremity pain.

The additional extremity movement may cause strain, tension, and/or over-activation, which may increase pressure (Valsalva) and, thus, symptoms. Any of these scenarios may cause pain. If none of these attempts successfully eliminate the pain, then this exercise is beyond the current limit capacity and should not be done. [932, 940, 941, 942, 943, 944, 945, 946, 947]

BIRD DOG SERIES

The Bird Dog Series Progression continues to build on the foundational concept of achieving Full Spinal Control while creating movement from the hips, shoulders, arms, and legs.

The Bird Dog movement control exercise is like the Dead Bug flipped upside down in the quadruped position (on all fours). This reverses muscular activation, working the hip extensor muscles instead of the hip flexors and the shoulder flexor muscles instead of the extensor group.

Beginning in the quadruped position, achieve Full Spinal Control by running through your checklist of the three main pieces: pelvic neutral, set scapular position, and DNF neck position. This may not be easy at first since this is the first time you are doing this in free space, without the support of the ground or a wall.

Once you achieve full spinal neutral, turn the core "on" to maintain the position, at which point you have achieved Full Spinal Control. You are now ready to begin moving from the extremities. Like the Dead Bug progression, the Bird Dog progression begins with the arms only in Stage I, progresses to the legs only in Stage II, and puts arms and legs together in Stage III.

Bird Dog stage I begins in the quadruped starting position with Full Spinal Control. The next step is to move the shoulder into further flexion, lifting the arm up, out, and in front of the body overhead, one side at a time, back and forth. If shoulder or neck pathology is present, then special attention is needed regarding the shoulder movement, set scapular position, and DNF position.

Stage II involves only hip movement, as you extend the hip out of the 90-degree flexed position, as the leg is lifted up behind the body, as far as Full Spinal Control will allow. As with the gluteal bridge exercise, correct lumbopelvic hip mechanics require that hip motion be separated from pelvic and spinal motion. As the leg reaches back through hip extension by way of glute activation, no pelvic or spinal motion should occur. Do not allow the lower back to extend and lose its neutral position.

In Stage III, the movement progresses to include the upper and lower extremities together, as arms flex and legs extend contralaterally. Again, maintaining spinal control while the major motion is occurring in the extremities is critical, as this mimics many of life's everyday tasks.

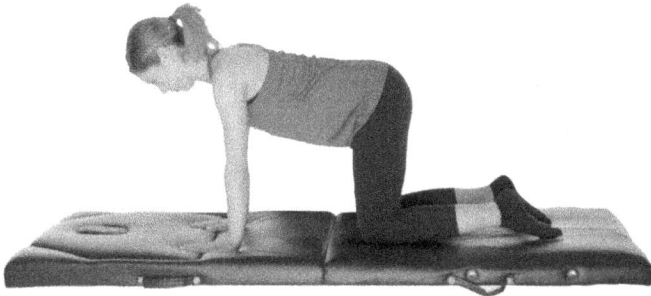

Beginning Position for I, II, and III

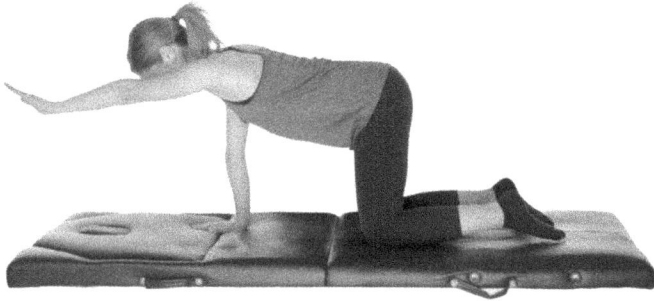

Bird Dog Movement Position I

Bird Dog Stage I
Goal/Purpose:

- Integration of upper extremity movement with increased core activation to maintain pelvic neutral and / or Full Spinal Control.

Beginning Position:

- Quadruped (hands and knees).
- Achieve Full Spinal Control with Pelvic, Scapular, and C/S neutral.
- Keep head, face, and neck relaxed.

Movement/Action:

- Core stability is already "on" to a certain extent just to maintain the starting position. Begin the exercise movement by further increasing core stability "on" to maintain pelvic neutral. Next, reach one arm out into further shoulder flexion,

then complete the arm movement back to the starting position. To end the movement, ramp core stability down (not low enough to allow loss of pelvic neutral and/or spinal neutral).
- Repeat 10 reps, alternating side to side.

Key Notes/Common Faults:

- Pain/discomfort/straining of any kind.
- Faulty breathing pattern.
- Loss of Full Spinal Control.
- Loss of pelvic neutral position, seen mainly as <u>lower back arching</u>. Do not allow the lower back to arch.
- Other body region compromise.

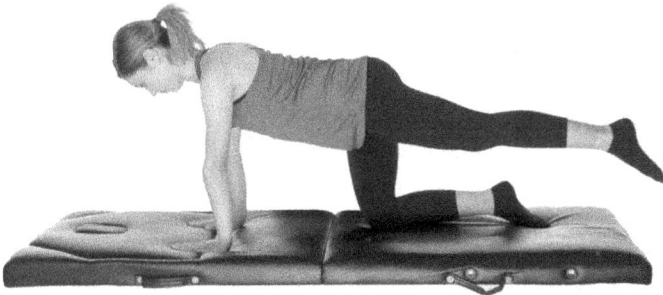

Bird Dog Movement Position II

Bird Dog Stage II
Goal/Purpose:

- Integration of lower extremity movement with increased core activation to maintain pelvic neutral and/or Full Spinal Control.

Beginning Position:

- Quadruped (hands and knees).
- Achieve Full Spinal Control with Pelvic, Scapular, and C/S neutral.
- Keep head, face, and neck relaxed.

Movement/Action:

- Core stability is already on to a certain extent just to maintain the starting position. Begin the exercise movement by further increasing core stability "on" to maintain pelvic neutral. Next, reach one leg out by way of hip extension, then complete the leg movement back to the starting position. To end the movement, ramp core stability down (not low enough to allow loss of pelvic neutral).
- Repeat 10 reps, alternating side to side.

Key Notes/Common Faults:

- Pain/discomfort/straining of any kind.
- Faulty breathing pattern.
- Loss of Full Spinal Control.
- Loss of pelvic neutral position, seen mainly as <u>lower back arching</u>. Do not allow the lower back to arch as the hip extends.
- Other body region compromise.

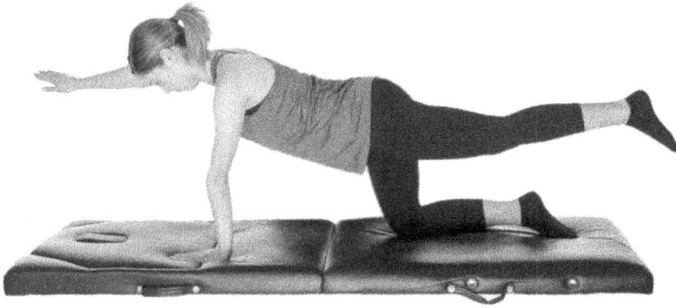

Bird Dog Movement Position III

Bird Dog Stage III Goal/Purpose:

- Integration of upper and lower extremity movement with increased core activation to maintain pelvic neutral and/or Full Spinal Control.

Beginning Position:

- Quadruped (hands and knees).
- Achieve Full Spinal Control with Pelvic, Scapular, and C/S neutral.
- Keep head, face, and neck relaxed.

Movement/Action:

- Core stability is already on to a certain extent just to maintain the starting position. Begin the exercise movement by further increasing core stability "on" to maintain pelvic neutral. Next, reach one leg out while reaching the opposite side arm out, then complete the leg and arm movement back to the starting position, then ramp core stability down (not low enough to allow loss of pelvic neutral).

- Repeat 10 reps, alternating side to side.

Key Notes/Common Faults:

- Pain/discomfort/straining of any kind.
- Faulty breathing pattern.
- Loss of Full Spinal Control.
- Loss of pelvic neutral position, seen mainly as <u>lower back arching</u>. Do not allow the lower back to arch as the arms and legs move.
- Other body region compromise.

As in all exercises and movements learned until now, no pain should be experienced. All the same pathologies and pain generators explained throughout the spinal control series may be accentuated here and must be kept in mind. In the quadruped position, increased difficulty in maintaining Full Spinal Control may occur. For one, the support and tactile cues of the floor are no longer there for the spine. The posterior spinal musculature, especially the spinal erector group, has increased activity and workload in this position, especially in the cervical spine. These changes in position and workload increase the chance of certain pathology being aggravated.

The extremities are bearing the weight of the torso now. This may create compression in the shoulder and hip joints. Common pathologies that may cause pain here can be specific to the hip or shoulder joints. Examples include degenerative joint disease, arthritis, labral tears, tendinitis, and other joint lesions. If this is the case and the exercise is causing pain, first attempt to change the pelvic position, set scapular position, and/or DNF neck position, as these may not be in the correct neutral position. If this does not work, attempt to change the angle of motion at the hip or shoulder joint to allow for increased or decreased flexion, rotation, abduction, and/or adduction during the movement. If this does not work, next attempt to limit the range of motion to a pain-free range.

If the pain is not originating from the actual hip or shoulder joint, it could be coming from the sacroiliac joints, or the spine, including the neck. If this is the case, more attention to maintaining pelvic neutral, the set scapular position, and the C/S DNF neck position should be attempted. The hip flexor muscle group is no longer very active here, but with the hip extending and/or shoulder flexing, it is quite common also to create excessive movement in the spine. This is incorrect and may cause excessive torque, rotation, extension, or compression of the spine, thus causing pressure to the facet joints in the spine, mechanical stenosis to the IVF space/s or the central spinal canal causing radicular or myelopathic complications, and/or increased pressure on the discs of the spine.

If pain is caused by cervical spine pathology, special attention must be given to the DNF position. Remember that cervical spine pathology can cause anything from local pain to upper and even lower extremity pain and/or other signs and symptoms.

Also, remember that the additional extremity movement and difficulty of the exercise may cause strain, tension, and over-activation, which may increase pressure (Valsalva) and, thus, symptoms. If pain is present and no attempts are successful at eliminating it, this particular exercise is beyond current limit capacity and thus should not be done. (932, 940, 941, 942, 943, 944, 945, 946, 947)

WALL ANGEL SERIES

The Wall Angel Series continues to build off the concept of maintaining Full Spinal Control while creating movement from the extremities. In this exercise, the beginning position is upright, with the back against a wall. This is a key transitional exercise because it moves the supine starting position to an upright position. The tactile cue for the spine is still present in the wall. This is a big progression because this is the first time Full Spinal Control will be achieved in the vertically loaded position.

Begin by positioning the pelvis in neutral, setting the scapula, and then achieving a DNF neutral neck position. Core stability is then turned "on" to maintain the full spinal neutral position while the shoulders and hips perform movement control exercises. If you look at the exercise illustrations, you will see that the elbows, wrists, and hands are also positioned back against the wall. This can actually be a very difficult position for many people to achieve. It takes a certain amount of mobility and flexibility in several different places to achieve this position correctly.

For this reason, the Wall Angel is also a very good test of proper body mobility, as discussed in that section of the key concepts at the beginning of the book. If you have trouble achieving the Wall Angel position correctly, you most likely have some basic human mobility issues. Not to worry. Remember, moving correctly is one of the best ways to achieve and maintain proper human functional mobility. This just happens to be exactly what this program is teaching you. So if you are having mobility difficulties, don't worry, just keep practicing staying strict to the fundamentals. As you progress through the program, your mobility will improve over time.

The Wall Angel Series has two basic stages. Stage I involves shoulder movement, and Stage II consists of both shoulder and hip movement.

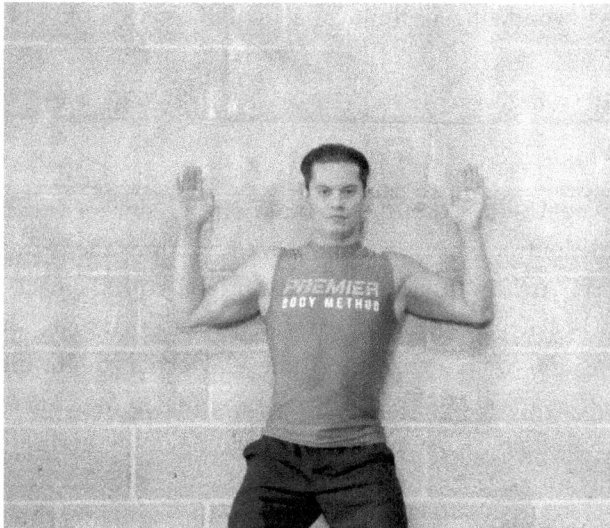

Wall Angel Stage I Beginning Position

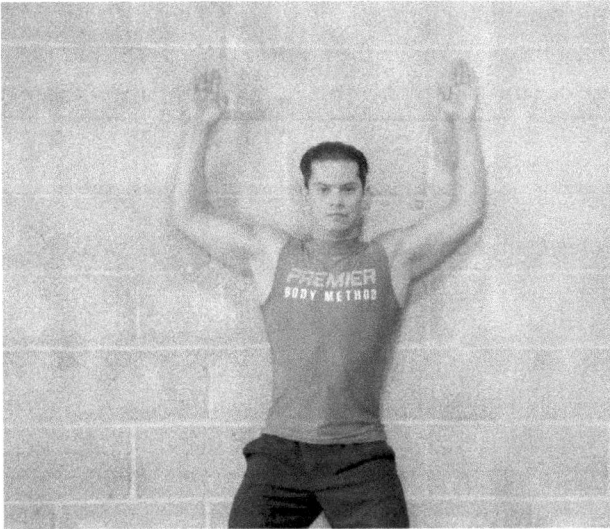

Wall Angel Stage I Movement Position

Wall Angel Stage I
Goal/Purpose:

- Integration of upper extremity movement while maintaining Full Spinal Control (core-shoulder-neck!).

Beginning Position:

- Standing with back against the wall.
- Achieve Full Spinal Control with pelvic neutral, set scapular position, and C/S DNF neutral.
- Feet flat on the ground, hip-width apart, with knees slightly flexed.
- Upper extremity externally rotated at the shoulder with the elbow flexed to 90 degrees (W position). The elbow and back of the wrist and hand should be flat against the wall.

Movement/Action:

- While maintaining Full Spinal Control with the back flat against the wall, move the arms up and down, but not so far as to lose the set scapular position (do not allow the shoulder to shrug or hike up).
- Repeat 10 reps.

Key Notes/Common Faults:

- Pain / discomfort / straining of any kind.
- Faulty breathing pattern.
- Loss of Full Spinal Control.
- Loss of pelvic neutral position, seen mainly as <u>lower back arching</u> away from the wall.
- Other body region compromise.

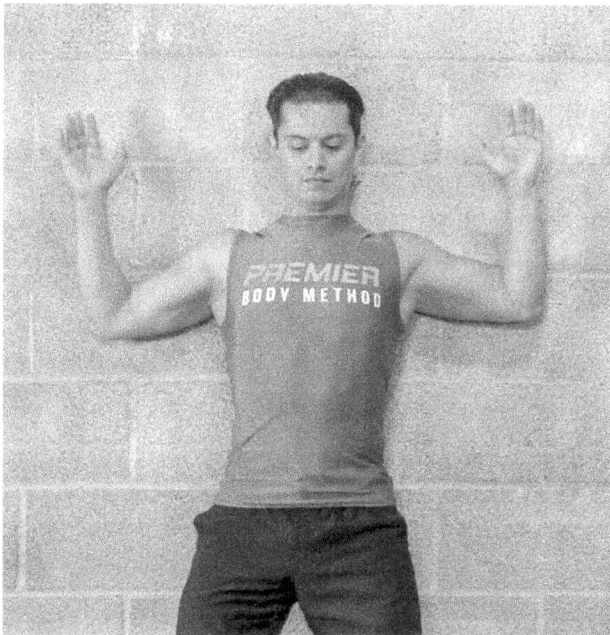

Wall Angel Stage II Beginning Position

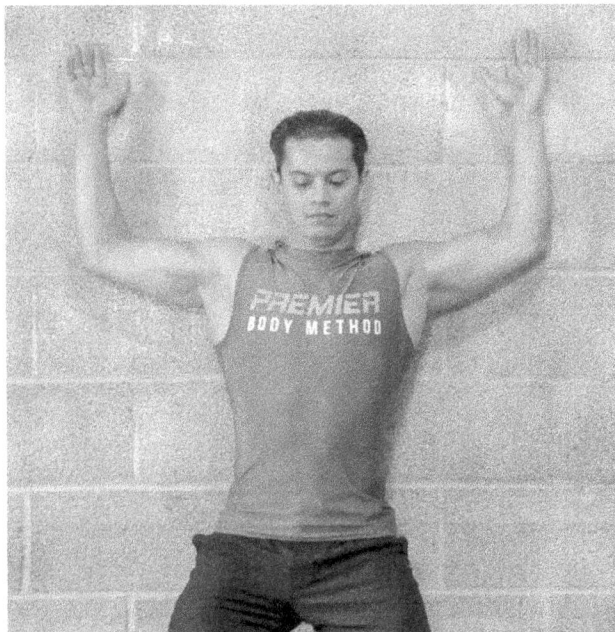

Wall Angel Stage II Movement Position

Wall Angel Stage II
Goal/Purpose:

- Integration of upper and lower extremity movement while maintaining Full Spinal Control (core-shoulder-neck!).

Beginning Position:

- Standing back against the wall.
- Achieve Full Spinal Control with pelvic neutral, set scapular position, and C/S DNF neutral.
- Feet flat on the ground, hip-width apart, with knees slightly flexed.
- Upper extremity externally rotated at the shoulder with the elbow flexed to 90 degrees (W position). The elbow and back of the wrist and hand should be ideally flat against the wall.

Movement/Action:

- While maintaining Full Spinal Control with the back flat against the wall, perform a wall squat motion by bending at the hips and knees as the torso slides down and then back up the wall. Keep the hands tacked to the wall in the original starting position.
- Repeat 10 reps.

Key Notes/Common Faults:

- Pain/discomfort/straining of any kind.
- Faulty breathing pattern.
- Loss of Full Spinal Control.
- Loss of pelvic neutral position, seen mainly as <u>lower back arching</u> away from the wall.
- Other body region compromise.

The purpose of the Wall Angel exercise is to fine-tune spinal control while gaining the ability to move from the extremities. If you've been following carefully, you may be starting to notice a trend in these exercises. Full Spinal Control is a commonality in everything we have done so far, and this focus will continue up to the highest level. This is why I keep saying that the biggest key to all of this is to master the basic fundamentals. Mastering Full Spinal Control and applying it to everything you do is the ticket to movement, performance, strength, speed, power, reducing injury risk, and anything else you want to do. **Always continue to practice and focus on the basic fundamentals.**

No pain should be experienced in the Wall Angel series, just as in all exercises. All the same pathologies and pain generators explained thus far can occur here and must be kept in mind. The trainee may experience increased difficulty in Full Spinal Control in the vertical position. Axial loading also increases in this position. These alterations in position increase the chance of aggravation of pathology.

The lower extremity bearing the body's weight may create compression in the hip, knee, and ankle/foot joints. Common pathologies that may cause pain here can be specific to any of these joints, including degenerative joint disease, arthritis, labral tears, tendinitis, and other joint lesions. If this is the case and the exercise is causing pain, first attempt to change the pelvic position, set scapular position, and/or DNF neck position, as these may not be in the correct neutral position. If this does not work, attempt to change the angle of motion at the hip or shoulder joint to allow for increased or decreased flexion, rotation, abduction, or adduction during the movement. If this does not work, next attempt to limit the range of motion to a pain-free range.

If the pain does not originate from the hip, knee, ankle/foot, or shoulder joints, it may be coming from the sacroiliac joints or the spine, including the neck. If this is the case, more attention to maintaining pelvic neutral, the set scapular position, and DNF position should be attempted. Failure to maintain Full Spinal Control may cause excessive torque, rotation, extension, or compression of the spine, thus causing pressure to the facet joints, mechanical stenosis to the IVF space/s or the central canal, causing radicular or myelopathic complications, and/or increased pressure on the discs of the spine.

Also, remember that the additional extremity movement and increased exercise difficulty may cause strain, tension, and over-activation, which may increase pressure (Valsalva) and, thus, symptoms. If pain is present and no attempts are successful at eliminating the pain, then this particular exercise is beyond current limit capacity and thus should not be done. [932, 940, 941, 942, 943, 944, 945, 946, 947]

LEVEL I SUMMARY

The main goal of level I of The PREMIER Body Method's movement education course is to learn the fundamental pieces of human movement mechanics, to understand how movement is created in the human body, and to lay the groundwork for producing proper movement. The first fundamental involves understanding that the muscles of the spinal column, core, and torso are designed to prevent motion and provide a solid foundation for the larger muscles of the hips, legs, shoulders, and arms to pull from. The job of the muscles in the extremities is to create movement. These muscles are the prime movers.

Understanding the roles of muscles in preventing and creating movement permits understanding of Full Spinal Control, which consists of pelvic neutral held in place by correct core activation, set scapular and thoracic spine (upper back) position, and cervical spine (neck) neutral by way of DNF activation. You first master each piece of spinal control individually and then combine them at the same time to achieve Full Spinal Control.

The second key to fundamental human movement is to now apply and maintain Full Spinal Control during slightly larger motions, as you begin to master movement in the hips, legs, shoulders, and arms. Full

Spinal Control must be maintained throughout all movement of the extremities to let the body achieve correct fundamental movement. Full Spinal Control provides the stable base of the body, thus allowing the prime movers of the extremities to do their job of moving us around this world.

I simply cannot stress the importance of Full Spinal Control enough. All other movement depends on it. Without mastery of Full Spinal Control, nothing else will work nearly as well. This concept can apply all the way up to the highest level of human performance, in fact, even more so at the highest levels of human performance. If you learn nothing else from this program besides achieving Full Spinal Control and applying it to all movements, you are well on your way to a healthy physical life for years to come.

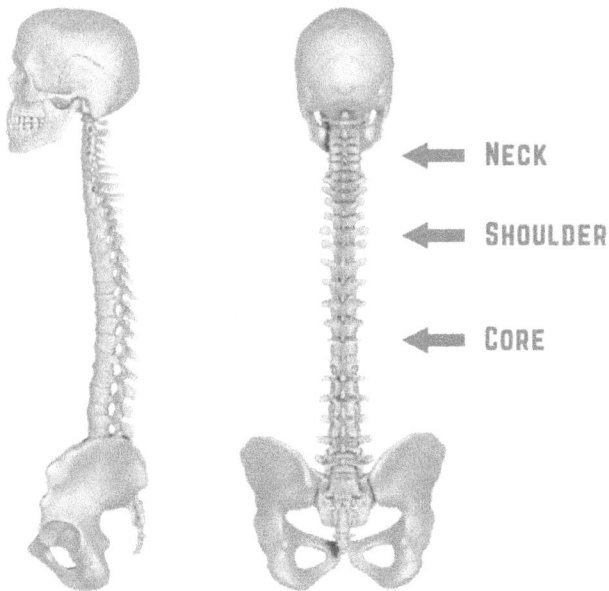

NECK

SHOULDER

CORE

LEVEL II: BASIC FUNCTIONAL HUMAN MOTION

In Level I of The PREMIER Body Method, we learned the fundamentals of biomechanics. We first learned individual pieces and then began adding the pieces together to achieve Full Spinal Control and the beginnings of hip and shoulder movement. Now, in Level II, we will continue to put pieces together in a loaded position (upright standing position) and apply them to the larger functional movements of the human body. The hard, focused work from Level I will pay off in Level II.

Level II applies the details of Level I to larger real-world mechanics and exercise performance. Let's face it: as stimulating as the Level I training was, it's not doing us much good if we can't apply it to the real world. Recall that there are essentially three major motions of the human body: Hip Hinging, pulling, and pressing motions. Level II works on the large biomechanics of Hip Hinging, deadlifting, squatting, pushing, pulling, balance, coordination, and gait pattern training.

HIP HINGE SERIES

L evel II of Human Movement Education begins with the Hip Hinge movement pattern, which may be the single most important movement learned in the entire program. It is the pivotal transition between all the pelvic, hip, and spinal control pieces learned lying down in the unloaded setting of Level I and the advanced movements you will get to in Level III. Hip Hinging puts the Level I movements together in a loaded, standing, and functional position/movement.

The Hip Hinge is also essential because it is the single most functional movement pattern the human body can produce. The Hip Hinge takes the detailed mechanics of lumbopelvic hip control, core stability, and spinal control and puts them all together in the standing position to create the beginnings of a squatting and/or deadlifting movement pattern. Learning this movement pattern correctly opens the door to the squat, deadlift, lunge, step-up, lateral squat/lunge, and many more movement patterns and exercises. It also helps to train proper walking, running, sprinting, and jumping mechanics, as well as higher-level athletic agility, explosive power movement, and sports performance training. Whether you're an athlete or someone interested in being

pain-free and healthy, the Hip Hinge lets you perform all of this.
(948, 949)

A correct Hip Hinge movement pattern lets the body efficiently utilize its most powerful muscles. If you want to improve athletic performance, there is no better place to start than to improve your hip-hinging mechanics. You can never be good enough at the fundamentals. Your squats and deadlifts may already be good, but doing them with proper movement can take them and your athletic training to a new level. So many athletes have come to me over the years thinking they are already strong enough, only to discover how much stronger they can be when they go through one of my training programs and learn to move correctly.

A Hip Hinge is also crucial because it is your most functional (useful) movement pattern. You need it for countless routine daily tasks and activities. You use a Hip Hinge movement pattern every time you sit on and get up from a chair, the bed, and the toilet, bend over to pick up or put down something, go up or down stairs, lift and carry, and run, jump, and walk.

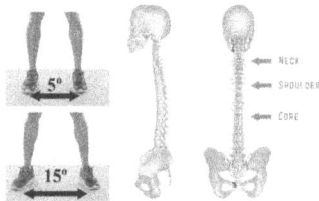

The Hip Hinge Series progressions begin with learning the basic Hip Hinge pattern and then progressing this basic movement pattern into several larger movements and compound exercises. The starting position for the Hip Hinge is standing with feet hip-width apart or slightly wider than hip-width, depending on one's specific dimensions and comfort. Somewhere between 5 and 15 degrees of lower extremity external rotation (feet turned out) is typical, as long as it is equal from side to side. Then achieve Full Spinal Control by first achieving a neutral pelvic position, then achieving a set scapular position, then achieving a DNF neutral neck position. This is the first time the trainee will achieve Full Spinal Control in an upright axial loaded position in free space (not supported by the ground or a wall). Once the correct Full Spinal Neutral standing position is achieved, the next step is to activate core stability "on" to lock this neutral spinal position in place and ensure it is maintained throughout the movement.

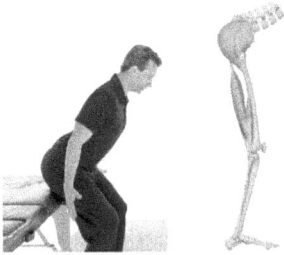

The movement of the Hip Hinge is done by utilizing the posterior chain mechanics of the body, mainly the gluteus maximus and hamstring, to eccentrically control hip flexion as the body's weight is shifted back and down. Eccentric muscle contraction is when a muscle contracts and gains length simultaneously, like a bicep curl on the way down. The bicep contracts and gets longer at the same time in order to lower the weight. This is opposed to concentric muscle contraction, when a muscle is contracting and shortening at the same time, as in the bicep curl on the way up. For the Hip Hinge, imagine you are going to sit back and down on a chair that is just a little too far behind you, so you have to reach your hips (butt) back to it. The challenge is maintaining Full Spinal Control while doing this.

The weight distribution through the soles of the feet should be towards the foot's posterior (back) aspect, ideally straight through the Navicular bone, not towards the foot's anterior (front) end or through the toes. We commonly tell trainees to sit the body's weight back on the heels, just for simplicity. Most people with poor hip-hinging mechanics shift far too much weight to the front of the foot and body, so getting the weight back towards the heels can be a significant improvement. Allowing the body's weight to shift too far forward causes many mechanical dysfunctions and can lead to increased stress in the ankles, knees, and spine. This can predispose the body to injuries in these areas and can also lead to accelerated degenerative changes and other chronic pain conditions.

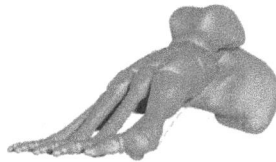

The Hip Hinge exercise focuses only on the initiation of the movement of the hips back and down, so once this movement is engaged, the gluteus should concentrically begin to contract to create hip extension, thus returning the movement back to the standing starting position. The best way to typically teach and practice the basic Hip Hinge is in front of a table or high bench (something about mid-thigh level). The table or bench serves as a target for the trainee to sit the hips back to during the motion and limits the motion to a small range. Going low is not the goal at this point.

The hip and hip musculature should be doing nearly all of the work to create this motion. The spine, spinal musculature, and core are also doing work, but their job is to prevent motion. There should be no spinal (back) movement during the Hip Hinge. The knee, ankle, and the rest of the lower extremity anatomy also move and create motion as secondary support to the hip musculature.

There are a few main faults to be aware of. Many people try to initiate the movement with the knees and quads, which is incorrect. The hips must control the movement. The knees are moving, and the quads are working, but the hip should initiate and control the movement. The knees are just going along for the ride,

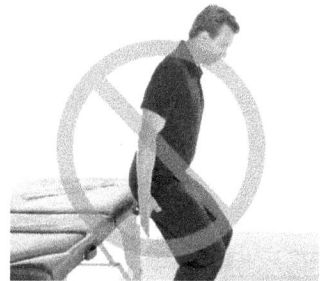

assisting the hips. So, as the hip hinging movement occurs, the hips should (correct) move back and down towards the target (the bench you are standing in front of), the knees should NOT (incorrect) shoot forward.

Also, the knees must not be allowed to cave inward. Our basic rule of knee width being just as wide or slightly wider than foot width is more valid than ever here. Push the legs (entire leg) out and wide from the heels as though you were standing over the center of a crack in the ground, and you were going to push the earth apart to make a canyon between your legs. The feet should not roll or cave out as this lower extremity push-out occurs. Instead, keep the feet flat and think about pushing out from the inside of the heels. This push-out is essential not only to activate lateral hip strength and stability and protect the knees but also to prepare for correct squatting mechanics later. That being said, this is still just a slight push out. We do not need to be excessive here.

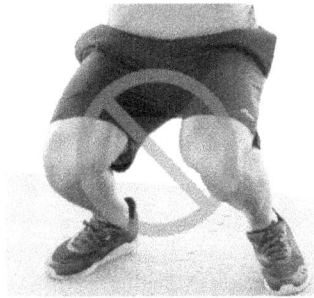

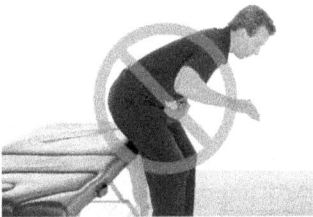

Another common problem is breaking spinal control. One way this can happen is if the spine rounds and caves forward into slight flexion. This usually occurs when the second piece of Full Spinal Control, the set scapular position, is lost. If the shoulder girdle begins to hike up and round over the top, the rest of the spine tends to topple over with it. This creates flexion in both the thoracic and lumbar spine, which forces more weight towards the front half of the body, putting more stress on the knees, lower back, and even neck. This fault is usually fairly obvious and needs to be corrected. The correction is usually resolved with more attention to maintaining the proper set scapular position. A **strong upper back protects the lower back.** This will be accomplished with correct practice and continued focus on the fundamentals.

The other common hip-hinging fault also deals with the loss of spinal control due to the creation or allowance of excessive lumbar spine extension resulting from loss of pelvic control. It is not quite as obvious but can be even more detrimental than letting the spine roll forward. The neutral pelvic position is lost, and an anterior pelvic tilt is created, forcing the lower back to hyperextend. This causes two main problems.

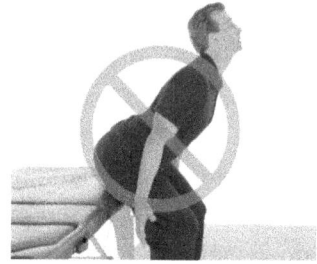

The first problem is that losing a neutral pelvic position shifts the workload that should be done by the core musculature to the joints of the lumbar spine. This goes against the definition of proper mechanics, which states that **whenever possible, workload production can and should be performed by muscles, not the passive joint structures. Whenever that workload that can and should be done by muscles is not done, and therefore that workload is transferred to joints, cartilage, ligaments, and/or tendons, the movement should be considered tissue wasting and thus biomechanically "unsafe."** And we wonder why so many of us end up with back pain and degenerative disease (arthritis) when we get older. So, from the standpoint of lowering the risk of injuries, not allowing any of these faults is crucial.

This can cause pain later in life, but losing the pelvic neutral position is just as detrimental from a performance standpoint. Remember, muscles pull on bones. The torque angle and lever arm are critical for proper force production. Loss of pelvic neutrality during any hip-hinging movement will shut down and inhibit full-force production for our most powerful muscles, such as the gluteal muscles and other muscles of the hip. These are the very muscles we are trying to train when we perform exercises like squats and deadlifts, so limiting their force production is certainly limiting our performance gains.

Again, why keep beating your body up for minimal gains? Stop training harder and start training smarter. If you understand how your body is supposed to work and can better control it, you will see better strength, speed, power, and other performance gains. Learning how to perform the Hip Hinge movement pattern is a must for athletic performance and pain-free everyday existence.

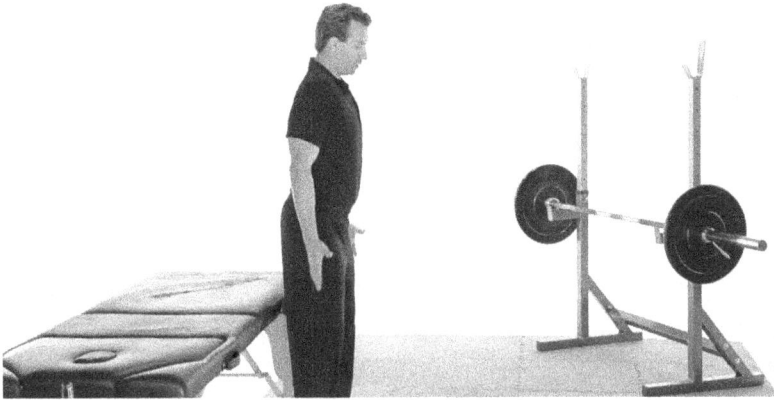

Hip Hinge Beginning Position

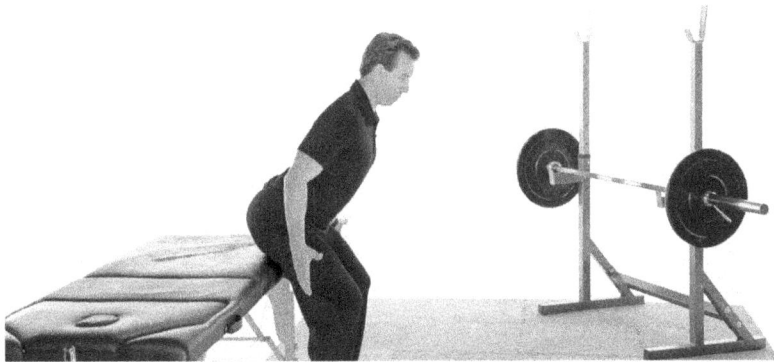

Hip Hinge Movement Position

Hip Hinge
Goal/Purpose:

- Achieve Full Spinal Control in a freestanding position while initiating the hip-hinging movement pattern.

Beginning Position:

- Standing with Full Spinal Control posture, including pelvic neutral, set scapular position, and C/S DNF neutral.
- Feet hip-width apart, feet slightly turned out (between 5-15 degrees of external lower extremity rotation is considered normal).

Movement/Action:

- Activate core stability "on" by way of Core Bracing I, then perform a Hip Hinge motion by sitting the hips back and down by way of hip flexion. The knees should bend slightly as the hips move, but the hips should control the movement (the knees just go along for the ride). Hinge the hips back and down just slightly, then reverse the motion back to the standing starting position, then relax core stability "off." As the Hip Hinge motion is being performed, push the legs apart from the heels, as if you were trying to spread the earth apart under your feet to make a canyon.
- Repeat 10 reps.

Key Notes/Common Faults:

- Pain/discomfort/straining of any kind.
- Faulty breathing pattern.
- Loss of pelvic neutral, set scapular position, or neutral neck position.
- Initiating the motion, or excessively moving, from the knees.
- Excessive weight towards the front of the foot rather than through the heels.

Once you master the basic initiation of the Hip Hinge movement pattern, you can open up this movement and progress to various more complex compound movement patterns. The basic Hip Hinge will first progress into two main movements: the squat and the deadlift patterns. The main mechanical difference between these two movement patterns concerns the axis of rotation of the thorax (pelvis and spinal column) at the hip joint.

The squat form movement pattern continues the Hip Hinge in a vertical fashion. Once the basic Hip Hinge position is achieved, the torso will be at a certain angle, approximately 5 to as much as 45 degrees, depending on the type of squat (such as Olympic Back, Power Back, Front, Overhead, or other variations) being performed and the specific dimensions, or structural anatomy, of the person performing it, relative to the ground. This initial hinged angle will not change as the torso moves in a vertical plane of motion up and down as the hips, knees, and ankles move respectively into greater flexion, flexion, and dorsiflexion. This vertical movement of the torso puts greater emphasis on the knee and quadriceps muscle group than does the deadlift pattern, which we will discuss in the next section.

The squat's stance width should be slightly wider than hip-width for most people, again, depending on individual anatomy. Feet, again, should have 5-15 degrees of external rotation. Once the basic hip hinge is initiated, the movement continues as one fluid motion, and the hips and body continue to move down in a vertical fashion.

Maintaining Full Spinal Control and avoiding all the faults mentioned above is very important. The upper back and shoulders should not cave forward. Remember, a strong upper back protects the lower back. Do not lose the set scapular position. Also, maintain pelvic neutrality. Do not allow the pelvis to roll forward and create lower back arching/extension. Pay attention to the neck as well. Many people have a habit of extending the neck and tilting the head up while squatting, but when the neck is out of place, it can pull the rest of the spine with it because the spine works as a single unit. The knees should not shoot forward or cave in. Push the earth wide.

At this point, it is important to discuss the purpose of pushing the legs open during the squatting motion. It allows for a greater range of motion and depth during the squat movement pattern. If the legs do not open up during the squat, at some point, the femurs will run into the pelvis. Your legs will literally run into your body. The only way to go lower is either to break spinal alignment and move from your spine (back) or shift the majority of your weight forward (anterior weight-bearing problem again!). Both of these are examples of faulty mechanics. If, instead, the legs open up by pushing the ground apart, the pelvis has room to drop between the femurs, and the body will have room to drop through the legs. This allows for a much greater range of motion without sacrificing Full Spinal Control or other mechanics.

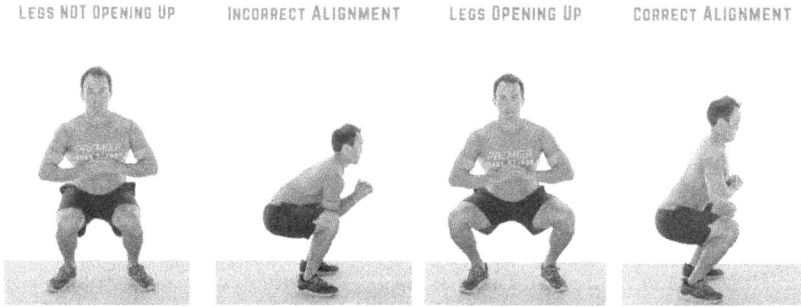

LEGS NOT OPENING UP   INCORRECT ALIGNMENT   LEGS OPENING UP   CORRECT ALIGNMENT

This brings up another critical topic regarding squatting mechanics. How low should you go? This is a constant debate. Some say thighs should be parallel to the floor, while others say the thighs need to go past parallel to count. Some say pushing the thighs past parallel is bad for the knees, although no concrete research backs that up. I have a different view: it does not matter *how* low the squat goes. The only thing that matters is correct mechanics, from maintaining Full Spinal Control to all the other specifics already discussed. How low you go with proper form is determined by two things: body mobility (mainly hip, ankle, and T/S mobility) and your ability to master and maintain spinal alignment and Hip Hinge mechanics. If you are squatting, and your Full Spinal Control breaks six inches above your thighs parallel to the ground, that is as deep as your squat should go. If you are squatting and maintain the correct alignment and mechanics to parallel, then your squat goes to parallel. If you can maintain Full Spinal Control and correct mechanics past parallel, your squat can go past parallel. Squat depth is determined by correct mechanics and the ability to maintain alignment, not some arbitrary range that is predetermined by some dude at the local gym. It is different for everyone based on individual anatomy/structure (physical capability limits!) and the ability to control movement. As long as the mechanics are correct (for you as an individual), the back, knees, and everything else will be perfectly safe, regardless of the squat depth. The strength gains will also be better because the muscles will be doing the work.

If your squat depth is not very low to start, don't sacrifice the mechanics to gain greater range. You will only be getting false range this way, and you will be putting your body at risk for injury and increased wear and tear. You will also get fewer performance gains this way since your muscles will not work as well as they could. Stick to correct mechanics, and do not worry about depth. Increased depth will come naturally over time if you stick to correct mechanics. Moving correctly is the best way to gain a quality functional range of motion (mobility). **Never sacrifice Full Spinal Control and correct mechanics for an increased ("false") range of motion.** This is a general rule for all movements and exercises, not just squats.

The squat pattern includes three main sub-groups: the power back squat, the Olympic back squat, and the front squat. The main difference between these squatting patterns is the torque angle at the hip. This hip torque angle is determined by the angle of the torso (the spine) relative to the ground (the line of force created by gravity). The front squat has the greatest torso angle relative to the ground, as the torso is the most vertical. Out of all the squatting patterns, this puts the greatest emphasis on the quadriceps, although the hips are still doing much of the work.

FRONT SQUAT TORQUE ANGLE   OLYMPIC BACK SQUAT TORQUE ANGLE   POWER BACK SQUAT TORQUE ANGLE

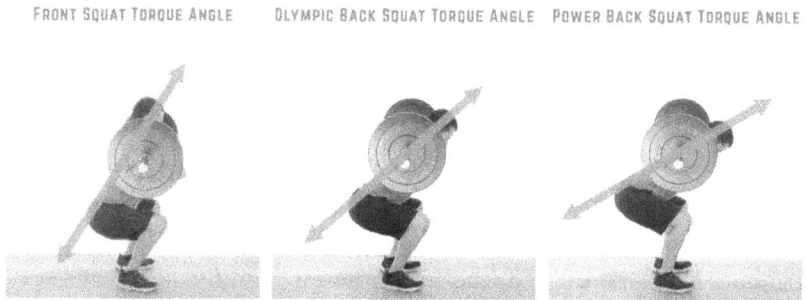

The Olympic back squat has a slightly smaller angle, and the Power back squat will have the smallest angle relative to the ground and the shortest lever arm. A smaller angle of the torso relative to the ground places less emphasis on the quadriceps and more on the hamstring. Therefore, the power back squat is the least quad-dominant of all the squatting movement patterns. The power back squat is often the squatting pattern that will produce the highest overall strength due to the decreased lever arm.

Please remember that these squatting patterns can have grey areas and sometimes blend together. Also, these variations in patterns can vary due to an individual's specific anatomical structure and physical capability limits, thus creating predispositions for certain people to be better at certain patterns over others. Some patterns may also be more beneficial and mechanically safer for certain individuals.

The squatting movement pattern can be further progressed into a variety of angles and applied to many movement exercises, including overhead squats, split squats, lateral squats, multidirectional squats, forward lunges, backward lunges, lateral lunges, step-ups, and single-leg squats, among other variations.

There is a basic squat form and several variations as described below:

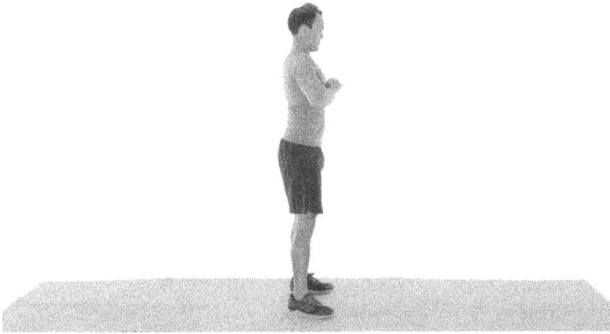

The Basic Squat Pattern Beginning Position

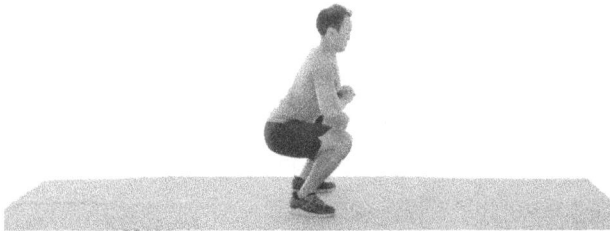

The Basic Squat Pattern Movement Position

Hip Hinge Stage II – The Squat Pattern
Goal/Purpose:

- Progress the Hip Hinging Movement pattern to a full-range
  squat pattern for the purpose of functionally getting up and
  down and increasing hip/leg strength.

Beginning Position:

- Standing with Full Spinal Control posture including pelvic
  neutral, set scapular position, and C/S DNF neutral.
- Feet slightly wider than hip-width apart, feet slightly turned

out (between 5-15 degrees of external rotation of the lower extremity is considered normal).

Movement/Action:

- Activate core stability "on" by way of Core Bracing I, then, using a Hip Hinge motion, continue to move the torso down vertically into a squat by sitting the hips back and down by way of hip and knee flexion. Continue to squat as low as correct mechanics (i.e., maintenance of Full Spinal Control) allows. Then reverse the motion to return to the standing starting position, then relax core stability "off." Remember to push the legs apart as if you were trying to spread the earth apart as the squat motion occurs.
- Repeat 10 reps.

Key Notes/Common Faults:

- Pain/discomfort/straining of any kind.
- Faulty breathing pattern.
- Loss of pelvic neutral, set scapular position, or neutral neck position.
- Initiating the motion from the knees.
- Allowing the knees to cave inward.
- Excessive weight towards the front of the foot instead of through the heels.

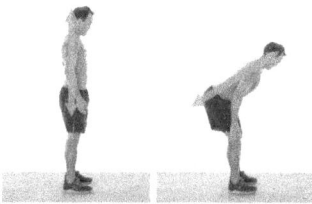

Deadlift Movement Pattern

The deadlift movement pattern continues the Hip Hinge in the horizontal plane, thus creating an arched motion for the torso with the hip as the axis of rotation/torque. The torso, which starts in the vertical position, will continue to angle closer and closer to parallel with the ground as the hips move into greater flexion. Unlike the squat pattern, where the angle of the torso (spine) relative to the ground is constant once the initial Hip Hinge angle has been achieved as it is moved vertically up and down, the torso (spine) angle relative to the ground during the deadlift pattern is continually changing.

This continual change in spinal angle makes it more challenging to maintain Full Spinal Control during the deadlift pattern. This motion also increases the shear force on the spine due to the increasing angle of the spine away from vertical. Finally, the change in spinal angle increases the internal load force (the force created on the structures of the body by the musculature of the body itself due to muscle contraction) on the spine because the core and spinal musculature will have to be ramped "on" to a greater degree to maintain spinal neutral. These aspects of the deadlift may make it a risky movement pattern for persons suffering from more severe spinal pathology. That being said, faulty hip hinging and deadlifting mechanics have most likely contributed to the spinal pathology over time, so learning how to perform these movement patterns correctly can still have tremendous value for someone suffering from back and spinal pain.

The starting position for the deadlift is very close to the squat. The foot width is typically slightly narrower, and the lower extremity external rotation generally is slightly less for the deadlift than the squat. However, this can vary depending on individual anatomy and structure, as well as the type of deadlift you are performing (power, RDL, stiff, sumo, among others). The force production should still be ideally through the Navicular bone in the foot, with more emphasis shaded even further back towards the heels with the deadlift. Once the stance is set, Full Spinal Control must be achieved and maintained throughout the deadlift. The deadlift motion begins with the basic Hip Hinge motion and then continues the hinge as the hips are pushed further back and the torso (spinal column) is angled forward to counterbalance. The same faults discussed regarding the basic Hip Hinge can be accentuated here, so watch out for them, especially the shoulder/upper back (set scapular) position caving. Here, a strong upper back truly protects the lower back!

The deadlift movement pattern includes three main sub-groups: the power deadlift, the Romanian deadlift (commonly referred to as the RDL), and the straight or stiff leg deadlift. The main difference between these variations is the amount of knee and quadriceps involvement in the movement pattern. The straight or stiff leg deadlift has no knee motion, essentially taking the quadriceps out of the movement altogether, making this purely a hamstring and glut movement exercise. It also makes this pattern variation the most challenging and risky movement to perform correctly while maintaining Full Spinal Control for the reasons stated above.

The power deadlift involves the most knee and quadriceps, thus making this pattern closer to a hybrid between the deadlifting and squatting patterns. In fact, the two patterns, deadlift and squat, can occur at the same time. If the torso is rotating (hinging), a deadlift pattern occurs. If the torso is moving up and down vertically, a squat pattern occurs. These can happen together.

The power deadlift may be the most important exercise a human being can do. It is a full-body lift. It produces the best, most efficient performance gains. It is far and away the most real-world functional exercise. If you told me I was only allowed to do one exercise for the rest of my life and nothing else, I would choose, without question, the power deadlift. It is used to get up and down, pick up, lift, carry things, jump, sprint, and even walk.

The third basic type of deadlift is the Romanian deadlift (RDL). The RDL involves the knee and quadriceps, but not to the extent the power deadlift does, thus putting it in between the straight leg and power forms. There is slight knee motion occurring during the RDL, unlike the straight leg deadlift, but not nearly as much knee motion as with the power deadlift. The RDL is still mainly a posterior chain exercise. We start with this deadlift form because it is usually the easiest for people to learn. Still, the deadlift movement pattern can be quite challenging for many people, including athletes, to get right.

POWER DEADLIFT   ROMANIAN DEADLIFT   STIFF/STRAIGHT LEG DEADLIFT

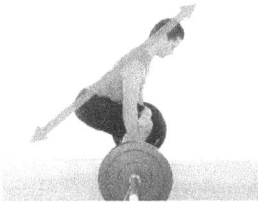

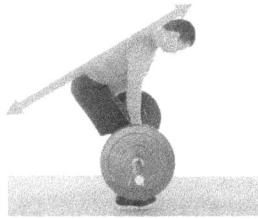

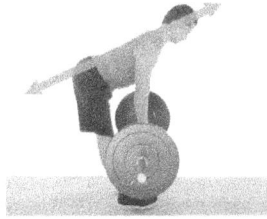

Please remember that there is a broad grey area with all these variations in squatting and deadlifting movement patterns. Many of these forms can blend together. However, learning to distinguish between them is vital to understanding how the human body works mechanically. The RDL is the form of choice when first learning the deadlift pattern. This is where we begin in the PREMIER Body Method's Movement Education Course. Once learned correctly, the deadlift movement pattern, as well as the squat pattern, can be applied and progressed to a variety of exercise movements.

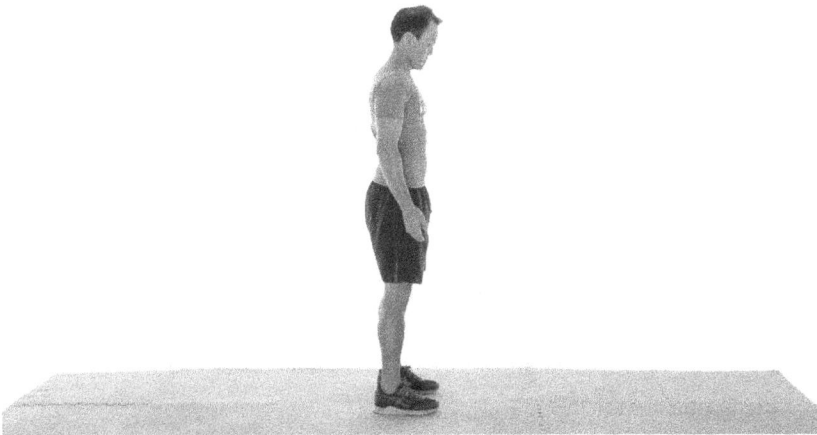

Deadlift Pattern Beginning Position

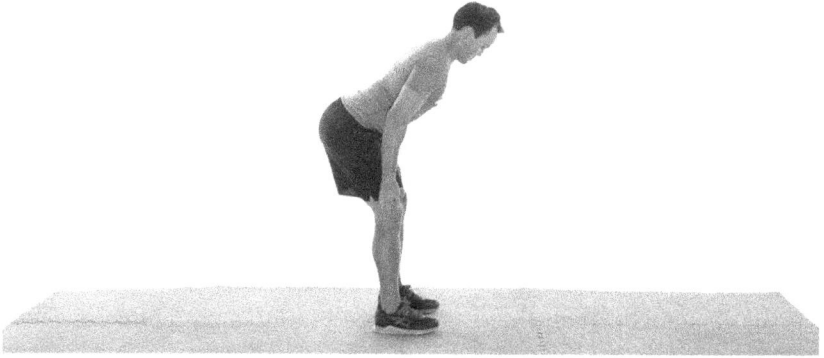

Deadlift Pattern Movement Position

Hip Hinge Stage III – The Deadlift Pattern
Goal/Purpose:

- Progressing the Hip Hinging Movement pattern to a full range deadlifting pattern (RDL) for the purpose of functional lifting and increasing hip/leg/full body strength.

Beginning Position:

- Standing with Full Spinal Control posture including pelvic neutral, set scapular position, and C/S DNF neutral.
- Feet hip-width apart, feet slightly turned out (between 5-15 degrees of external lower extremity rotation is considered normal). Typically, a deadlift pattern has less turn out of the feet and a slightly narrower stance width than the squatting pattern.

Movement/Action:

- Activate core stability "on" by way of Core Bracing I. Then, using a Hip Hinge motion, continue to hinge the torso over into a deadlift by continuing to sit the hips back and down by way of hip flexion. Continue to hinge as low as correct mechanics (i.e., maintaining Full Spinal Control) will allow. This will typically be limited by hamstring flexibility. Then reverse the motion back to the standing starting position, then relax core stability "off."

- Repeat 10 reps.

Key Notes/Common Faults:

- Pain/discomfort/straining of any kind.
- Faulty breathing pattern.
- Loss of Full Spinal Control.
- Initiating the motion from the knees.
- Allowing the knees to cave inward.
- Excessive weight towards the front of the foot instead of through the heels.

We conclude the Hip Hinge Level II Series with Stage IV - Crab Walks.

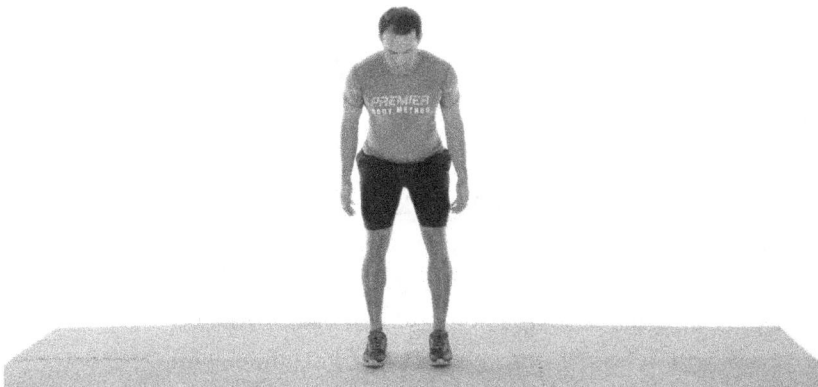

Crab Walks Beginning Position

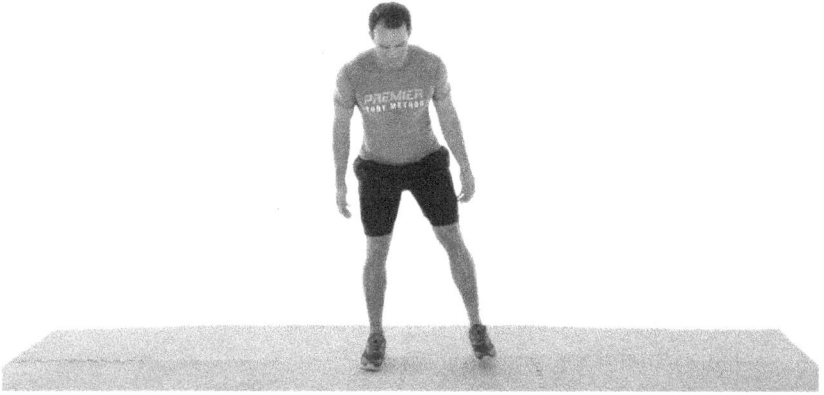

Crab Walks Movement Position I

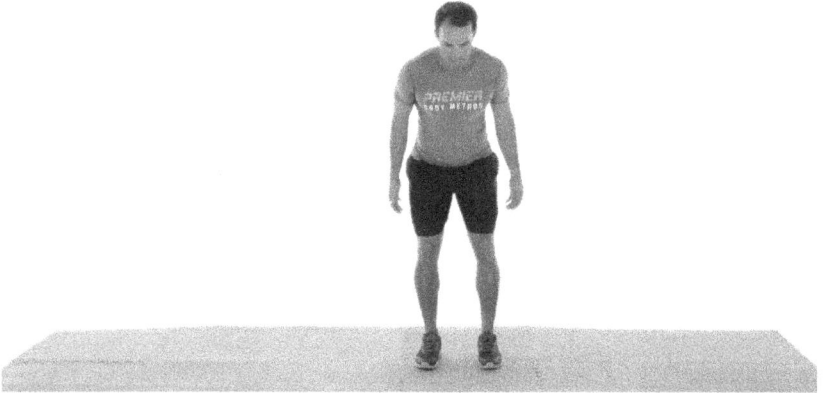

Crab Walks Movement Position II

Hip Hinge Stage IV – Crab Walks
Goal/Purpose:

- Progressing the Hip Hinging Movement pattern in a lateral direction for the purpose of functional side-to-side movement, and increasing lateral hip strength and stability.

Beginning Position:

- Standing with Full Spinal Control in a Hip Hinged position, including all specifics as noted in the basic Hip Hinge.

Movement/Action:

- Core stability will already be on to a certain extent just to maintain the starting position. Begin the exercise movement by ramping up core stability "on" more to maintain pelvic neutral, then move one leg out laterally by stepping out to the side further than normal Hip Hinge / squat width. Then move the opposite side leg/foot in, thus returning body to the Hip Hinged starting position.
- Repeat 10 steps to the side, then reverse the steps back in the other direction. 10 steps down and 10 steps back completes one set.

Key Notes/Common Faults:

- Pain/discomfort/straining of any kind.
- Faulty breathing pattern.
- Loss of Full Spinal Control.
- Allowing the knees to cave inward.
- Excessive weight towards the front of the foot (weight should be through the heels).

Remember, as with all exercises and movements learned, ideally, no pain should be experienced. The same pathologies and pain generators explained throughout Level I may be accentuated here and must be kept in mind. In the vertical freestanding position, increased difficulty in achieving and maintaining Full Spinal Control may be experienced. There will also be increased axial loading in this position. These alterations in position may increase the chance of pathology being aggravated.

The lower extremity is bearing the weight of the body now as well. This may create compression in the joints: hip, knee, ankle, and foot. Common pathologies that may cause pain here can be specific to any of these joints, such as degenerative joint disease, arthritis, labral tears, meniscus lesions, tendinitis, ligament pathology, or other joint and soft tissue lesions. If this is the case and the exercise is causing pain, first attempt to change the pelvic position, set scapular position, and/or DNF neck position, as these may not be in the correct neutral position.

If this does not work, attempt to change the angle of motion at the hip, knee, or ankle joint to allow for increased or decreased flexion, extension, rotation, abduction, and/or adduction during the movement. If this still does not work, next attempt to limit the range of motion to a pain-free range.

If the pain does not originate in the hip, knee, or ankle/foot, it may come from the sacroiliac joints or the spine, including the neck. If this is the case, more attention to maintaining pelvic neutrality, the set scapular position, and the DNF position should be attempted. If Full Spinal Control is not maintained, it may cause excessive torque, rotation, extension, or spine compression. This may cause pressure to the Facet joints and mechanical stenosis to the IVF space/s or the central canal, in turn causing radicular or myelopathic complications and/or increased pressure on the spine's discs. Also, a deadlift pattern creates more posterior to anterior (back to front) shear force on the spine due to the angle of the spine (torso) relative to gravity. For spinal pathology, especially instability, this may increase the chance for aggravation by increasing loading stress to the spine's structures, even if ideal Full Spinal Control is maintained. It may just be beyond the physical capability limits for some people with severe pathology.

It should also be noted that performing any unilateral, single-leg, lateral, split, or multidirectional movement pattern progressions will increase the difficulty of maintaining spinal neutrality. This may increase the chance of loading stress in multiple planes of motion and thus aggravate certain pathologies, especially sacroiliac (SI joint) pathology.

Also, remember that the additional extremity movement may cause strain, tension, and over-activation, which may increase pressure (Valsalva) and cause symptoms. Any of these scenarios may cause pain. If pain is present and no attempts are successful at eliminating the pain, the particular exercise is beyond the current limit capacity and thus should not be done. [932, 940, 941, 942, 943, 944, 945, 946, 947]

BALANCE AND UNILATERAL STABILITY SERIES

Now that we have achieved the loaded, upright, standing position of The PREMIER Body Method's Level II, we will progress the movement education towards continued functional abilities. Balance plays a significant role at all levels of large human movement. Maintaining stability and control during complex movements is more difficult without the ability to maintain balance. Unilateral and single-leg activities involve many daily tasks, such as walking. Balance is critical for athletic training and performance as well. The unilateral stability series is designed to address and train this aspect of human movement.

This series begins simply with a single-leg stance/single-leg balance exercise. Proper body position during the single-leg stance involves all the mechanical details learned thus far in the course. Full Spinal Control must be maintained, with particular attention paid to the pelvic position. While balancing on one leg, all planes of motion are involved. The lateral/coronal plane seems to be a weak area of stability for many. This will show up here as hip hiking or an un-leveling of the pelvis (known in orthopedics as a Trendelenburg sign). The pelvis should remain level and in a neutral position, as should the rest of the spine all the way to the neck and head.

One should be in a slight hip-hinged position so the body's weight is on the gluteus and other active muscular structures. We do not want the hip and knee locked out since that places the majority of the force through the passive structures of the joints, cartilage, and ligaments. The force at the sole of the foot should be through the Navicular (back towards the heel), just as it is with proper Hip Hinge mechanics. It is important to be in the correct Hip Hinge position; do not let the knee shoot forward.

The single-leg stance can be progressed in many ways to increase difficulty and further improve balance. One advanced technique is to perform it with eyes closed. Adding perturbations, either externally using wobble boards, Airex stability pads, Bosu balls, and other unstable surfaces, or internally, as in the standing hip stability exercise, can improve balance. That being said, it is important to be able to sufficiently balance on flat ground before progressing on to unstable surfaces. Level 2 of the Premier Body Method continues this training next with the Standing Hip Stability exercise, followed by Single Leg Stance with eyes closed. The detailed descriptions for these specific training exercises are below. The goal is to maintain Full Spinal Control and correct hinging details no matter how difficult the challenge. If the challenge is so great that control cannot be maintained, training is not accomplishing its intended goal and should not be done.

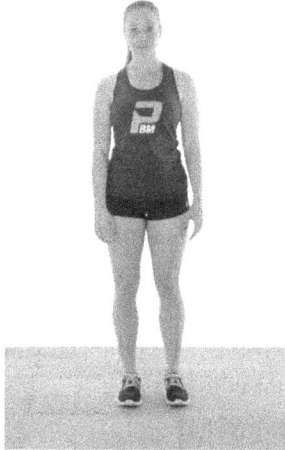

Single Leg Balance Begin

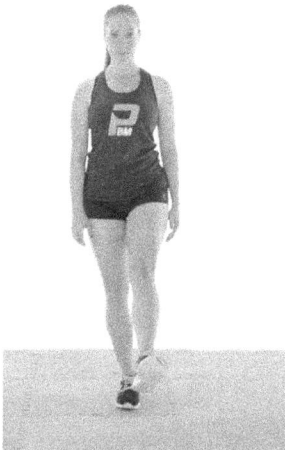

Single Leg Balance 30-Second Hold Position

Single Leg Balance
Goal/Purpose:

- Learning to feel comfortable and stable in a single-leg unilateral position. Many normal daily activities require unilateral efforts and single-leg stability.

Beginning Position:

- Standing with Full Spinal Control in a slightly Hip Hinged position, including all specifics as noted in the basic Hip Hinge.

Movement/Action:

- Begin the exercise by ramping up core stability "on" more to maintain spinal control; lift one leg while balancing on the other. Maintain all fundamental positions, postures, and mechanics, including Full Spinal Control, a slight Hip-Hinged position on the standing leg, and weight back on the hip and the heel.
- Hold the position for 30 seconds, then switch to the other side.

Key Notes/Common Faults:

- Pain/discomfort/straining of any kind.
- Faulty breathing pattern.
- Loss of Full Spinal Control.
- Un-leveling of the pelvis.
- Loss of slight Hip Hinge position.
- Allowing the knee to cave inward.
- Excessive weight towards the front of the foot (weight should be through the heels).

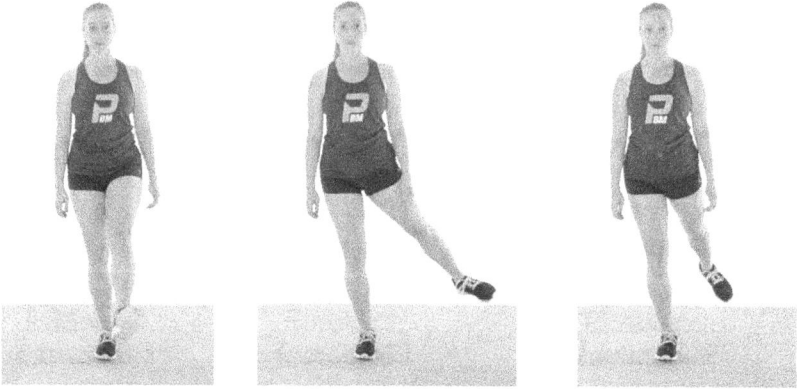

Standing HIp Stability Movement Positions Front (Flexion), Side (Abduction), and Back (Extension)

Standing Hip Stability
Goal/Purpose:

- To continue to progress unilateral stability in a more 'real-world' manner with the addition of functional movements in the single-leg position.

Beginning Position:

- Standing with Full Spinal Control in a slightly Hip Hinged position, including all specifics noted in the basic Hip Hinge.

Movement/Action:

- Begin the exercise by ramping up core stability "on" more to maintain spinal control. Lift one leg while balancing on the other. Maintain all fundamental positions, postures, and mechanics described in the single-leg balance exercise. Once in the single-leg stance, begin to move the opposite leg 10 times to the front (hip flexion), then 10 times to the side (hip abduction), and then 10 times back (hip extension). Do not allow any loss of pelvic neutrality as the leg moves.
- Repeat with the other side.

Key Notes/Common Faults:

- Pain/discomfort/straining of any kind.
- Faulty breathing pattern.
- Loss of Full Spinal Control.
- Loss of slight Hip Hinge position.
- Allowing the knee to cave inward.
- Excessive weight towards the front of the foot (weight should be through the heels).

Single Leg Balance with Eyes Closed
Goal/Purpose:

- Continued progression of single leg stability. The purpose of eyes closed is to increase the body's proprioceptive abilities.

Beginning Position:

- Standing with Full Spinal Control in a slight Hip Hinged position, including all specifics as noted in the basic Hip Hinge (refer to page 295).

Movement/Action:

- Begin the exercise movement by ramping up core stability "on" more to maintain spinal control, and lift one leg up to stand on one leg. Maintain all fundamental positions, postures, and mechanics including Full Spinal Control, slight Hip Hinged position on the standing leg, weight back on the hip and the heel. Once in the correct single leg stance position, close the eyes for the duration of the 30 seconds. If balance is lost, open the eyes, regroup and get back into the single leg position, and then close the eyes again.

- Hold the position for 30 seconds, and then switch to the other side.

Key Notes/Common Faults:

- Pain/discomfort/straining of any kind.
- Faulty breathing pattern.
- Loss of Full Spinal Control.
- Loss of slight Hip Hinge position.
- Allowing the knee to cave inward.
- Excessive weight towards the front of the foot (weight should be through the heels).

Remember, as with all exercises and movements learned, ideally, no pain should be experienced during the balance and unilateral stability series. The pathologies and pain generators explained throughout the spinal control series may be accentuated here and must be kept in mind. Remember that the vertical freestanding position increases difficulty in maintaining Full Spinal Control. This position also leads to increased axial loading. These alterations in position may increase the chance of pathology being aggravated.

The lower extremity is now unilaterally bearing the body's weight, possibly further compressing the hip, knee, and ankle/foot joints. Common pathologies that may cause pain here can be specific to any of these joints. Examples include degenerative joint disease, arthritis, labral tears, meniscus lesions, tendinitis, ligament pathology, and other joint and soft tissue lesions. If the exercise is causing pain, first attempt to change the pelvic position, set scapular position, and/or DNF neck position, as these may not be in the correct neutral position. Ensure the correct slight Hip Hinge position is maintained to load the force on the musculature, not the joints.

If the pain does not originate from any structure in the lower extremity, it may be coming from the sacroiliac joints or the spine, including the neck. For any unilateral positions or movements, the load may be unbalanced across the pelvis, SI joint, and spine. If this is the case, try to focus on maintaining pelvic neutrality, the set scapular position, and the DNF position. Core stability may need to be ramped up "on" to a high degree. Failure to maintain Full Spinal Control may cause excessive torque, rotation, extension, or compression of the spine. This may cause increased pressure to the Facet joints, mechanical stenosis to the IVF space(s) or the central canal, radicular or myelopathic complications, and/or increased pressure on the spine's discs.

Also, remember that with increased difficulty comes increased strain, tension, and over-activation, which may increase pressure (Valsalva) and cause symptoms. It is essential to remain calm and controlled, especially as the difficulty level increases.

Any of these scenarios may cause pain. If pain is present and no attempts are successful at eliminating the pain, the particular exercise being performed is beyond the limit capacity for now and thus should not be done. (932, 940, 941, 942, 943, 944, 945, 946, 947)

ADVANCED SPINAL CORE CONTROL SERIES

The advanced Spinal Core Control series is designed to continue the Full Spinal Control learned in detail in Level I of the program and progress this control by applying a variety of new body positions and movement challenges. Greater strength and endurance are necessary to perform the advanced progressions in this series. For some trainees, this series may be beyond physical capability limits, and is unnecessary to perform. It may do more harm than good.

However, a greater level of Core Control is necessary for many trainees, especially those looking to progress to a higher level of athleticism or improve sports performance. The forces and demands placed on the body during most sports activities, both recreational and certainly competitive, are great enough to warrant more advanced core training. Remember, at any level of sport, we must prepare the body to perform. We cannot expect to have the sport itself be the training. In other words, if athletes cannot perform the progressions in this advanced Core Control Series correctly, they may have difficulty in improving their sports performance ability.

The series begins with the basic plank exercise, first from the knees to learn the correct form and then from the feet as the trainee gains strength of control. The series then progresses to more advanced planks by adding various extremity movements and body positions. As the strength and endurance of Full Spinal Control continue to improve, these skills can be advanced to more functional movements and exercises like the chop and the push/pull exercises. Remember that, above anything else, the goal is to maintain perfect Full Spinal Control throughout all progressions. Any sacrifice in pelvic position, set scapular position, and/or DNF neck position is not only defeating the purpose of the training but also increasing the risk of injury aggravation or causing a new injury.

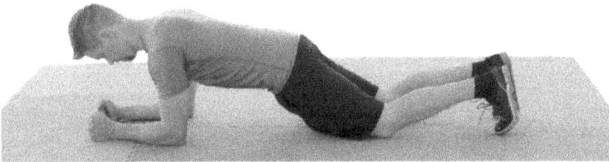

Front Plank Knee Position

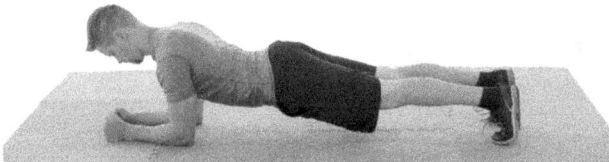

Front Plank Feet Position

Front Plank (Knees or Feet)
Goal/Purpose:

- Further progression of pelvic control (as well as Full Spinal Control) and core stability, mainly for athletes or people who need to achieve above-average core strength.

Beginning Position:

- Face down, supporting the body's weight equally on the elbows and knees (or elbows and feet as shown, when ready). Full Spinal Control, especially pelvic neutral, must be achieved and maintained.

Movement/Action:

- Hold the position for 30 seconds. While holding, continue to mentally review the fundamentals checklist, including pelvic position, scapular position, neck position, and core stability (kegel-abs-breathing).

Key Notes/Common Faults:

- Pain/discomfort/straining of any kind.
- Faulty breathing pattern.
- Loss of Full Spinal Control, especially the neutral pelvic position, manifesting as anterior pelvic tilt and low back extension.
- Do not allow the lower back to extend.
- Any stressing or straining, especially in the face and neck, should not be allowed.

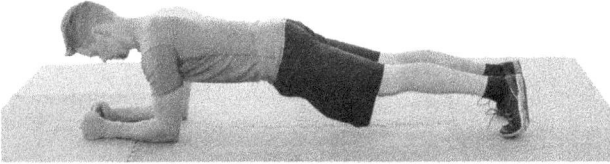

Front Plank Starting Position (Feet)

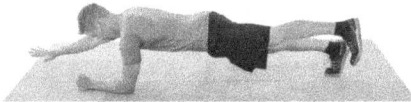

Front Plank Movement Position 1

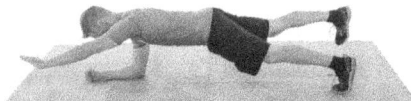

Front Plank Movement Position 2

Front Plank (Knees or Feet) with Extremity movement
From the Beginning Position:

- Face down, supporting the body's weight equally on the elbows and knees (or elbows and feet as shown). Full Spinal Control, especially pelvic neutral, must be achieved and maintained.

Movement/Action:

- While maintaining the correct front plank position, begin with lifting one knee (leg) at a time off the ground by way of hip extension. Hold the leg lifted momentarily, then place the knee back down into the starting plank position. Repeat with the opposite leg. Perform 10 reps.
- Once ready, this can be repeated with arm movement instead of leg movement, and eventually, arms and legs can be moved in unison by lifting the opposite arm and leg at the same time.

Key Notes/Common Faults:

- Pain/discomfort/straining of any kind.
- Faulty breathing pattern.
- Loss of Full Spinal Control.
- Do not allow the lower back to extend.
- No stressing or straining allowed, especially in the face and neck.

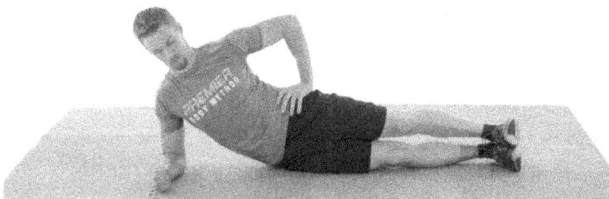

Side Plank from Knees - Hold Position

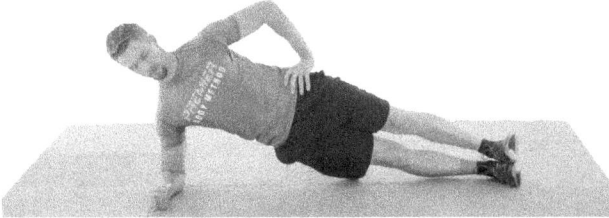

Side Plank from Feet - Start from Knees, Then Hold Position

Side Plank (Knees or Feet)
Goal/Purpose:

- Further progression of pelvic control (as well as Full Spinal Control) and core stability, mainly for athletes or persons who need to achieve above average core strength.

Beginning Position:

- Side-lying, supporting the body's weight equally on the elbow and knee (or elbow and feet with top foot in front as shown). Full Spinal Control, especially pelvic neutral, must be achieved and maintained.

Movement/Action:

- Hold the position for 30 seconds. During this time, mentally review the fundamentals checklist, including Pelvic position, scapular position, neck position, and core stability (kegel-abs-breathing).
- Repeat on the opposite side.

Key Notes/Common Faults:

- Pain/discomfort/straining of any kind.

- Faulty breathing pattern.
- Loss of Full Spinal Control, especially the neutral pelvic position manifesting as anterior pelvic tilt and low back extension.
- Do not allow the lower back to extend.
- Any stressing or straining, especially in the face and neck, should not be allowed.

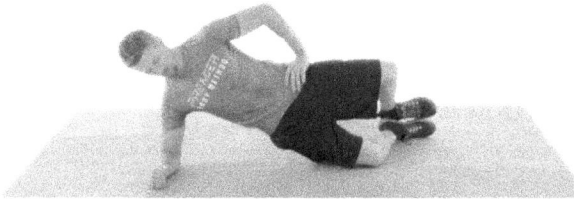

Side Plank from Knees with Clamshell Hip Abduction

Side Plank from Knees with Hip Abduction
Goal/Purpose:

- Further progression of pelvic control (as well as Full Spinal Control) and core stability, mainly for athletes or persons who need to achieve above average core strength.

Beginning Position:

- Side-lying, supporting the body's weight equally on the elbow and knee. Full Spinal Control, especially pelvic neutral, must be achieved and maintained.

Movement/Action:

- While maintaining the correct side plank position, perform a clam motion by way of hip abduction. Perform 10 reps.
- Repeat on the opposite side.
- Note that if you begin with a side plank from the feet, your hip abduction will be with a straight leg lift, not a clamshell.

. . .

Key Notes/Common Faults:

- Pain/discomfort/straining of any kind.
- Faulty breathing pattern.
- Loss of Full Spinal Control, especially the neutral pelvic position manifesting as anterior pelvic tilt and low back extension.
- Do not allow the lower back to extend.
- Any stressing or straining, especially in the face and neck, should not be allowed.

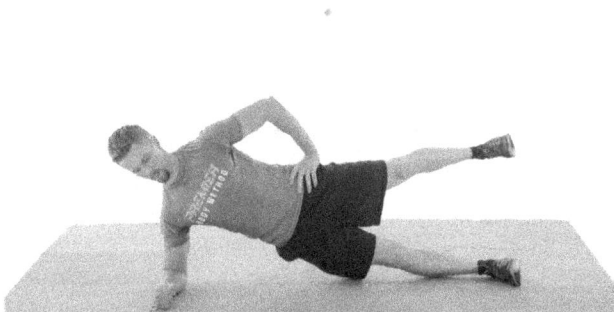

Side Plank from Feet with Hip Abduction (Straight Leg)

Side Plank from Feet with Hip Abduction
   Goal/Purpose:

- Further progression of pelvic control (as well as Full Spinal Control) and core stability, mainly for athletes or persons who need to achieve above average core strength. from the feet is increasingly more difficult than from the knees.

Beginning Position:

- Side lying supporting the weight of the body equally on the elbow and feet with the top foot in front of the bottom foot. Full Spinal Control, especially pelvic neutral, must be achieved and maintained.

Movement/Action:

- While maintaining the correct side plank position, perform a side lying hip abduction motion by way of hip abduction. Perform 10 reps.
- Repeat on the opposite side.

Key Notes/Common Faults:

- Pain / discomfort / straining of any kind.
- Faulty breathing pattern.
- Loss of Full Spinal Control, especially the neutral pelvic position as seen by anterior pelvic tilt and low back extension.
- Do not allow the lower back to extend.
- Any stressing or straining of any kind, especially in the face and neck should not be allowed.

Remember, as with all exercises and movements learned, ideally, no pain should be experienced. All the same pathologies and pain generators explained so far may be accentuated here. Remember that an advanced quadruped position (all four extremities bearing the body's weight) or variations of it increase the difficulty of Full Spinal Control. Any loss of Full Spinal Control will cause excessive loading in the spine. The most common fault when performing the exercises in this series is the loss of pelvic neutral, usually into an increased anterior pelvic tilt causing increased lower back extension.

This places increased loading stress on the facet joints, IFV spaces, nerve roots, and other posterior elements of the spine. This is another

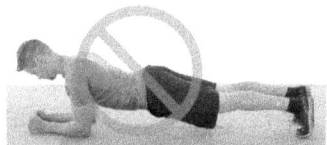

perfect example of a shift in active to
passive tissue stress according to the Law of 100% Motion. By allowing loss of spinal and pelvic control, you are taking workload from the core musculature and re-directing it into the facet joints of the lower spine. This violates proper biomechanics because now you have trans-ferred the workload from active tissues to passive tissues. Don't let it happen to you!

When done correctly, the core and spinal control musculature have increased activity and workload in this position. These alterations in position and workload may increase the chance of pathology being aggravated due to increases in intra-abdominal and intra-thecal pres-sure, even if the position and form are perfect. It is for this reason that the exercises in this series may be beyond the physical capability limits for some with severe spinal pathology. For most people, though, the exercises in this series are fine as long as they are done correctly.

The extremities bear the body's weight in the exercises in this series. This may create compression in the shoulder and hip joints. Common pathologies that may cause pain here can be specific to the hip and/or shoulder joints, such as degenerative joint disease, arthritis, labral tears, tendinitis, or other joint lesions. If any of these are present and the exercise is causing pain, first attempt to change the pelvic position, set scapular position, and/or DNF neck position, as it may not be in the correct neutral position. If this does not work, attempt to change the angle of motion or load position at the hip or shoulder joint to allow for increased or decreased flexion, rotation, abduction, and/or adduction during the movement or reduced load in the position. If this does not work and the exercise involves movement, next attempt to limit the range of motion to a pain-free range.

If the pain does not originate from the hip or shoulder joint, it may be from the sacroiliac joints or the spine, including the neck. If this is the case, more attention to maintaining pelvic neutral and the set scapular position should be attempted. Some of the more advanced exercises in this series involve extremity movement. As the hip and/or shoulder extend and flex, respectively, excessive movement in the spine is common. This may cause excessive torque, rotation, extension, or compression of the spine. This may then cause pressure to the Facet joints in the spine, mechanical stenosis to the IVF space(s) or the spinal central canal, causing radicular or myelopathic complications, and/or increased pressure on the spine's discs.

If pain is caused by cervical spine pathology, special attention must be given to the DNF position. Remember that cervical spine pathology can cause anything from local pain to upper and even lower extremity pain or other signs and symptoms.

Also, remember that the additional extremity movement may cause strain, tension, and overactivation, which may increase pressure (Valsalva) and, thus, symptoms.

Any of these scenarios may cause pain. If pain is present and no attempts are successful at eliminating the pain, the particular exercise is beyond the limit capacity at this point and, therefore, should not be done. [932, 940, 941, 942, 943, 944, 945, 946, 947]

ADVANCED SCAPULAR CONTROL SERIES

The advanced scapular control series is designed to continue the set scapular position control learned in Level I of the program by progressing it to various new and increasingly challenging body positions and movements. This continues to advance the control of the set scapular position and improves the strength and endurance of that control. This series also adds larger pieces of movement together as we continue the concept of building movement. The exercises and shoulder movements in this series involve a proper Hip Hinge and deadlift position. Thus, learning the proper progressions in the Hip Hinge Series is necessary before this Advanced Scapular Control Series can be learned. This is another example of building movement!

The series picks up where the scapular setting series from Level I left off. Further progressions include more advanced body and upper extremity positions with the introduction of the W, T, and Y shoulder positions and movements. Full Spinal Control is still mandatory throughout all the progressions. While important for everyone, this series is most pertinent for persons suffering from cervical and/or shoulder/upper extremity pathology. This is because faulty scapular setting is usually a big hole in the system for these trainees, so they need extra work in this area of control to correct these dysfunctions. The exercises in the series can also be extremely valuable for athletes, especially overhead and/or throwing athletes, such as athletes whose sports largely depend on the use of the shoulder and arm in high/above head ranges of motion, such as pitchers, weight lifters, gymnasts, and javelin throwers. The increased demands of overhead and throwing sports require proper and more advanced training.

W's, T's, & Y's
Goal/Purpose:

- Progression Scapular control beyond the Scapular Setting Series by increasing the control level required for the shoulder girdle while combining several major movement control pieces, including Full Spinal Control, Hip Hinge position, and scapular setting, with upper extremity movement.

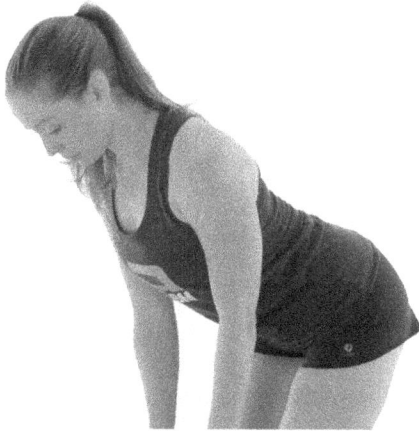

Beginning Position for W's, T's, and Y's.

Beginning Position for all three movements:

- Standing with Full Spinal Control, achieve a Hip Hinge

and/or deadlift (RDL) position as discussed in the Hip Hinge Series.

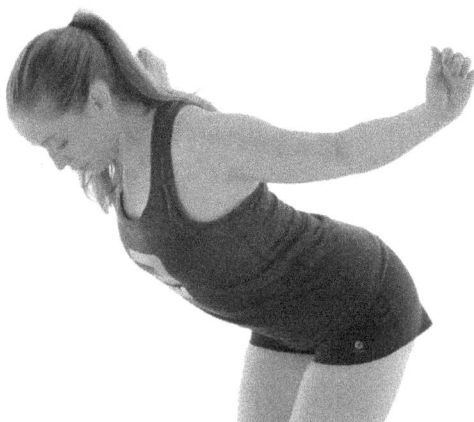

The W Movement Position

W's
Movement/Action:

- While maintaining the correct hip-hinged position, perform the W motion with the upper extremity by pulling the shoulder blades back and down as the elbows are pulled back with the elbows bent as if one were attempting to touch the elbows together behind the back. Then, relax the arm motion without losing the Hip Hinge position.
- Repeat 10 reps.

Key Notes/Common Faults:

- Pain/discomfort/straining of any kind.
- Faulty breathing pattern.
- Loss of Full Spinal Control.
- Loss of correct hip-hinged position.
- Overexertion or straining of any kind.

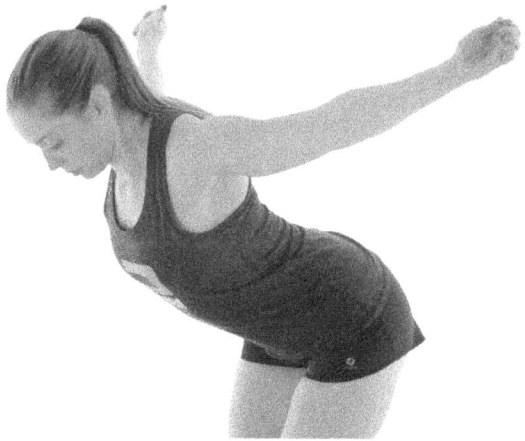

The T Movement Position

T's
Movement/Action:

- While maintaining the correct hip-hinged position, perform the T motion with the upper extremity by pulling the shoulder blades back and down as the arms are pulled back with the elbows straight, as if one were attempting to form the letter "T" with the arms and torso. Then, relax the arm motion without losing the Hip-Hinged position.
- Repeat 10 reps.

Key Notes/Common Faults:

- Pain / discomfort / straining of any kind.
- Faulty breathing pattern.
- Loss of Full Spinal Control.
- Loss of set scap position; do not allow the shoulders to hike up.
- Loss of correct hip-hinged position.
- Overexertion or straining of any kind.

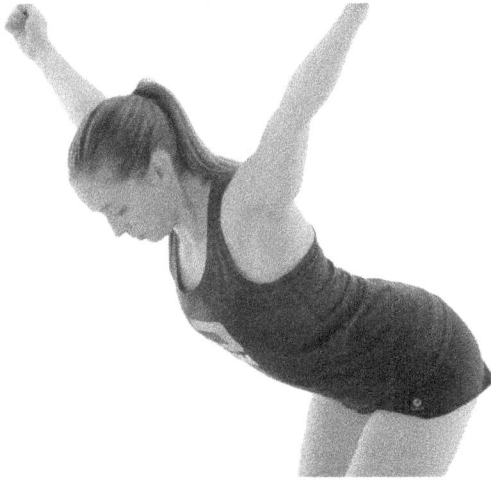

The Y Movement Position

Y's

Movement/Action:

- While maintaining the correct hip-hinged position, perform the Y motion with the upper extremity by pulling the shoulder blades back and down as the arms are pulled up overhead with the elbows straight as if one were attempting to form the letter "Y" with the arms and torso. Then, relax the arm motion without loss of the hip-hinged position.
- Repeat 10 reps.

Key Notes/Common Faults:

- Pain/discomfort/straining of any kind.
- Faulty breathing pattern.
- Loss of Full Spinal Control. Special attention to loss of pelvic neutral and lower back extension.
- Loss of correct hip-hinged position.
- Overexertion or straining.

Remember, as with all exercises and movements learned, ideally, no pain should be experienced. All the same pathologies and pain generators explained throughout must be kept in mind. As body positions and movements become increasingly challenging, increased difficulty in maintaining Full Spinal Control may be experienced. These changes in position and workload may increase the chance of pathology being aggravated.

The shoulder joint is advancing in movement and control difficulty throughout this series. Common pathologies that may cause pain specific to the shoulder joint are degenerative joint disease, arthritis, labral tears, tendinitis, and other joint lesions. If any of these are present and the exercise is causing pain, first attempt to change the pelvic position, set scapular position, and/or DNF neck position, as it may not be in the correct neutral position. If this does not work, attempt to change the angle of motion at the shoulder joint to allow for increased or decreased flexion, extension, rotation, abduction, and/or adduction during the movement. If this does not work, next attempt to limit the range of motion to a pain-free range.

If the pain does not originate from the shoulder joint, it may be coming from the neck, spine, or even the Sacroiliac joints. If this is the case, more attention to DNF neck position, set scapular position, and pelvic neutral position should be attempted.

Also, remember that increasing the difficulty of exercise movement may cause strain, tension, and overactivation, which may increase pressure (Valsalva) and cause increased symptoms.

Any of these scenarios may cause pain. If pain is present and no attempts are successful at eliminating the pain, the particular exercise is beyond the limit capacity at this point and thus should not be done.
(932, 940, 941, 942, 943, 944, 945, 946, 947)

ROTATOR CUFF CONTROL SERIES

T he Rotator Cuff Control Series is designed to provide extra stability to the shoulder's glenohumoral joint (GHJ). The GHJ (ball and socket) of the shoulder has one of the largest ranges of motion in the entire human body, but this range of motion comes with a price. It leaves the shoulder joint susceptible to stability issues, usually resulting in joint damage, cartilage and labral lesions, and various forms of tendinitis and bursitis.

The positioning of the entire shoulder girdle plays a huge part in overall shoulder health or lack thereof. Creating a good mechanical position and a stable base for the muscles of the GHJ of the shoulder to work from sets the stage for proper shoulder and upper extremity mechanics. The Scapular Setting Series and the Advanced Scapular Control Series already covered these mechanics. However, even with superior shoulder girdle mechanics, certain athletic movements may put the GHJ of the shoulder in jeopardy. By strengthening the active component of GHJ stability, the rotator cuff, we can achieve a higher level of dynamic stability and lower the risk of shoulder damage in the future. If damage is already present, strengthening the rotator cuff is almost certainly necessary.

Recall that loading stress is taken up by one of two types of body tissues: active tissues or passive tissues. Active tissues (muscles) should take as much of that load as possible, so if there is a way to get more out of the active tissues by training them correctly, I'm all for it, and you should be, too! From another perspective, if an injury to the shoulder is already present, by training the active stability components and proper biomechanics of the shoulder, we can take pressure off the damaged passive tissues to allow them to heal correctly or at least prevent them from suffering further chronic damage.

This series begins with internal and external rotator cuff exercises with the GH joint held at zero degrees. Remember that all of the mechanical details learned thus far still apply here. Although the GH joint is the only joint moving when the rotator cuff creates the motion, many muscles are working to prevent motion. This combination of motion and holding will give the rotator cuff the stable base required to produce the force necessary for proper mechanics and control of the GH joint. This requires achievement and maintenance of set scapular position. To achieve the correct set scapular position, pelvic neutral and Core Control must be achieved and maintained. Also, remember the DNF neck position, as many shoulder muscles are attached to the neck. If the cervical spine (neck) is out of position, the function of these muscles decreases, and mechanics change. This could increase the loading stress on various passive structures. Full Spinal Control must be maintained.

The series continues by advancing the GH joint position to 90 degrees and then 120 degrees as necessary for the trainee's ability and performance goals. For many people, remaining at 0 degrees should suffice for most functional and fitness goals. For more advanced athletes, especially overhead athletes, higher angles should be achieved within tolerance, as these are the demands of the sport.

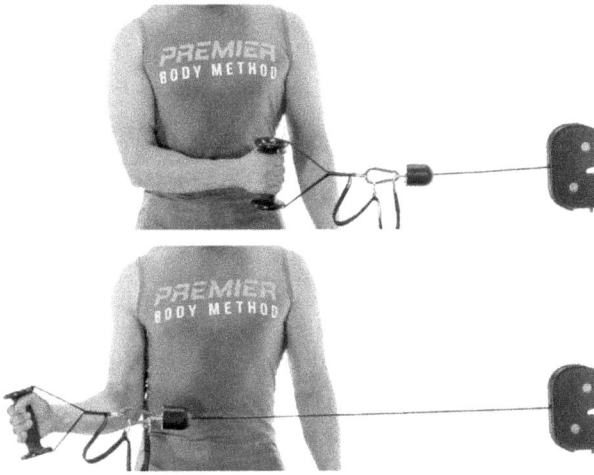

External Rotation at 0-degrees

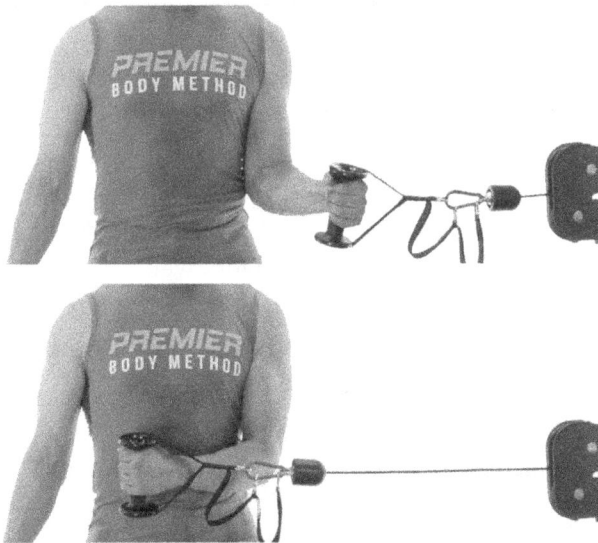

Internal Rotation at 0-degrees

External/Internal Rotation at 0°
Goal/Purpose:

- Progression of shoulder stability as well as continued reinforcement of Full Spinal Control mechanics.

Beginning Position:

- Standing with Full Spinal Control in a slightly hip-hinged position, as discussed in the Hip Hinge Series.

Movement/Action:

- While maintaining the correct standing position, perform shoulder (GH joint) rotations in both internal and external directions using a Theraband or cable machine. Make sure to keep the elbow tight against the side of the torso.
- Repeat 10 reps for external rotation and then 10 reps for internal rotation.
- Repeat with the opposite shoulder.

Key Notes/Common Faults:

- Pain / discomfort / straining of any kind.
- Faulty breathing pattern.
- Loss of Full Spinal Control, especially the set scapular position. The rotator cuff needs the solid foundation of the set scapular position in order to work well.
- Do not allow the arm to drift away from the body during the rotational movement.
- Overexertion or straining of any kind.

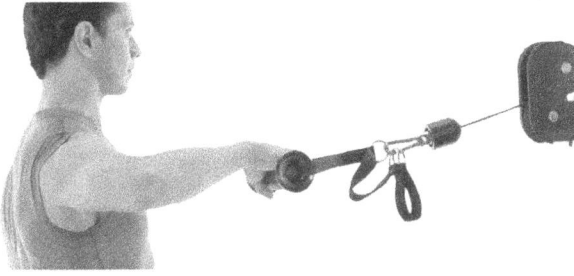

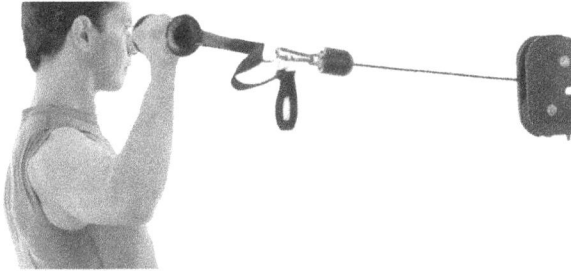

External Rotation at 90-degrees

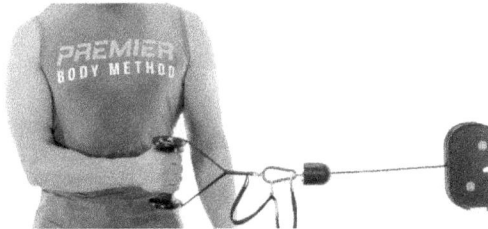

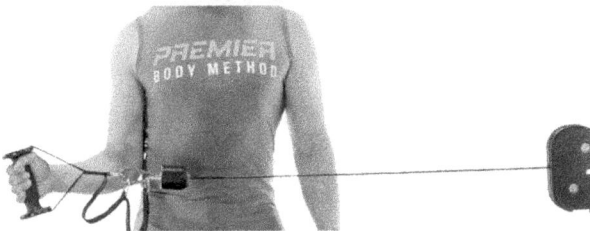

Internal Rotation at 90-degrees

External/Internal Rotation at 90°
Goal/Purpose:

- Progression of shoulder stability, mainly in the overhead

athlete or persons who need to work overhead in increased amounts.

Beginning Position:

- Standing with Full Spinal Control in a slightly hip-hinged position, as discussed in the Hip Hinge Series.

Movement/Action:

- While maintaining the correct standing position, perform shoulder (GH joint) rotations in both the internal and external directions using a Theraband or cable machine with the arm (shoulder joint) up at 90 degrees of abduction. Make sure to maintain the correct 90-degree shoulder position throughout the rotational movement.
- Repeat 10 reps for external rotation and then 10 reps for internal rotation.
- Repeat with the opposite shoulder.

Key Notes/Common Faults:

- Pain / discomfort / straining of any kind.
- Faulty breathing pattern.
- Loss of Full Spinal Control, especially the set scapular position. The rotator cuff needs the solid foundation of the set scapular position in order to work well.
- Do not allow the arm to waver from the 90-degree abducted position during the rotational movement.

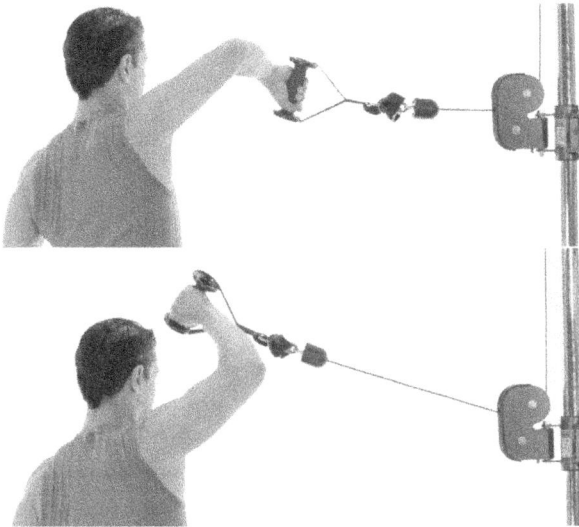

External Rotation at 120-degrees

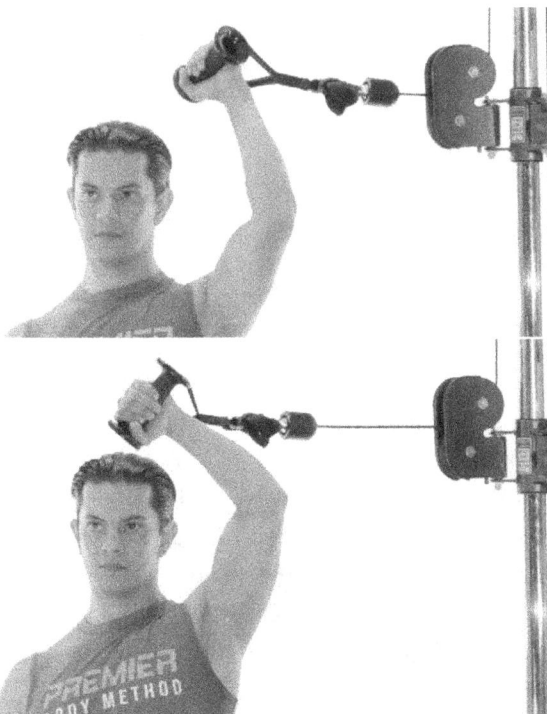

External Rotation at 90-degrees

External/Internal Rotation at 120°
Goal/Purpose:

- Progression of shoulder stability, mainly in the overhead athlete or persons who need to work overhead in increased amounts.

Beginning Position:

- Standing with Full Spinal Control in a slightly hip-hinged position, as discussed in the Hip Hinge Series.

Movement/Action:

- While maintaining the correct standing position, perform shoulder (GH joint) rotations in both the internal and external directions using a Theraband or cable machine with the arm (shoulder joint) up at 120 degrees of abduction. Make sure to maintain the correct 120-degree shoulder position throughout the rotational movement.
- Repeat 10 reps for external rotation and then 10 reps for internal rotation.
- Repeat with the opposite shoulder.

Key Notes/Common Faults:

- Pain / discomfort / straining of any kind.
- Faulty breathing pattern.
- Loss of Full Spinal Control, especially the set scapular position. The rotator cuff needs the solid foundation of the set scapular position in order to work well.
- Do not allow the arm to waver from the 120-degree abducted position during the rotational movement.

Remember, as with all exercises and movements learned, ideally, no pain should be experienced. All the same pathologies and pain generators explained thus far may be accentuated here. The shoulder joint will be advancing in movement and control difficulty throughout this series. Common pathologies that may cause pain specific to the shoulder joint are degenerative joint disease, arthritis, labral tears, tendinitis, and other joint lesions. If these are present and the exercise is causing pain, first attempt to change the pelvic position, set scapular position, and/or DNF neck position, as it may not be in the correct neutral position. If this does not work, attempt to change the angle of motion at the shoulder joint to allow for a smaller range of motion at the GH joint within tolerance. The range of motion can be reduced or limited to an isometric exercise with no actual movement, if necessary. This is still very effective at activating and strengthening the rotator cuff without the risk of joint irritation due to motion. Once the rotator cuff and scapular stabilizers have gained enough stability and strength, it may be easier to regain range of motion.

If the pain is not originating from the shoulder joint, it may be coming from the neck. Remember that many of the shoulder's muscles are anchored to the neck. A faulty position of the cervical spine may lead to faulty mechanics of the shoulder and thus create pain. Also, remember that the neurology controlling all the shoulder muscles originates in the cervical spine as the nerves exit the spinal column. A faulty neck position may be causing complications leading to various pathologies such as facet pain, mechanical stenosis to the IVF space(s) or the central canal causing radicular or myelopathic complications, and/or increased pressure on the spine's discs. The thoracic spine, lumbar spine, or sacroiliac joints may be aggravated if position and mechanics are not given full attention and pathology is present.

Remember that increases in the difficulty of exercise movement may cause strain, tension, and over-activation, which may increase pressure (Valsalva) and cause increased symptoms.

Any of these scenarios may cause pain. If pain is present and no attempts are successful at eliminating the pain, the particular exercise is beyond the present limit capacity and, therefore, should not be done. (932, 940, 941, 942, 943, 944, 945, 946, 947)

PULL SERIES

The Pull Series is designed to continue all the shoulder girdle mechanics learned so far and apply them in the functional manner of pulling. Pulling is one of the three fundamental movements of the human body. Just as the Hip Hinge movement pattern is vital for countless functional, exercise, and higher-level athletic movements, pulling mechanics are essential for a wide variety of normal daily activities as well as exercise and higher-level sports performance. You use pulling mechanics whenever you pick something up, carry something in your arms, or even open a car door. The countless exercises and sports training movements that involve pulling mechanics include pull-ups, rows, running, sprinting, jumping, and climbing.

The Pull Series begins with the set scapular pull exercise. This picks up where the Scapular Setting Series and the Advanced Scapular Control Series left off. Continuing to build scapular control, this movement is designed to improve the strength of the scapular control muscles, particularly the mid and lower trapezius. Scapular control and the ability to control and maintain the set scapular position are critical for proper pulling mechanics.

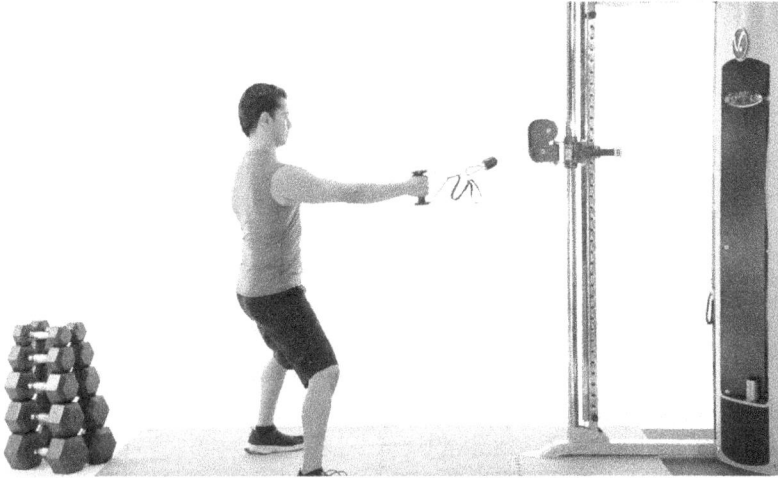

Set Scap Pull Beginning Position

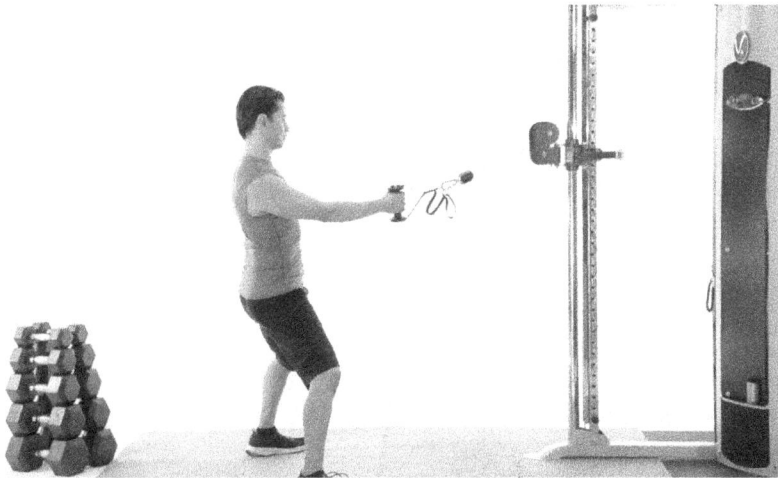

Set Scap Pull Movement Position

Set Scap Pull
Goal/Purpose:

- Progression and preparation of the shoulder girdle for
  Pulling motions, the second major category of movement.

Beginning Position:

- Standing with Full Spinal Control in a slightly hip-hinged position, as discussed in the Hip Hinge Series, with one arm flexed at the shoulder out in front of the body, grasping a cable or band.

Movement/Action:

- While maintaining the correct standing position, perform a set scapular pull by first allowing the cable or Theraband to pull the shoulder blade and the shoulder blade only out of the set scapular position. Then, pull the shoulder blade back into position by setting the shoulder back and down, as discussed in the Scapular Setting Series.
- Repeat 10 reps, then repeat with the opposite shoulder.

Key Notes/Common Faults:

- Pain/discomfort/straining of any kind.
- Faulty breathing pattern.
- Loss of Full Spinal Control.
- Be sure the scapula (shoulder blade) is the only moving body part. Do not allow the spine to rotate with the scapular movement. This can be a common fault because this is meant to be a small motion, and the tendency is to overdo it.
- Overexertion or straining of any kind.

Remember that the way muscles work is by pulling on bones. The positions of those bones relative to each other largely determine how effectively the muscles can produce the necessary force to pull on them. If the muscles that work to create motion have a solid, well-positioned base to pull from, they can generate the force they need to produce proper mechanics. If the base from which these muscles pull is not held in the proper stable position, the muscles working to create the motion will not be able to function effectively. This will create mechanical dysfunction. The loading stress that the muscles should do will be transferred, in part, to passive structures. By now, we all know where that can lead. A properly maintained set scapular position is crucial for correct pulling mechanics. To have a proper set scapular position, we must have a biomechanically correct spinal position. We must have a neutral pelvic position for the spine to function properly. Once again, Full Spinal Control is a must for correct pulling mechanics. As you can see, we are building movement now and adding fundamental control pieces together! To keep the fundamentals proper, stick to the checklist strategy and continue to review and repeat every detail of every piece all the way from the beginning, every rep, every exercise, every time.

The pull series continues to full-range pulling motions, beginning first with the basic mid-row exercise. We have already added the pelvic control piece, with core stability, scapular control, and DNF control, to create Full Spinal Control. From there, we add the pulling mechanism of the row while maintaining scapular control in addition to Full Spinal Control.

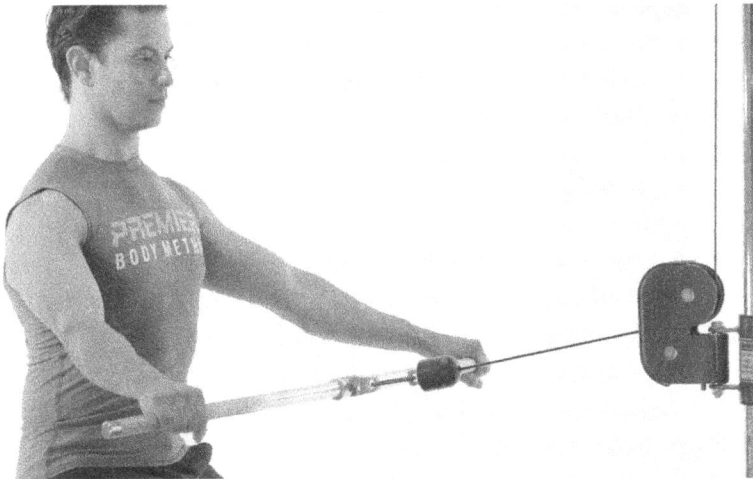

Mid Row Beginning Position

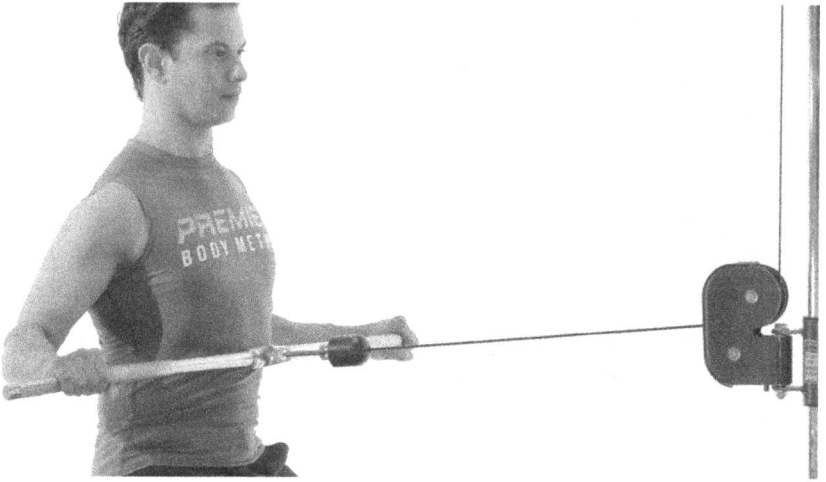

Mid Row Movement Position

Mid Rows
Goal/Purpose:

- Progression of the shoulder girdle to full pulling motions. This is the first progression for a full, complete pull. Pulling motions are one of the three major motions of the human body.

Beginning Position:

- Standing with Full Spinal Control in a slightly hip-hinged position, as discussed in the Hip Hinge Series, with both arms flexed at the shoulder out in front of the body, grasping a cable or band from an angle at the height of the body's center of mass (the navel).

Movement/Action:

- While maintaining the correct standing position, perform a row by pulling the cable or Theraband back towards the mid-belly just above the navel. Keep the elbows/arms tight to the body during the pulling motion.

- Repeat 10 reps.

Key Notes/Common Faults:

- Pain/discomfort/straining of any kind.
- Faulty breathing pattern.
- Loss of Full Spinal Control.
- Ensure the scapulae (shoulder blades) remain in their set scapular position. Now that a full pull is being performed, the scapulae should not move in and out of the set scapular position as with the Set Scap Pull exercise. Full Spinal Control, including the set scapular position, must be maintained throughout all pulling motions.

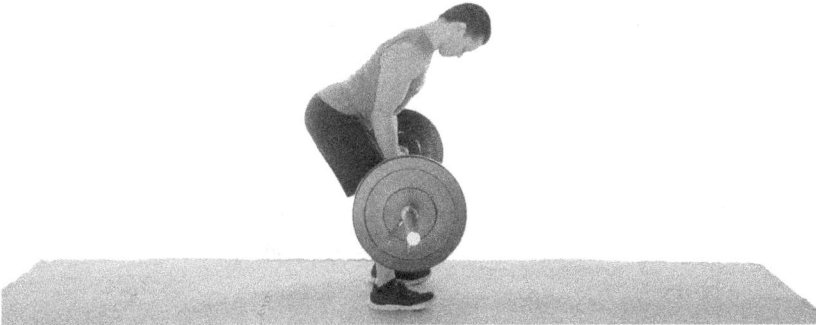

Bent-Over Row Beginning Position

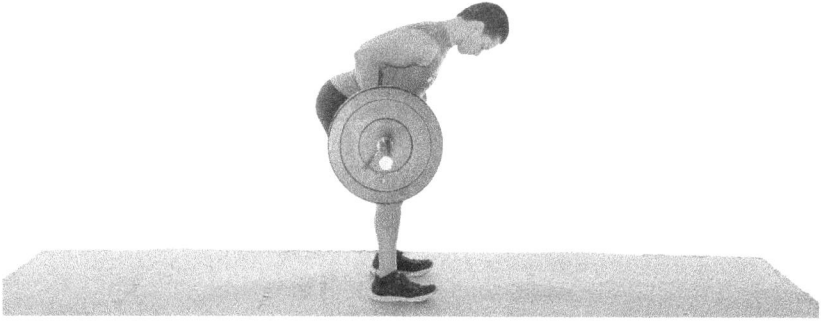

Bent-Over Row Movement Position

Bent-Over Rows
Goal/Purpose:

- Progression of the shoulder girdle for Pulling motions to one of the most functional movement mechanics the human body can perform, the bent-over row. This is how you pick things up!

Beginning Position:

- Standing with Full Spinal Control, achieve a deadlift (RDL) position as discussed, holding weights (either dumbbells or a barbell).

Movement/Action:

- While maintaining the correct deadlift position, perform a row by pulling the weights back towards the mid-belly just above the navel. Keep the elbows/arms tight to the body during the pulling motion. Think of this pull as similar to the

W exercise, and imagine trying to tap the elbows back behind the body.

- Repeat 10 reps.

Key Notes/Common Faults:

- Pain/discomfort/straining of any kind.
- Faulty breathing pattern.
- Loss of Full Spinal Control.
- Loss of the correct deadlift position. Please review deadlifts.
- Ensure the scapulae (shoulder blades) remain in their set scapular position. The set scapular position must be maintained throughout all pulling motions.
- Overexertion or straining of any kind.

It is important to mention that once a full pulling motion begins, the set scapular position should remain set. In the first exercise of this series, the set scapular pull exercise, as with all scapular positioning exercises learned thus far, we continued moving the scapula in and out of the set scapular position. All this movement of the scapula in and out of position was simply to provide awareness of this motion so you can recognize when you are in and out of the set scapular position. Most people do not even realize they have a scapula, let alone understand how it moves.

Now that we are actually ready to create the functional movement of a full pulling motion, the scapula should no longer move in and out of the set position. The scapula should remain locked in its set position as the pulls take place, thereby providing a stable base for the large prime moving pulling muscles, such as the lats and the posterior deltoid, to pull from. One of the main reasons we see so many shoulder problems like rotator cuff issues, labral issues, impingement, tendinitis, bursitis, and degenerative joint disease in the shoulder is that most people have no awareness of scapular control.

This series progresses further to multiple variations of the pulling mechanism and various pulling exercises, including low rows, high rows, lat pulls, pull-ups, and various unilateral versions of the same. Grip and hand positions can also be varied to give the pull series a more well-rounded training experience in Level III and the exercise conditioning part of the program.

As with all exercises and movements learned, ideally, no pain should be experienced. All the same pathologies and pain generators explained throughout are possible here. Since the shoulder joint advances in movement and control difficulty throughout this series, common pathologies that may cause pain specific to the shoulder joint are degenerative joint disease, arthritis, labral tears, tendinitis, or other joint lesions. If these are present and the exercise is causing pain, first attempt to change the pelvic position, set scapular position, and/or DNF neck position, as it may not be in the correct neutral position.

If this does not work, attempt to change the angle of motion at the shoulder joint to allow for greater or lesser flexion, extension, abduction, adduction, or rotation at the GHJ. This usually can be done easily by changing elbow width during the pull motion. A smaller range of motion at the GHJ can also be used to stay within pain tolerance. Always stay within a pain-free range.

If the pain is not originating from the shoulder joint, it may be coming from the neck. Remember that many of the shoulder's muscles are anchored to the neck, as discussed above. A faulty position of the cervical spine may lead to faulty mechanics of the shoulder and thus create pain. Also, keep in mind that the neurology controlling all the muscles of the shoulder originates in the cervical spine. A faulty position of the neck may be causing complications leading to various pathologies such as facet pain, mechanical stenosis to the IVF space(s) or the central canal causing radicular or myelopathic complications, and/or increased pressure on the discs of the spine.

Even the Thoracic spine, Lumbar spine, and Sacroiliac joints may be aggravated if position and mechanics are incorrect and pathology is present. The rest of the upper extremity is now involved as well. Aggravation is common with the elbow, with injuries such as lateral epicondylitis (tennis elbow) or medial epicondylitis (golfer's elbow). If this is the case, focus on maintaining a neutral wrist position. The wrist and hand can also cause pain if certain conditions exist.

Remember that the Cervical spine can also cause referral pain anywhere in the upper extremity, so the pain felt in the arm may have nothing to do with the arm itself. If this is the case, more attention must be given to the DNF position. Also, remember that increasing the difficulty of exercise movement may cause strain, tension, and overactivation, which may increase pressure (Valsalva) and cause increased symptoms.

Any of these scenarios may cause pain. If pain is present and no attempts are successful at eliminating the pain, the exercise is beyond the current limit capacity and thus should not be done. [932, 940, 941, 942, 943, 944, 945, 946, 947]

PRESS SERIES

The Press Series is designed to continue all the shoulder girdle mechanics learned so far and apply them to a pressing motion. Pressing is one of the three fundamental movements of the human body. Just as the Hip Hinge and pull mechanics are vital for countless functional, exercise, and higher-level athletic movements, pressing mechanics are essential for a wide variety of normal daily activities and higher-level sports performance. Every time you reach over your head, push a shopping cart, or wash a dish, you use pressing mechanics. Countless exercises and sports training movements involve pressing mechanics, such as push-ups, bench presses, overhead presses, dips, running, sprinting, jumping, and punching.

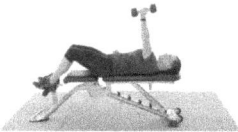

The Press Series begins with the serratus push. This picks up where the advanced scapular control series left off. Continuing to work with scapular control, this movement is designed to improve the strength of the scapular control muscles, particularly the serratus anterior. This exercise movement is very similar to the set scapular pull exercise that begins the pull series, but in this serratus push exercise, the resistance is reversed. The trainee is in the supine starting position, holding a weight in hand to create resistance towards the body as the scapula is moved in and out of the set position.

The series progresses this movement next to a more functional loaded
position with the push-up plus exercise and then to a full press movement
pattern with the push-up exercise.
The push-up starts from an angulated

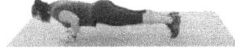

position so the trainee can learn and practice the correct movement pattern before progressing the angle closer to parallel with the ground as strength of control is gained. Keep in mind that we are still building movement. All of the foundational mechanics learned thus far still apply here. Full Spinal Control is a must. The fundamental pieces added together here come from the Advanced Spinal Core Control Series; if you cannot perform a plank, you cannot perform a push-up. We are also employing all of the Full Spinal Control pieces; if you cannot achieve pelvic control, set scapular position, and DNF neutral, you cannot perform a plank.

The Advanced Scapular Control Series is also in effect. If the scapular control cannot be maintained, the powerful muscles creating the press motion will not have the solid foundation they need to perform correct pressing mechanics. The GHJ and shoulder are defi-nitely working hard during a pressing motion so the Rotator Cuff Series had better be working as well. All of these pieces are necessary to create a biomechanically correct press movement pattern. Keep reviewing that checklist every time!

Similar to pulling motions, keeping the elbows and arms close to the body with pressing motions is important. Many people allow the arms to float too far away from the body during pressing motions. High school and college football players are the worst! I know because I used to be one of them. They are all in the weight room doing heavy, wide-grip bench presses, but they don't get much out of it. That's because football players do not hit with really wide arms. If you are going to hit someone, you keep your arms and hand in tight so you can punch straight through your opponent! If these football players are lifting weights because they want to become better football players, they should lay off the wide-grip bench and start doing close-grip pressing exercises with the arms and elbows held tight to the body. This is how you will get the functional strength you need for your sport. Wide-grip bench pressing can put more stress on the shoulder joint, which can cause increased wear and tear and possibly lead to injury or predisposition to injury. Train smarter, not harder!

Once the basic press movement pattern is learned, it opens the door to a wide variety of movements and exercises that will continue progressing in Level III of the program. These include the bench press, incline press, decline press, overhead press, dips, cable presses, other push-up variations, and many more!

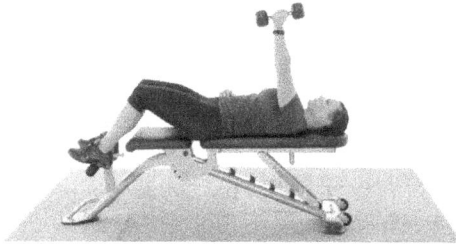

Serratus Push Beginning Position

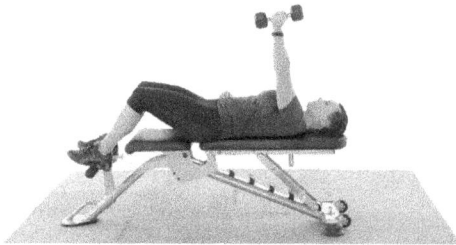

Serratus Push Movement Position

Serratus Push
Goal/Purpose:

- Progression and preparation of the shoulder girdle for Pressing motions, the third major category of movement.

Beginning Position:

- Supine (face up).
- Achieve Full Spinal Control with Pelvic, Scapular, and C/S neutral with hips and knees flexed to 90 degrees.
- One shoulder at 90 degrees of flexion up in the air holding a light dumbbell weight.

Movement/Action:

- While maintaining Full Spinal Control, perform a serratus push motion by moving only the shoulder blade out of the set scapular (set scap) position and pressing the weight up toward the ceiling. Then, pull the shoulder blade back into position by setting the shoulder back and down, as discussed in the Scapular Setting Series.
- Repeat 10 reps, and then switch to the opposite side.

Key Notes/Common Faults:

- Pain/discomfort/straining of any kind.
- Faulty breathing pattern.
- Loss of Full Spinal Control.
- Be sure to keep the arm straight. Do not bend at the elbow to perform the motion. Only the scapula (shoulder blade) should provide the motion.

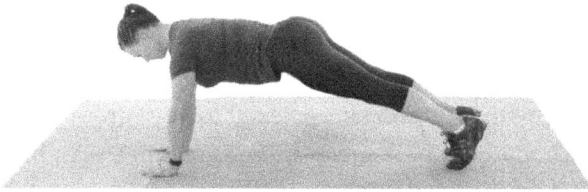

Push-up Plus Beginning Position

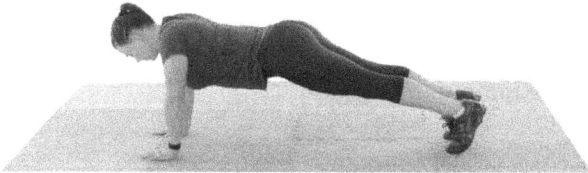

Push-up Plus Movement Position

Push-up Plus
Goal/Purpose:

- Further functional progression and preparation of the shoulder girdle for Pressing motions, the third major category of movement.

Beginning Position:

- Quadruped position supporting the body's weight equally on the hands and feet with arms/elbows straight (push-up position). Full Spinal Control, especially pelvic neutrality, must be achieved and maintained. This is a plank position from the hands.

Movement/Action:

- While maintaining the correct starting position, perform a push-up plus motion by pressing with the shoulder blades only, not the elbows, up out of the set scapular position, then return to the set scapular position. It is the same motion as in the serratus push, set scap pull, and scapular setting exercises, just now applied in a push-up/plank from hands position, using the hands rather than the forearms (not a plank position).

Key Notes/Common Faults:

- Pain/discomfort/straining of any kind.
- Faulty breathing pattern.
- Loss of Full Spinal Control.
- Do not allow the lower back to extend.
- Faulty scapular motion. The elbows should not bend. It is not a full push-up! Keep the arms straight and move the shoulder blades back and forth only.

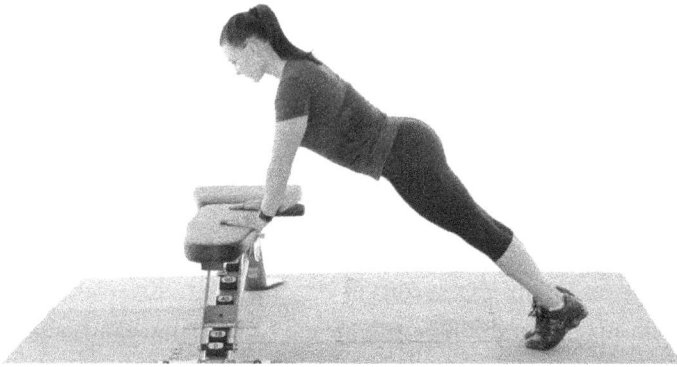

Push-ups (Angle) Beginning Position

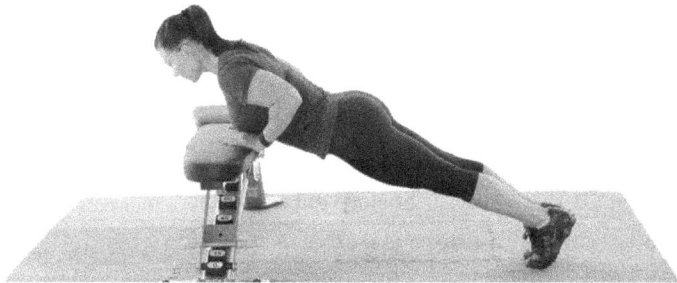

Push-ups (Angle) Movement Position

Push-ups (Angle)
Goal/Purpose:

- Progression of the shoulder girdle to full pressing motions. This is the first progression for a complete press. Pressing motions are one of the three major types of motion of the human body.

Beginning Position:

- Quadruped position supporting the body's weight equally on the hands and feet with arms/elbows straight (push-up position). Full Spinal Control, especially pelvic neutral, must be achieved and maintained. Keep in mind this is a plank position from the hands (not the forearms). This exercise should begin by pushing from a counter or bench before progressing to a floor position.

Movement/Action:

- While maintaining the correct starting position, perform a push-up motion by slowly lowering the torso/body down towards the ground/counter by way of shoulder extension and elbow flexion. Then press the torso/body back away from the ground/counter, returning to the starting position. The arms/elbows should remain tight/close to the body during the push-up motion. Do not allow the elbows to flair out away from the body.

Key Notes/Common Faults:

- Pain/discomfort/straining of any kind.
- Faulty breathing pattern.
- Loss of Full Spinal Control.
- Do not allow the lower back to extend.
- Now, when performing the full press, maintain the set scap position.

As with all exercises and movements learned, ideally, no pain should be experienced. All the same pathologies and pain generators explained throughout can be possible here. The shoulder joint will be advancing in movement and difficulty of control throughout this series. Common pathologies that may cause pain specific to the shoulder joint are degenerative joint disease, arthritis, labral tears, tendinitis, and other joint lesions. If these are present and the exercise is causing pain, first attempt to change the pelvic position, set scapular position, and/or DNF neck position, as it may not be in the correct neutral position.

If this does not work, attempt to change the angle of motion at the shoulder joint to allow for greater or lesser flexion, extension, abduction, adduction, or rotation at the GH joint. This can usually be done easily by changing elbow width during the press motion. Maintaining a narrow elbow/arm width is usually preferable to keep excessive loading stress off the GH joint. However, this may depend on one's individual anatomy. Thus changing the hand and elbow width may benefit certain individuals. A wider elbow/arm width can put the GH joint in a provocative position, such as an anterior apprehension position. A smaller range of motion at the GHJ can also be used to stay within pain tolerance. Always stay within a pain-free range.

If the pain is not originating from the shoulder joint, it may be coming from the neck. Remember that many of the shoulder's muscles are anchored to the neck. A faulty position of the cervical spine may lead to faulty mechanics of the shoulder and thus create pain. Also, keep in mind that the neurology controlling all the muscles of the shoulder originates in the cervical spine. Faulty position of the neck may be causing complications leading to various pathologies such as Facet pain, mechanical stenosis to the IVF space(s) or the central canal causing radicular or myelopathic complications, and/or increased pressure on the discs of the spine. Decreases in neurological function can lead to decreased force output by the muscles affected and, thus, mechanical changes.

The Thoracic spine, Lumbar spine, or Sacroiliac joints may be aggravated if attention to position and mechanics is inadequate and pathology is present. This may be more or less pertinent, depending on the exercise. For example, during the push-up exercise, the correct plank position must be maintained with Full Spinal Control as described in the Advanced Spinal Core Control Series. If the trainee cannot perform this spinal control correctly, he or she will be better off (safer) performing a bench press exercise with greater spinal support.

Full Spinal Control must still be maintained either way, but this is much easier during the bench press than during the push-up.

The rest of the upper extremity is now involved as well. The elbow is a common place for aggravation, as explained in the Pull Series section. Be mindful of a neutral wrist position. Using dumbbells or various handgrips to help maintain a neutral wrist/hand position may be beneficial.

Remember that the Cervical spine can also cause referral pain anywhere in the upper extremity, so pain felt in the arm may have nothing to do with the arm itself. If this is the case, more attention must be given to the DNF position. Also, remember that increasing the difficulty of exercise movement may cause strain, tension, and overactivation, which may increase pressure (Valsalva) and cause increased symptoms.

Any of these scenarios may cause pain. If pain is present and no attempts are successful at eliminating the pain, the exercise is beyond the current limit capacity and thus should not be done. [932, 940, 941, 942, 943, 944, 945, 946, 947]

LEVEL III: ADVANCED EXERCISES

In Level I of The PREMIER Body Method's Human Movement Education course, we learned the key fundamental pieces of biomechanics. In Level II, we learned how to add the pieces together to create a large fundamental human movement. Now, in Level III, we will apply strength and endurance to these mechanics. By adding strength and endurance, we will be able to perform our new mechanics consistently throughout the day and during each of our activities and sports. We will not only have the control we need but also the strength and endurance to maintain that control. This is a critical step because it is not enough just to know how to move correctly; you also must be able to physically move that way in the real world. This requires a certain amount of physical ability, strength, and endurance.

Level III applies everything you learned in Levels I and II to an exercise training program. Whether you are a high-level competitive athlete looking to improve overall performance or the average person recovering from an injury and wanting to get back in shape, Level III of Human Movement Education will give you the basic strength and conditioning foundation you need to succeed. You will be ready to make a smooth transition back to higher-level sports training or simply to continue training for the sport of life. Being happy, healthy, and fit is what it is all about.

ADVANCED HIP HINGE SERIES (A CONTINUATION OF THE HIP HINGE SERIES FROM LEVEL II)

Several of the basic series progressions that began in Level II continue in Level III with more advanced movements and exercises. In the Hip Hinge Series, squat and deadlift patterns continue to advance with progression to weighted versions and greater variety, such as front squats, overhead squats, power deadlifts, and so on. Level III also adds a wide variety of unilateral squat patterns, such as split squats, lateral squats, multidirectional squats, step-ups, and single-leg squats. These progressions continue with more dynamic versions of the Hip Hinging pattern by adding various lunge exercises such as forward lunges, lateral lunges, and reverse lunges. The dead-lifting pattern also progresses with weighted and unilateral versions, such as the single-leg RDL.

The same basic Hip Hinging mechanics still apply all the way through to the highest progressions. Just as we learned the basic pieces of spinal control in Level I, then added those pieces together to create Full Spinal Control, and then learned to apply Full Spinal Control to larger-scale basic movements in Level II, now in Level III, we must apply all the basic body mechanics learned in Level II to more advanced movements.

For example, consider a split squat exercise. Once in the correct

split stance position (this will be
discussed in the individual exercise
progression sheets), all the basic
squatting mechanics are the same. The
fundamentals don't change. Achieve
and maintain Full Spinal Control,
drive the squatting leg heel (Navicu-
lar) through the floor, hinge the hip back and down utilizing mainly
the gluteal muscle group to do the work of creating the movement, do
not allow the leg/knee to cave inward, and so forth – just as you practiced before with a two-legged squat.

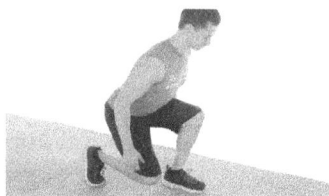

This is why I have been stressing the idea of focusing on the fundamentals throughout this program. If you understand the basic fundamentals, you have the knowledge to do any kind of movement you
want, whether in daily life or as part of a sport or fitness routine. The
only challenge is your ability to apply the fundamentals to whatever
you are doing. Take climbing a flight of stairs, for example. This is basically the step-up exercise. The basic mechanics are still the same.
Whether you are actually climbing a flight of stairs or doing this
motion as a step-up exercise, they are both hip-hinging / squatting
motions. All the basic Hip Hinge mechanics apply. Maintain Full
Spinal Control, drive your heel down through the step, make the hip
musculature do the work by hinging correctly, and don't let your leg
cave in. **Focus on and master the basic fundamentals, and apply them
to everything you do.**

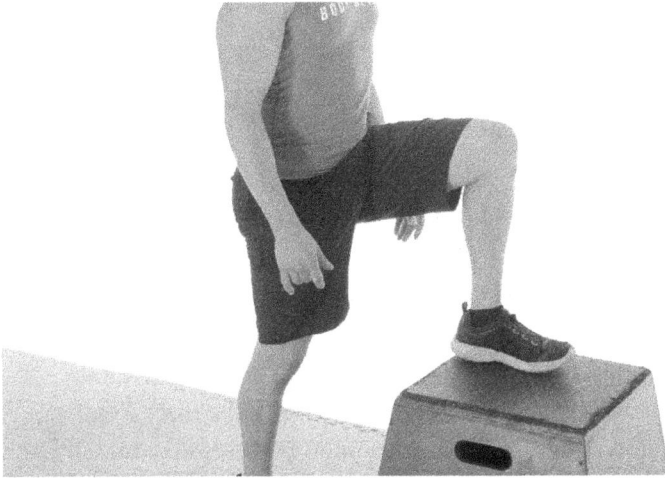

Step-ups Beginning Position

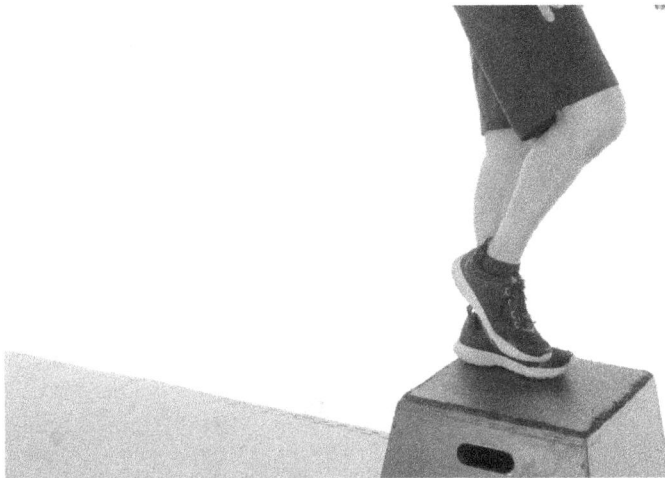

Step-ups Movement Position

Step-ups
Goal/Purpose:

- Progressing the Hip Hinging Squatting Movement pattern in a unilateral (single leg) fashion for the purpose of increasing hip stability and strength in all three planes of motion for stairs, climbing, etc.

Beginning Position:

- Standing with Full Spinal Control with one foot/leg secure up on at step. The step height should ideally be around the height of one's knee, but use a smaller step if necessary to maintain correct mechanics (Full Spinal Control).

Movement/Action:

- Ramp up core stability "on" by way of Core Bracing I, then initiate a unilateral Hip Hinge motion with the front step leg to drive the body up. The force should be driven through the heel (Navicular) of the stepping leg. Then complete the movement back to the starting position, then ramp down core stability.
- Repeat 10 reps. Then, switch to the other side.

Key Notes/Common Faults:

- Pain/discomfort/straining of any kind.
- Faulty breathing pattern.
- Faulty Hip Hinging Mechanics.
- Loss of Full Spinal Control.
- Now, in the single-leg position, all three planes of motion need to be accounted for. Make sure the body (pelvis) remains neutral.

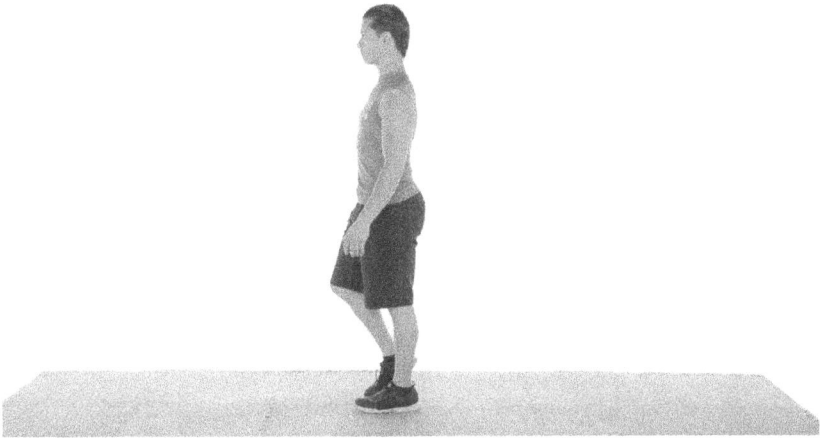

Single Leg RDL Beginning Position

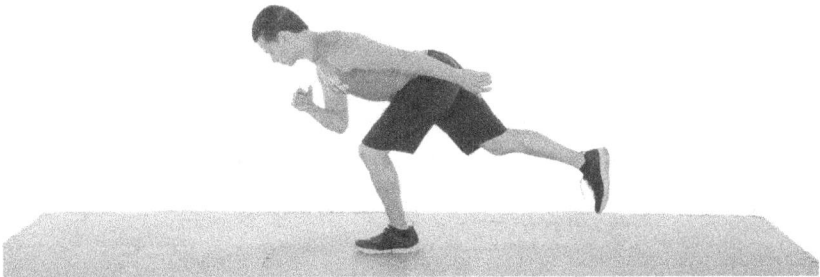

Single Leg RDL Movement Position

Single Leg RDL's
  Goal/Purpose:

- Progressing the Hip Hinging Romanian Deadlift (RDL) Movement pattern in a unilateral (single leg) fashion for the purpose of increasing hip stability and strength in all three planes of motion.

Beginning Position:

- Standing with Full Spinal Control in a single-leg stance.

Movement/Action:

- Ramp up core stability "on" by way of Core Bracing I, then using a unilateral Hip Hinge motion, continue to hinge the torso over into a single-leg deadlift by continuing to sit the stance hip back and down as the off leg reaches back long and straight. Then reverse the motion back to the single-leg stance starting position, then ramp down core stability "off."
- Repeat 10 reps. Then, switch to the other side.

Key Notes/Common Faults:

- Pain / discomfort / straining of any kind.
- Faulty breathing pattern.
- Faulty Hip Hinging Mechanics.
- Loss of Full Spinal Control.
- Now, in the single-leg position, all three planes of motion need to be accounted for. Ensure the body (pelvis) remains neutral, flat, and level during the motion.
- Make sure to sit the hip back; do not shoot the knee forward.
- Do not allow the knee to cave inward.

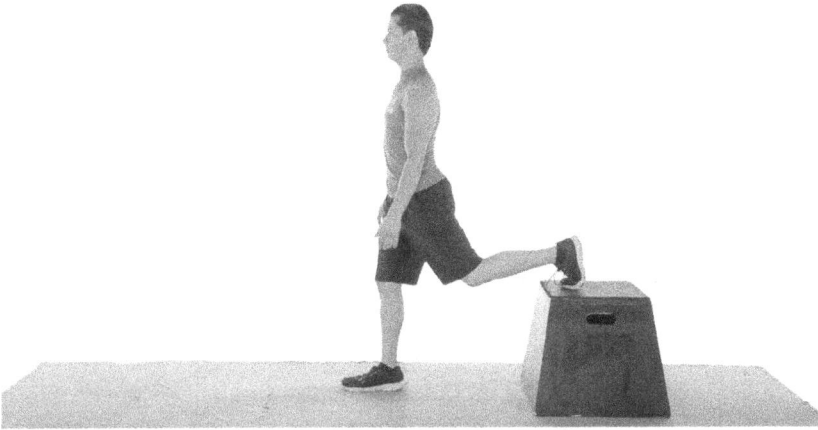

Single Leg (Bulgarian) Squat Beginning Position

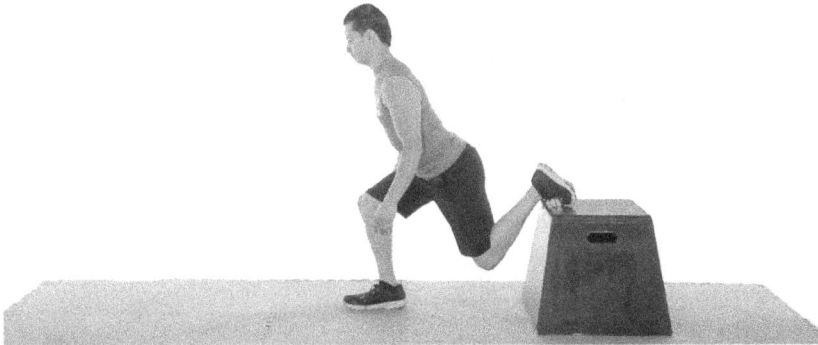

Single Leg (Bulgarian) Squat Movement Position

Single Leg (Bulgarian) Squats
Goal/Purpose:

- Progressing the Hip Hinging Squat Movement pattern in a unilateral (single leg) fashion for the purpose of increasing hip stability and strength in all three planes of motion.

Beginning Position:

- Standing with Full Spinal Control in a single-leg stance with the off leg extended back with the foot on a step (ideally knee height for the step).

Movement/Action:

- Ramp up core stability "on" by way of Core Bracing I, then using a unilateral Hip Hinge motion, continue to squat by sitting hip back and down, just as a full squat only on one leg. Then reverse the motion back to the single-leg stance starting position, then ramp down core stability.
- Repeat 10 reps. Then, switch to the other side.

Key Notes/Common Faults:

- Pain / discomfort / straining of any kind.
- Faulty breathing pattern.
- Faulty Hip Hinging Mechanics.
- Loss of Full Spinal Control.
- Now, in the single-leg position, all three planes of motion need to be accounted for. Ensure the body (pelvis) remains neutral, flat, and level during the motion.
- Make sure to sit the hip back; do not shoot the knee forward.
- Do not allow the knee to cave inward.

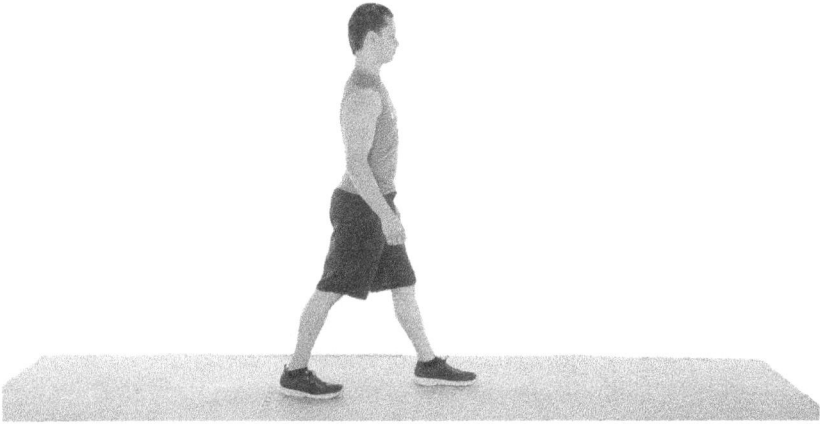

Split Squat Beginning Position

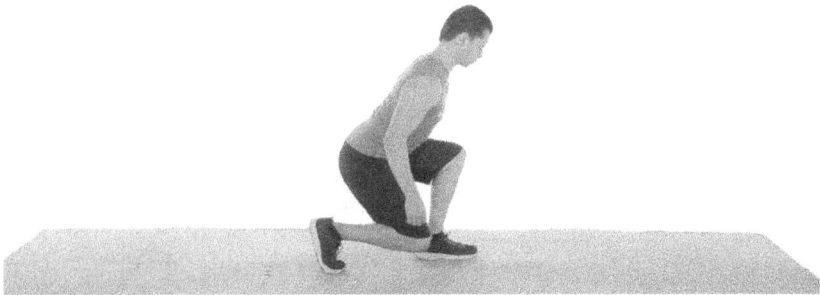

Split Squat Movement Position

Split Squats
  Goal/Purpose:

- Progressing the Hip Hinging Squat Movement pattern in a unilateral (single leg) fashion for the purpose of increasing hip stability and strength in all three planes of motion.

Beginning Position:

- Standing with Full Spinal Control in a split stance.

Movement/Action:

- Ramp up core stability "on" by way of Core Bracing I, then using a unilateral Hip Hinge motion, continue to squat by sitting hip back and down, just as a full squat only on one leg. Then reverse the motion back to the single-leg stance starting position then ramp down core stability.
- Repeat 10 reps. Then, switch to the other side.

Key Notes/Common Faults:

- Pain/discomfort/straining of any kind.
- Faulty breathing pattern.
- Faulty Hip Hinging Mechanics.
- Loss of Full Spinal Control.
- Now, in the single-leg position, all three planes of motion need to be accounted for. Ensure the body (pelvis) remains neutral, flat, and level during the motion.
- Make sure to sit the hip back; do not shoot the knee forward.
- Do not allow the knee to cave inward.
- Make sure to sit the front hip back (Hip Hinge); do not shoot the knee forward. The body movement should translate up and down, not back and forth.
- Do not allow the knee to cave inward.

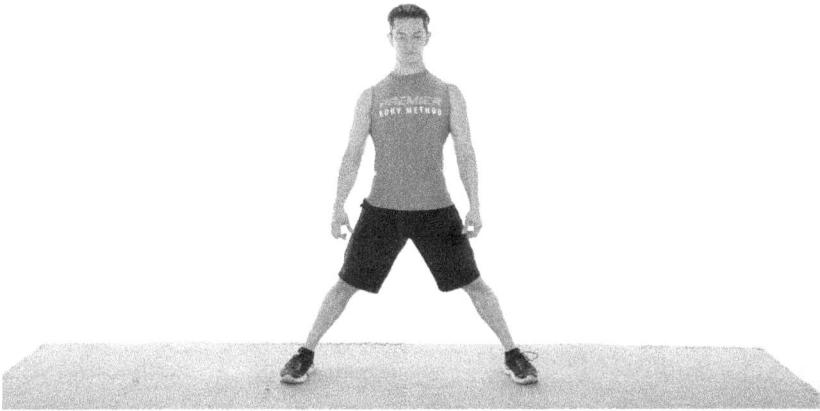

Lateral Squat Beginning Position

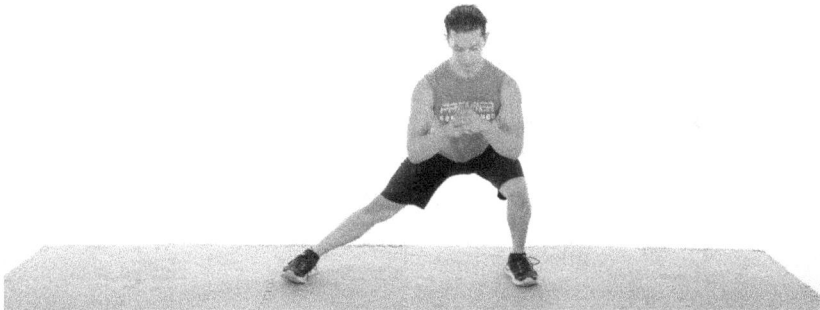

Lateral Squat Movement Position

Lateral Squats
  Goal/Purpose:

- Progressing the Hip Hinging Squatting Movement pattern in a unilateral (single leg) fashion for the purpose of increasing specifically lateral (side to side) hip stability and strength in all three planes of motion.

Beginning Position:

- Standing with Full Spinal Control in a wide squat stance with feet well beyond hip-width apart.

Movement/Action:

- Ramp up core stability "on" by way of Core Bracing I, then initiate a Hip Hinge movement with one leg (involved side) and continue into a squatting pattern through continued hip and knee flexion and ankle dorsiflexion as deep as proper form allows (maintain Full Spinal Control), then complete the movement back to the starting position, then ramp down core stability.
- The uninvolved leg should remain straight during the movement of the involved leg.
- Repeat 10 reps. Then, switch to the other side.

Key Notes/Common Faults:

- Pain/discomfort/straining of any kind.
- Faulty breathing pattern.
- Faulty Hip Hinging Mechanics.
- Loss of Full Spinal Control.
- Now, when moving with a single leg, all three planes of motion need to be accounted for. Make sure the body (pelvis) remains neutral.

As mentioned above, in addition to squats, there are three basic lunge patterns that can be used to vary the hip hinge movement., Forward Lunges, Lateral Lunges, and Reverse Lunges. The mechanics of these lunge patterns/exercises hold try to Hip Hinging mechanics just as all the rest of the hinging movement patterns and exercises and correspond to their stationary base mechanic. For example, a forward or backward lunge is basically the same as a split squat mechanic, but if you are lunging, that means you are ambulating (moving across the ground). A lateral lunge is essentially the same as a lateral squat but with ambulation. This takes these basic stationary movements and adds a more dynamic element to them to increase the challenge and create more variety for a better, more well-rounded physical outcome.

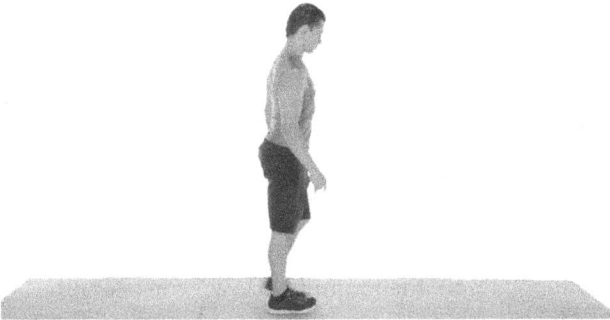

Forward Lunge Beginning Position

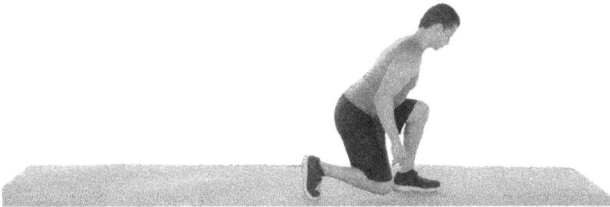

Forward Lunge Movement Position

Forward Lunges
   Goal/Purpose:

- Progressing the Hip Hinging Squatting Movement pattern in a unilateral (single leg) fashion with ambulation for the purpose of increasing hip stability, strength, and dynamic body control.

Beginning Position:

- Standing with Full Spinal Control.

Movement/Action:

- Ramp up core stability "on" by way of Core Bracing I, then step out to the front in a split squat position and initiate a Hip Hinge movement with the front leg and continue into a split squat movement pattern as deep as proper form will allow (maintain Full Spinal Control), then complete the movement by stepping forward with the back leg up to a standing position, then ramping down core stability.
- Then continue to step out and forward alternating legs each step.
- Repeat 10 steps/reps.

Key Notes/Common Faults:

- Pain/discomfort/straining of any kind.
- Faulty breathing pattern.
- Faulty Hip Hinging Mechanics.
- Loss of Full Spinal Control.
- Now, with dynamic movement, all three planes of motion need to be accounted for. Make sure the body (pelvis) remains neutral. Do not allow the body/torso to waver or wobble during the motion steps. Do not allow the knees to scissor or cave inward.
- This exercise should have the same basic mechanics as split squats, only with the added ambulation. Please review all the details involved with this movement pattern.

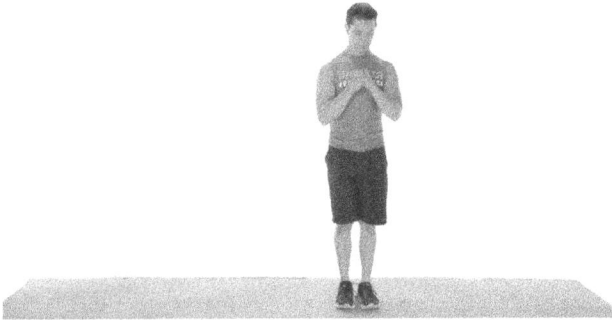

Lateral Lunge Beginning Position

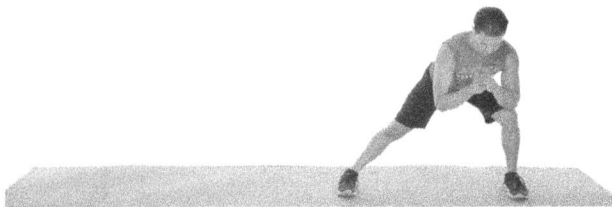

Lateral Lunge Movement Position

Lateral Lunges
Goal/Purpose:

- Progressing the Hip Hinging Squatting Movement pattern in a unilateral (single leg) fashion with ambulation laterally for the purpose of increasing hip stability, strength, and dynamic body control.

Beginning Position:

- Standing with Full Spinal Control.

Movement/Action:

- Ramp up core stability "on" by way of Core Bracing I, then step out to the side in a lateral squat position and initiate a Hip Hinge lateral squat movement with the involved leg as deep as the proper form will allow (maintain Full Spinal Control), then complete the movement by stepping medial with the uninvolved leg up to a standing position, then ramp down core stability.
- Continue to step lateral to lunge and medial to stand.
- Repeat 10 steps/reps in one direction, then 10 steps/reps back in the opposite direction.

Key Notes/Common Faults:

- Pain/discomfort/straining of any kind.
- Faulty breathing pattern.
- Faulty Hip Hinging Mechanics.
- Loss of Full Spinal Control.
- Now, with dynamic movement, all three planes of motion need to be accounted for. Make sure the body (pelvis) remains neutral. Do not allow the body/torso to waver or wobble during the motion steps.

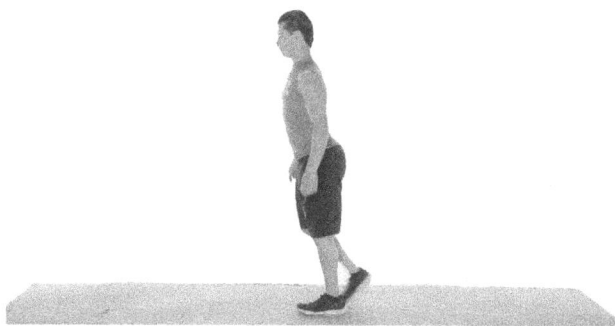

Reverse Lunge Beginning Position

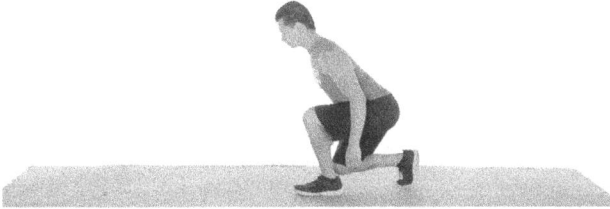

Reverse Lunge Movement Position

Reverse Lunges
Goal/Purpose:

- Progressing the Hip Hinging Squatting Movement pattern in a unilateral (single leg) fashion with ambulation for the purpose of increasing hip stability, strength, and dynamic body control.

Beginning Position:

- Standing with Full Spinal Control.

Movement/Action:

- Ramp up core stability "on" by way of Core Bracing I, then step backward in a split squat position and initiate a Hip Hinge movement with the front leg, and continue into a split squat movement pattern as deep as proper form will allow (maintain Full spinal Control), then complete the movement by stepping backward with the front leg up to a standing position, then ramping down core stability.
- Then, continue to step backward, alternating legs with each step.
- Repeat 10 steps/reps.

Key Notes/Common Faults:

- Pain/discomfort/straining of any kind.
- Faulty breathing pattern.
- Faulty Hip Hinging Mechanics.
- Loss of Full Spinal Control.
- Now, with dynamic movement, all three planes of motion need to be accounted for. Make sure the body (pelvis) remains neutral. Do not allow the body/torso to waver or wobble during the motion steps.
- Do not allow the knees to scissor or cave inward.

Remember, just as with all exercises and movements learned, no pain should be experienced. All the same pathologies and pain generators explained throughout the Hip Hinge Series in Level II may be accentuated here and must be kept in mind. It should also be noted that performing any of the unilateral, single-leg, lateral, split, or multidirectional movement pattern progressions increases the difficulty of maintaining correct Full Spinal Control due to the greater involvement of all three planes of motion. This also increases the difficulty of control for Hip Hinge mechanics, which increases the chance of loading stress in multiple planes of motion and thus may increase the chance of aggravating certain pathologies.

Also, remember that increases in the difficulty of exercise movement may cause strain, tension, and over-activation, which may increase pressure (Valsalva) and, therefore, symptoms. All of these scenarios may cause pain. If pain is present, attempts should be made to correct and adjust all the mechanics involved, as discussed before in the previous sections. If pain continues and no attempts are successful at eliminating the pain, the particular exercise being performed is beyond the limit capacity at this point in time and thus should not be done. [932, 940, 941, 942, 943, 944, 945, 946, 947]

ADVANCED PELVIC CORE CONTROL SERIES (A CONTINUATION OF THE ADVANCED PELVIC CORE CONTROL SERIES FROM LEVEL II)

T he Advanced Pelvic Core Control Series continues to progress in Level III in the same manner, adding a variety of new exercises and movements. As noted before, many higher levels of training and sport demand an increased ability to maintain core and spinal control. These increased demands justify the need for increased levels of training for the core.

This series continues to progress where the Level II core progressions left off. It continues to build on planking exercises with increasingly more challenging movements, and it introduces rotational components for the first time. Being able to control the core and the spine during rotational movements can be one of the most difficult tasks for the core, but rotational stability is one of the single most important factors in many high-level explosive power athletic movements. It is a key in effectively transferring power generated by the lower extremity to the upper extremity. This is pivotal for any sport involving throwing, hitting, cutting, and punching. Such as baseball, football, basketball, tennis, the shot put and javelin in track and field, golf, boxing, and/or mixed martial arts. Conversely, any sport in which power needs to be transferred from the upper extremity to the lower extremity must also have rotational stability; examples include gymnastics, dance, rock climbing, swimming, diving, and parkour. [(950)]

Remember, the core's job is to prevent motion. This is true for all planes of motion, especially the horizontal rotational plane, when discussing energy transfer between the arms and legs. This series introduces exercises such as the plank roll, the push-pull, and the chop exercises, which are designed specifically to address the rotational component of core stability. These are anti-rotation exercises since the core's job in the transverse plane is to prevent rotation, therefore providing a solid base for the transfer of energy/power/force between the upper and lower body.

Imagine a baseball player swinging a bat. The power to hit the ball is first generated in the legs. This power is transferred through the body, out to the arms, and then to the bat as the ball is struck. Suppose this player lacks rotational stability, and the core allows for excessive rotation to occur during the swing. In that case, much of the power generated by this player's legs will be dissipated and lost by the time it gets to the arms. The player will not be able to hit the ball as hard, and performance suffers.

Another problem also occurs. To make up for the loss in energy due to the insufficient core transfer, the back and upper extremities will compensate by working harder to pick up the slack. As you might guess, this forces the back and/or upper extremity to do more work than it should, increasing stress, wear and tear, and creating a predisposition to injury. Back, neck, shoulder, rotator cuff, and elbow problems are likely. These injuries aren't rare; we even call them by the name of the sports for which they are common: tennis elbow, golfer's elbow, and Little League shoulder. Unbelievable!

Even though these injuries are common, their causes are not hard to understand. Any hole in the system decreases performance ability and leaves the door open for injury to occur due to the compensation for that hole. What I suggest is that instead of waiting for the problem to occur and then trying to diagnose and correct it, we simply train the whole thing correctly from the beginning and lower the risk of developing problems in the first place. Even if a problem does occur, it will not be nearly as big of a deal because you will

already know what you are doing. **You will be able to recognize it light-years sooner and be able to correct it that much easier and faster.**

Rotational Core Control is not only important for athletes. Excessive rotational force is one of the top causes of damage to the vertebral discs in the spine. This can happen in everyday movements, even with something as simple as twisting your back as you reach to grab a glass of water off your nightstand. How many people on this planet suffer from disc-related injuries and pain? Way more than there should be! If we all understood that the job of the core is to prevent rotation, and we all trained our bodies to do so, I believe we would see a huge decrease in disc problems.

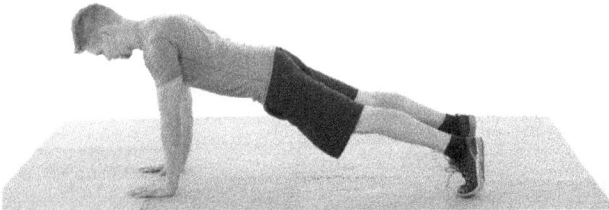

Plank Roll Beginning Position

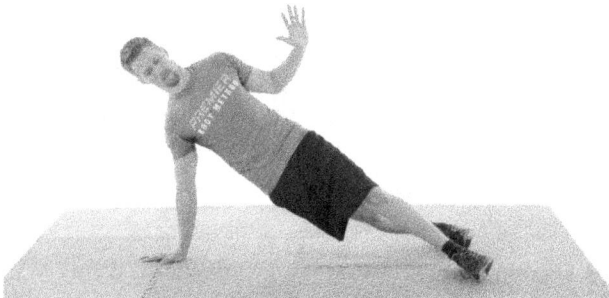

Plank Roll Movement Position

Plank Roll
Goal/Purpose:

- Further progression of pelvic control (as well as Full Spinal Control) and core stability with movement, mainly for athletes or persons who need to achieve above-minimal average core strength.

Beginning Position:

- Quadruped position supporting the weight of the body equally on the elbows and feet (Plank Position). Full Spinal Control, especially pelvic neutral, must be achieved and maintained.

Movement/Action:

- While maintaining Full Spinal Control, begin rolling the body to achieve a side plank position. Hold the side plank position for just a second and then roll back to the starting front plank position. Then, roll to the opposite side plank position.
- Repeat rolling 10 times / reps, alternating sides each time.

Key Notes/Common Faults:

- Pain / discomfort / straining of any kind.
- Faulty breathing pattern.
- Loss of Full Spinal Control, especially the neutral pelvic position, as seen by anterior pelvic tilt and low back extension.
- Do not allow the lower back to extend.
- The pelvis and torso (shoulders) should roll / rotate as one unit. No rotational disconnect should occur.

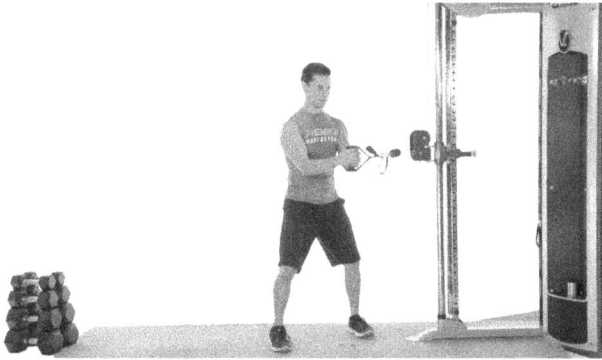

Chops (Neutral) Beginning Position

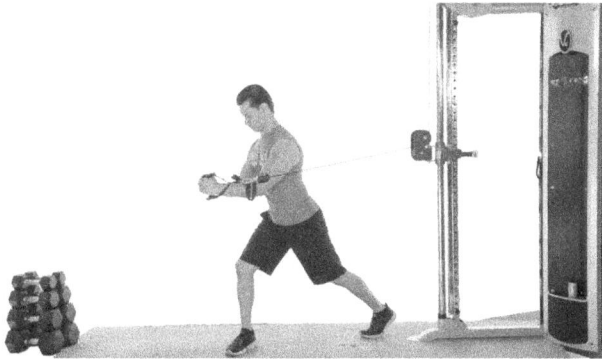

Chops (Neutral) Movement Position

Chops (Neutral) Goal/Purpose:

- Further progression of pelvic control (as well as Full Spina Control) and core stability with movement, and increased functional ability in a rotational manor. Many daily tasks require rotation of the body through space with resistance.

Beginning Position:

- Standing in a slight Hip Hinge position.
- Arms flexed to 75 degrees at the shoulder in front of the torso while grasping cable or Theraband with both hands.
- The cable/Theraband should be at mid-torso height.

Movement/Action:

- Ramp up core stability "on," then initiate the rotational movement by pivoting with the hips and legs while maintaining Full Spinal Control (shoulders should remain in line with the pelvis throughout the rotation), then rotate back to the starting position, then ramp down core stability.
- Repeat 10 reps, then switch to the opposite side.

Key Notes/Common Faults:

- Pain/discomfort/straining of any kind.
- Faulty breathing pattern.
- Loss of Full Spinal Control: The pelvis and torso (shoulders) should roll/rotate as one unit, and no rotational disconnect should occur.

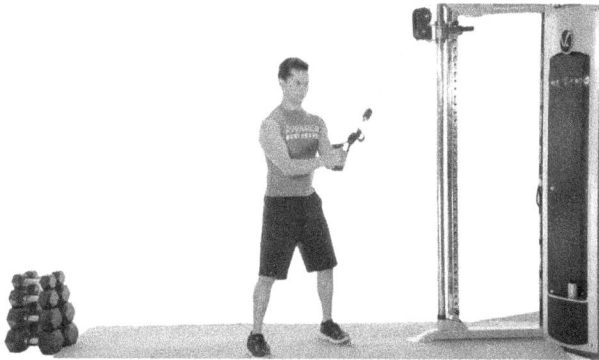

Chops (Down) Beginning Position

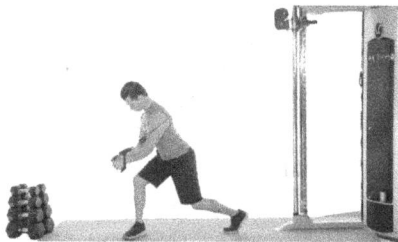

Chops (Down) Movement Position

Chops (Down)
Goal/Purpose:

- Further progression of pelvic control (as well as Full Spinal Control) and core stability with movement, and increased functional ability in a rotational manor. Many daily tasks require rotation of the body through space with resistance.

Beginning Position:

- Standing in a slight Hip Hinge position.
- Arms flexed to 75 degrees at the shoulder in front of the torso while grasping cable or Theraband with both hands.
- The cable/Theraband should be at a height above the head.

Movement/Action:

- Ramp up core stability "on," then initiate rotational movement in a slightly downward direction by pivoting with the hips and legs while maintaining Full Spinal Control (shoulders should remain in line with the pelvis throughout the rotation), then rotate back to the starting position, then ramp down core stability.
- Repeat 10 reps, then switch to the opposite side.

Key Notes/Common Faults:

- Pain/discomfort/straining of any kind.
- Faulty breathing pattern.
- Loss of Full Spinal Control,
- The pelvis and torso (shoulders) should roll/rotate as one unit. No rotational disconnect should occur.

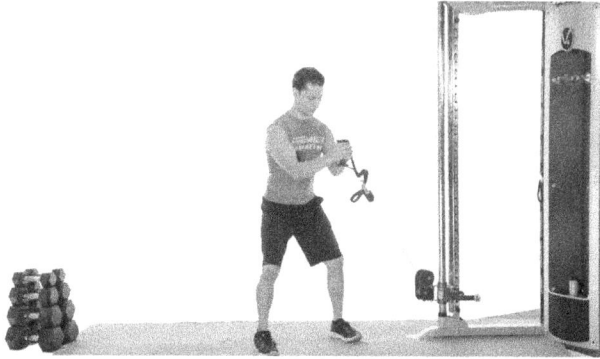

Chops (Up) Beginning Position

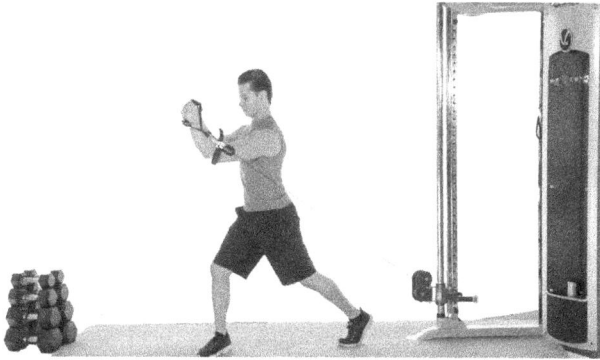

Chops (Up) Movement Position

Chops (Up)
Goal/Purpose:

- Further progression of pelvic control (as well as Full Spinal Control) and core stability with movement, and increased functional ability in a rotational manor. Many daily tasks require rotation of the body through space with resistance.

Beginning Position:

- Standing in a slight Hip Hinge position.
- Arms flexed to 75 degrees at the shoulder in front of the torso while grasping cable or Theraband with both hands.

- The cable/Theraband should be at a height below the hips.

Movement/Action:

- Ramp up core stability "on," then initiate rotational movement in a slightly upward direction by pivoting with the hips and legs while maintaining Full Spinal Control (shoulders should remain in line with the pelvis throughout the rotation), then rotate back to the starting position, then ramp down core stability.
- Repeat 10 reps, then switch to the opposite side.

Key Notes/Common Faults:

- Pain/discomfort/straining of any kind.
- Faulty breathing pattern.
- Loss of Full Spinal Control,
- The pelvis and torso (shoulders) should roll/rotate as one unit. No rotational disconnect should occur.
- Make sure the hips do the work to create the movement. This is an anti-rotational core exercise.
- Any stressing or straining of any kind, especially in the face and neck, should not be allowed.

Remember, just as with all exercises and movements learned, no pain should be experienced. All the same pathologies and pain generators explained throughout the Advanced Pelvic Core Control Series may be accentuated here and must be kept in mind. The difficulty of movement and control advances throughout this series, leading to an increased probability for pathology to be aggravated. Please refer back to the Advanced Pelvic Core Control Series section for any issues here. With the addition of rotational motion, the spine may be at increased risk for pathology aggravation, especially if excessive rotation is allowed. **Some of these exercises are what we would classify as** borderline exercises for some. **If these exercises are done correctly with proper control and biomechanics, they can be great exercises to help the situation. If, however, too many mistakes occur in the control of mechanics, the exercises may be detrimental and have the opposite effect.** This is a prime example of a borderline exercise, but you could argue that all exercises are borderline since their results depend on the correctness of their execution. Faulty execution can always cause injury.

If pain persists and no attempts are able to eliminate the pain, the particular exercise being performed should be considered beyond the limit capacity at this point in time and thus should not be done. [932, 940, 941, 942, 943, 944, 945, 946, 947]

ADVANCED BALANCE AND UNILATERAL STABILITY SERIES (A CONTINUATION OF THE BALANCE AND UNILATERAL STABILITY SERIES FROM LEVEL II)

The Advanced Balance and Unilateral Stability Series continues to progress in Level III by adding increased challenges with unstable surfaces such as airex pads and bosu balls, as well as training the ability to remain stable with the eyes closed.

Once the trainee has become stable in a single-leg position and can sufficiently balance on one leg on the flat earth during exercises like the Single Leg Balance and the Standing Hip Stability exercises, then he or she may be ready to try an unstable surface such as a Bosu ball, wobble board, or Airex pad. These unstable surfaces will provide an increased challenge to allow the trainee to improve balance and unilateral stability even more. That being said, you DO want to make sure you can proficiently balance on flat ground before moving on these unstable surfaces. If you can't balance on flat ground under your own power and control, then you simply have no business trying to do it on an unstable surface; sorry! Once you are ready, here are a few tips: Make sure always to have your

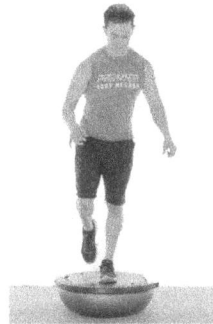

Bosu Ball

302 YOUR LIFE, PAIN-FREE

stance foot centered on the unstable surface you are using. Have a safety support by you to help you get on and off your unstable surface. When switching sides/feet, step off/down from your unstable surface first, then switch and reset on the other foot. Do not try to switch feet while staying up on the unstable surface. All of the progressions for the single-leg balance series in Level II, done on flat ground, can now be leveled up to an unstable surface, beginning with a basic single-leg balance, followed by Standing Hip Stability, etc....

Remember, just as with all exercises and movements learned, no pain should be experienced. All the same pathologies and pain generators explained throughout the Balance and Unilateral Stability Series may be accentuated here and must be kept in mind. Movement and control difficulty increases throughout this series, raising the probability of pathology aggravation, so please refer back to the Balance and Unilateral Stability Series section for any issues. If pain persists and no attempts are able to eliminate the pain, the particular exercise being performed should be considered beyond the limit capacity at this point in time and thus should not be done. [932, 940, 941, 942, 943, 944, 945, 946, 947]

Advanced Pull Series (A continuation of the Pull Series from Level II)

ADVANCED PULL SERIES (A CONTINUATION OF THE PULL SERIES FROM LEVEL II)

The Pull Series continues to progress in Level III in the same manner as all other Level III series, adding a variety of new exercises, movements, and increasing resistance. Once the basic movement pattern of the pull is learned in Level II, progression occurs through increasing weight/resistance and hitting a variety of angles for overall muscular and movement-control development. For the pull movement pattern, this can be achieved by changing the angle of the pull. The pull movement pattern was first learned as a mid-row exercise with the angle of pull perpendicular to the torso (pulling straight towards the body). By changing the angle of pull to low rows, high rows, and lat pulls, virtually any angle can be used.

Changes in body position can provide further challenges. Examples include standing utilizing a Hip Hinge position or squat position, seated, bent over utilizing an RDL position, and single-leg versions of these positions.

You can also change the grip and upper extremity position to add further angles and variety. Handgrips include supinated, pronated, and neutral grips, while possible upper extremity positions include anything from a wide grip position to a narrow grip position. If you are not getting it by now, variety is key!

The ultimate goal for the pulling motion category of human movement is to achieve the ability to do pull-ups. The pull-up is the single best upper body exercise for strength and mobility, and, when performed correctly, demonstrates superior functional human strength and movement control. The ability to pull oneself up, also known as climbing, has been a fundamental part of the human species from the beginning.

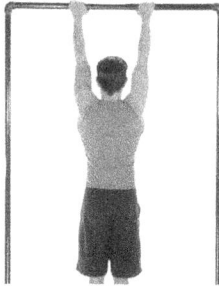

Pull-Up Beginning Position

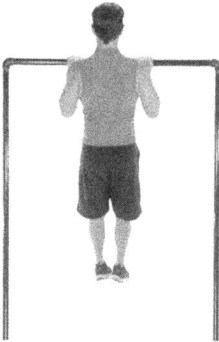

Pull-Up Movement Position

Pull-Ups
    Goal/Purpose:

- Progression of the shoulder girdle to full pulling motions above the head in the most functional manner possible.

Beginning Position:

- Hanging from a bar with the hands/arms just beyond shoulder width apart with an overhand (pronated) grip, achieve Full Spinal Control.

Movement/Action:

- While maintaining the correct body position, perform a pull-up by pulling the body up towards the bar so that the middle of the sternum (chest) touches or comes as close to the bar as possible. Keep the elbows/arms tight to the body during the pulling motion.
- Repeat 10 reps.

Key Notes/Common Faults:

- Pain/discomfort/straining of any kind.
- Faulty breathing pattern.
- Loss of Full Spinal Control.
- Do not allow the lumbar spine to extend out of neutral.
- Ensure the scapulae (shoulder blades) remain in their set scapular position. Now that a full pull is being performed, the scapulae should not move in and out of the set scapular position as with the Set Scap Pull exercise. Full Spinal Control, including the set scapular position, must be maintained throughout all pulling motions.

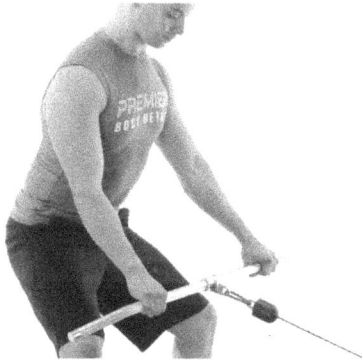

Low Row Beginning Position

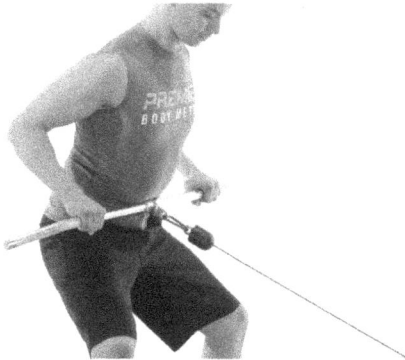

Low Row MovementPosition

Low Rows
   Goal/Purpose:

   • Progression of the shoulder girdle to full pulling motions
     with an added variety of pulling angles.

Beginning Position:

   • Standing with Full Spinal Control in a slight Hip Hinge
     deadlift position, as discussed in the Hip Hinge Series, with
     both arms flexed at the shoulder out in front of the body,

grasping a cable or band that is below the body's center of mass (the navel).

Movement/Action:

- While maintaining the correct standing position, perform a row by pulling the cable or Theraband back towards the mid-belly just above the navel. Keep the elbows/arms tight to the body during the pulling motion.
- Repeat 10 reps.

Key Notes/Common Faults:

- Pain/discomfort/straining of any kind.
- Faulty breathing pattern.
- Loss of Full Spinal Control.
- Ensure the scapulae (shoulder blades) remain in their set scapular position. Now that a full pull is being performed, the scapulae should not move in and out of the set scapular position as with the Set Scap Pull exercise. Full Spinal Control, including the set scapular position, must be maintained throughout all pulling motions.

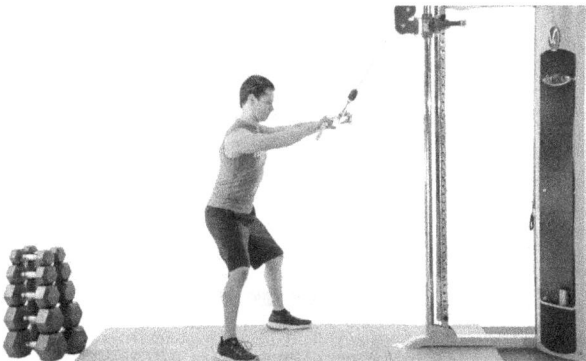

High Row Beginning Position

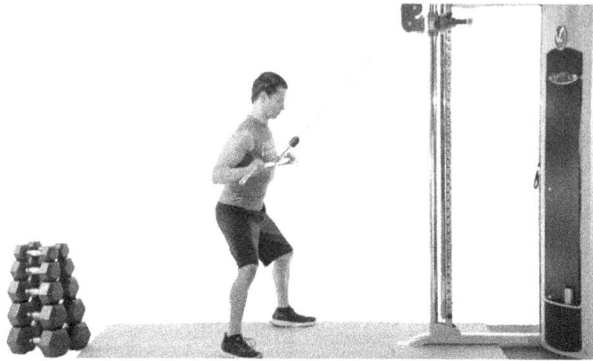

High Row Movement Position

High Rows
Goal/Purpose:

- Progression of the shoulder girdle to full pulling motions with added variety of pulling motions

Beginning Position:

- Standing with Full Spinal Control in a slight Hip Hinge deadlift position, as discussed in the Hip Hinge Series, with both arms flexed at the shoulder out in front of the body, grasping a cable or band that is above the body's center of mass (the navel).

Movement/Action:

- While maintaining the correct deadlift position, perform a row by pulling the weights back towards the center of the chest. Keep the elbows/arms tight to the body during the pulling motion.
- General pulling rule: if pulling from an angle above shoulder height, pull to the sternum. If pulling from below shoulder height, pull to the navel.

- Repeat 10 reps.

Key Notes/Common Faults:

- Pain/discomfort/straining of any kind.
- Faulty breathing pattern.
- Loss of Full Spinal Control.
- Make sure the scapulae (shoulder blades) remain in their set scapular position. Now that a full pull is being performed, the scpapulae should not move in and out of the set scapular position as with the Set Scap Pull exercise. Full Spinal Control, including the set scapular position, must be maintained throughout all pulling motions.
- Overexertion or straining of any kind.

Remember, just as with all exercises and movements learned, no pain should be experienced. All the same pathologies and pain generators explained throughout the Pull Series may be accentuated here and must be kept in mind. The shoulder joint and upper extremity will be advancing in movement and control difficulty throughout this series. As discussed before, with increases in exercise difficulty comes an increased probability for pathology to be aggravated, so please refer back to the Pull Series section for any issues here.

The basic rules of mechanics still apply no matter the level of exercise difficulty, and thus, all the fixes, adjustments, and alterations still apply. **In other words, regardless of the level of exercise difficulty, stick to the basic fundamentals!** As before, if pain persists and no attempts can eliminate the pain, the particular exercise being performed should be considered beyond the limit capacity at this point in time and thus should not be done. [932, 940, 941, 942, 943, 944, 945, 946, 947]

ADVANCED PRESS SERIES (A CONTINUATION OF THE PRESS SERIES FROM LEVEL II)

The Press Series continues to progress in Level III with more advanced progressions. Once the basic press pattern in learned in Level II, it can be applied to a variety of different angles, upper extremity positions, and handgrips. The push-up was used to teach the basic press pattern. This pattern can now be applied to the flat bench press, the incline press, the decline press, and dip exercises. Grips can be supinated, pronated, or neutral, and various weights or resistance, including barbells, dumbbells, medicine balls, kettlebells, rings, cables, or resistance bands, can be used. Once again, variety is the key to well-rounded muscular and movement-control development.

The overhead press is the most challenging movement pattern for the shoulder, upper extremity, cervical spine, and the human body in general. Thus, the overhead pressing motion will be reserved in its own series progression as the final piece of the pressing movement pattern. In the next section, overhead activity will be progressed in the Advanced Shoulder Control Series.

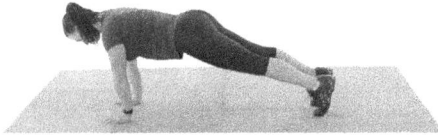

Push Up Beginning Position

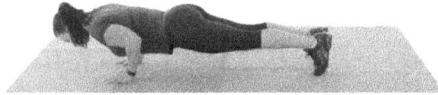

Push Up Movement Position

Push Ups
  Goal/Purpose:

- Progression of the shoulder girdle to full pressing motions. This is the first progression for a full, complete press. Pressing motions are one of the three major types of motion of the human body.

Beginning Position:

- Quadruped position supporting the weight of the body equally on the hands and feet with arms/elbows straight (push-up position). Full Spinal Control, especially pelvic neutral, must be achieved and maintained. Keep in mind this is a plank position from the hands.

Movement/Action:

- While maintaining the correct starting position, perform a push-up motion by slowly lowering the torso/body down toward the ground by way of shoulder extension and elbow flexion. Then, press the torso/body back away from the ground, returning to the starting position. The arms/elbows should remain tight/close to the body during the push-up motion. Do not allow the elbows to flair out away from the body.

Key Notes/Common Faults:

- Pain/discomfort/straining of any kind.
- Faulty breathing pattern.
- Loss of Full Spinal Control.
- Do not allow the lower back to extend.
- Now, when performing the full press, maintain a set scap position.

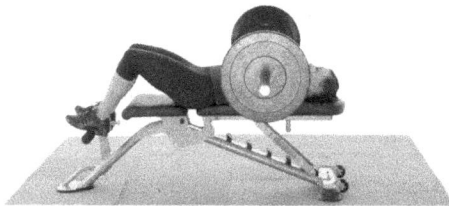

Bench Press (Flat) Beginning Position

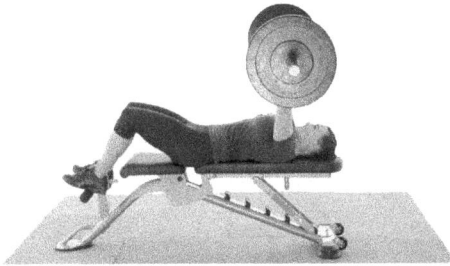

Bench Press (Flat) Movement Position

Bench Press (Flat)
  Goal/Purpose:

- Progression of the shoulder girdle to a greater variety of pressing motions as well as increasing pressing strength.

Beginning Position:

- Supine (face up) on a flat bench.
- Achieve Full Spinal Control with Pelvic, Scapular, and C/S neutral with hips and knees flexed to 90 degrees.
- Shoulder at 90 degrees of flexion up in the air holding dumbbells or barbell weight.

Movement/Action:

- While maintaining Full Spinal Control, perform a pressing motion by slowly lowering the weight down towards the body (center of the sternum) by way of shoulder extension and elbow flexion. Then, press the weight back away from the body, returning to the starting position. The arms/elbows should remain tight/close to the body during the press motion. Do not allow the elbows to flair out away from the body.

• Repeat 10 reps.

Key Notes/Common Faults:

• Pain / discomfort / straining of any kind.
• Faulty breathing pattern.
• Loss of Full Spinal Control.
• Remember, when performing a full press, maintain a set scap position.

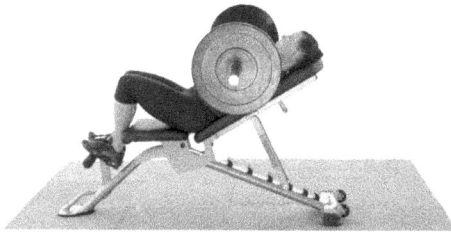

Bench Press (Incline) Beginning Position

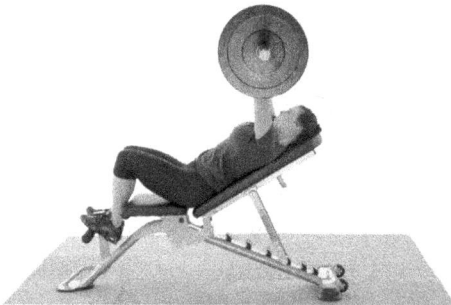

Bench Press (Incline) Movement Position

Bench Press (Incline)
  Goal/Purpose:

- Progression of the shoulder girdle to a greater variety of pressing motions as well as increasing pressing strength in various inclined angles of press.

Beginning Position:

- Supine (face up) on an incline bench.
- Achieve Full Spinal Control with Pelvic, Scapular, and C/S neutral with hips and knees flexed to 90 degrees.
- Shoulder degrees of flexion for holding dumbbells or barbell weights depend on the angle of the bench being utilized. Anywhere from 91 degrees to 189 degrees of GHJ (shoulder) flexion is technically possible here. Normal/average would be around 125 degrees.

Movement/Action:

- While maintaining Full Spinal Control, perform a pressing motion by slowly lowering the weight down towards the body (center of the sternum) by way of shoulder extension and elbow flexion. Then, press the weight back away from the body, returning to the starting position. The arms/elbows should remain tight/close to the body during the press motion. Do not allow the elbows to flair out away from the body.
- Repeat 10 reps.

Key Notes/Common Faults:

- Pain/discomfort/straining of any kind.
- Faulty breathing pattern.
- Loss of Full Spinal Control.

- Remember, when performing a full press, maintain a set scap position.

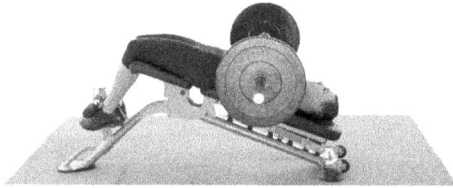

Bench Press (Decline) Beginning Position

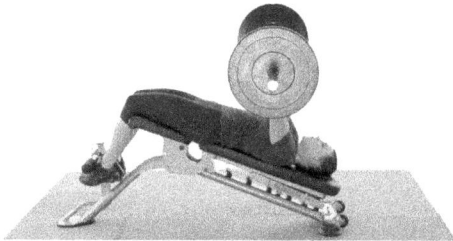

Bench Press (Decline) Movement Position

Bench Press (Decline)
  Goal/Purpose:

- Progression of the shoulder girdle to a greater variety of pressing motions as well as increasing pressing strength in various declined angles of press.

Beginning Position:

- Supine (face up) on a declined bench.
- Achieve Full Spinal Control with Pelvic, Scapular, and C/S neutral with hips and knees flexed to 90 degrees.
- Shoulder degrees of flexion for holding dumbbells or barbell weights are dependent on the angle of the bench being utilized. Anywhere from 1 degree to 89 degrees of GHJ (shoulder) flexion is technically possible here. Normal/average would be around 65 degrees.

Movement/Action:

- While maintaining Full Spinal Control, perform a pressing motion by slowly lowering the weight down towards the body (center of the sternum) by way of shoulder extension and elbow flexion. Then, press the weight back away from the body, returning to the starting position. The arms/elbows should remain tight/close to the body during the press motion. Do not allow the elbows to flair out away from the body.
- Repeat 10 reps.

Key Notes/Common Faults:

- Pain/discomfort/straining of any kind.
- Faulty breathing pattern.
- Loss of Full Spinal Control.
- Remember, when performing the full press, maintain a set scap position.

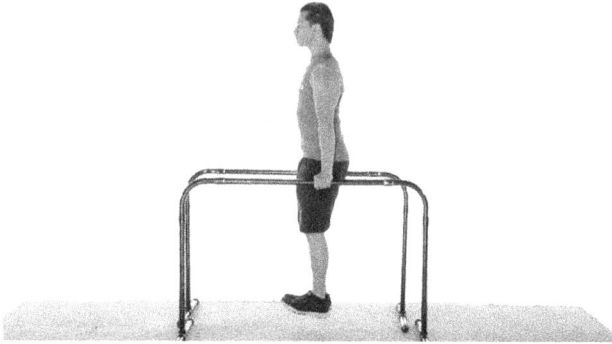

Dip Beginning Position

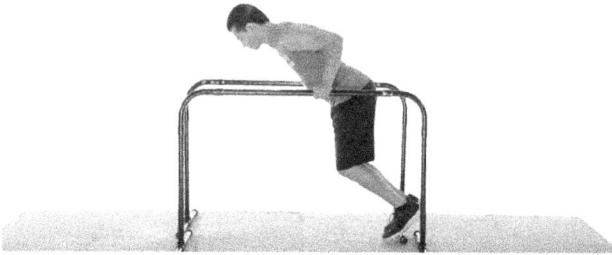

Dip Movement Position

Dips
Goal/Purpose:

- Progression of the shoulder girdle to a greater variety of pressing motions as well as increasing pressing strength. (This is a more advanced exercise, so be cautious.)

Beginning Position:

- Upright with arms at the sides holding the weight of the body up on two side-by-side parallel bars.

- Achieve Full Spinal Control with Pelvic, Scapular, and C/S neutral.

Movement/Action:

- While maintaining Full Spinal Control, perform a pressing dip motion by slowly lowering the body/torso down towards the parallel bars (center of the sternum) by way of shoulder extension and elbow flexion. Then, press the body back away from the bars, returning to the starting position. The arms/elbows should remain tight/close to the body during the press motion. Do not allow the elbows to flair out away from the body. Also, the forearms should remain perpendicular to the bar or ground. Do not let your forearms angle back during the dip-pressing motion.
- Repeat 10 reps.

Key Notes/Common Faults:

- Pain/discomfort/straining of any kind.
- Faulty breathing pattern.
- Loss of Full Spinal Control.
- Remember, when performing the full press, maintain a set scap position.

Remember, just as with all exercises and movements learned, no pain should be experienced. All the same pathologies and pain genera-tors discussed in the Press Series and all prior series' involved in the press series must be kept in mind. The shoulder joint and upper extremity advance in movement and control difficulty throughout this series. Remember that as the complexity of exercises increases, the ability to control the movement may be impaired. **In other words, the more complex the exercise, the more movement control pieces are involved.** This may be more or less pertinent depending on the partic-ular exercise being performed. For example, during the push-up exer-cise, the correct plank position must be maintained with Full Spinal

Control as described in the advanced Pelvic-Spinal Core Control series. If trainees are unable to perform this spinal control correctly, they are safer performing a bench press exercise with greater spinal support. Full Spinal Control must still be maintained, but this is much easier during the bench press than the push-up.

The rest of the upper extremity is now involved as well. You must be very aware of a neutral wrist position. Dumbbells or various hand-grips can help you maintain a neutral wrist/hand position. As with any exercise or movement, if pain is present and no attempts are successful at eliminating the pain, the particular exercise being performed should be considered beyond the limit capacity at this point in time and thus should not be done. [932, 940, 941, 942, 943, 944, 945, 946, 947]

ADVANCED SHOULDER CONTROL (OVERHEAD PRESS) SERIES

The advanced shoulder control series progresses the basic press series and all the pieces it is built from to achieve overhead activity for the upper extremity and human body. The ability to press weight overhead is the most challenging movement pattern for the shoulder, upper extremity, cervical spine, and possibly the whole body. True structural deficits in the GH joint of the shoulder or the cervical spine may put this movement pattern out of reach for some. This is the main reason this particular aspect of the pressing motion has been segregated out into its own series. Still, the ability to press weight overhead is an invaluable part of human functional ability. Imagine for a minute not being able to lift anything or reach to grab anything that is over the height of your head, and you will understand why.

This series begins with the overhead holdout exercise. This exercise is basically an isometric way to strengthen the stability and control needed to press weight overhead. The overhead holdout places a small amount of weight in the hand and has the trainee lock this weight out directly overhead with the GH

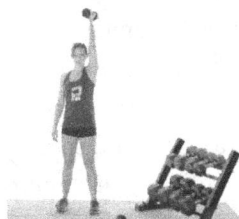

joint of the shoulder straight up overhead at 180 degrees of flexion/ab-
duction. This requires a full range of motion by the shoulder GH joint,
so if the trainee does not have this range, this exercise and, thus, this
series should not be done. Once this overhead holdout position is
reached, it is held without movement for 30 seconds. Holding weight
overhead is one of the best ways to train full shoulder girdle stability.

Just as with all exercises and movement patterns, Full Spinal Control,
including pelvic neutral, set scapular position, DNF neutral neck position, and core stability control, is a must. As long as one's structure
allows, the overhead holdout should be done in the standing position,
with a slight Hip Hinge stance to put the weight of the body on the
musculature of the hips. The lower extremities should never be locked
out, as this places the weight of the body on the passive structures of
the join.ts

[image: a person's profile holding weight overhead with anterior
pelvic neutral and increased L/S hyperextension.]

Again, a full 180-degree shoulder GH joint range of motion is absolutely necessary for this exercise. One of the most common compensation patterns seen for lack of proper shoulder range of motion during
overhead activity is loss of pelvic neutral and hyperextension of the
lumbar spine. This occurs when the body tries to cheat because it is
unable to reach up all the way overhead with the shoulder complex
itself. The compensation occurs when the trainee leans the whole
frame (torso) back to get that extra bit of range. To an untrained eye,
the person appears to have a full range of motion for the shoulder, so
be careful. Again, allowing this to occur is taking the workload off the
muscles of the core and placing that workload on the facet joints of the
lumbar spine. We all understand by now that this is unsafe faulty
biomechanics.

The overhead holdout exercise can be progressed by having the
trainee walk around while maintaining this holdout position. The
trainee can also be placed on an unstable surface to create advanced
challenges in stability.

Once the overhead holdout is mastered without negative effects, the series can progress to a full bilateral overhead press movement pattern. The overhead press can then be progressed further by adding a unilateral version of the movement. Unilateral movement requires added stability control because the weight will be unequal from side to side during movement. It requires increased control in all planes of motion.

The final progression is the addition of a curl to the overhead press for added functional ability training. Moving weight from the body's center of mass, around the midsection, to an overhead position is one of the most functional motions a human being can perform. Every time you put a box up on a shelf, change a light bulb in the ceiling light in the bedroom, or reach to get a glass out of the overhead kitchen cupboard, you are utilizing an overhead pressing movement pattern. Without the ability to overhead press, quality of life may depreciate to a large extent. The sad part for most is that instead of understanding this, and training the body to have the ability to go overhead correctly, they compensate by forcing too much overhead workload down to the lower back. This is yet another reason why low back pain is so prevalent in our society.

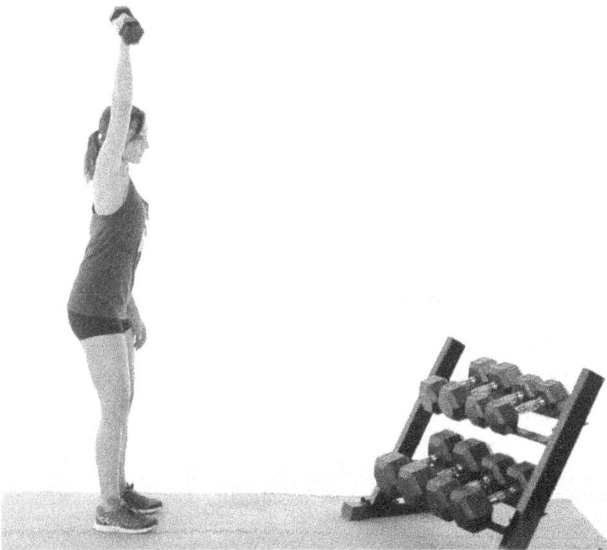

Overhead Holdout

. . .

Overhead Holdout
 Goal/Purpose:

- Further progression of the shoulder pressing motion to overhead activity. This exercise specifically prepares the body / shoulder for overhead activity with motion. No exercise can help the shoulder girdle gain overall stability more than holding weight out overhead.

Beginning Position:

- Standing in a very slight Hip Hinge position with Full Spinal Control.
- One arm / shoulder flexed to 180 degrees directly overhead.

Movement/Action:

- While maintaining Full Spinal Control, a light weight should be placed in the hand of the arm overhead. If possible, an assistant should help set and remove the weight.
- Hold this weighted overhead position as steady as possible for 30 seconds. Then repeat with the opposite side.

Key Notes/Common Faults:

- Pain / discomfort / straining of any kind.
- Faulty breathing pattern.
- Loss of Full Spinal Control.
- One of the most common faults during overhead activity is loss of pelvic neutral and increased lower back extension. This is usually due to a lack of mobility (tight lats) in the shoulder joint. Do not allow the lumbar spine to extend.

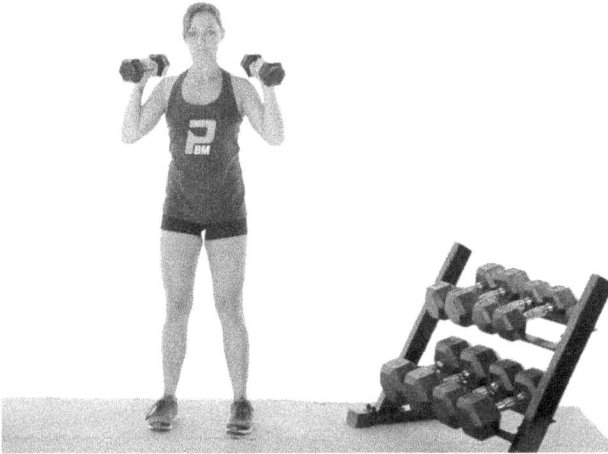

Overhead Press Beginning Position (Bilateral and Unilateral)

Overhead Press (Bilateral)
Goal/Purpose:

- Further progression of the shoulder pressing motion to overhead activity. Pressing weight or objects overhead is one of the most difficult activities the human body is asked to do, yet many daily tasks require overhead motions.

Beginning Position:

- Standing in a very slight Hip Hinge position with Full Spinal Control.
- Arms flexed at the elbow to allow one to hold dumbbell weights at the side of one's shoulder on either side of the head.

Movement/Action:

- While maintaining Full Spinal Control, perform an overhead press by pressing the weights up directly overhead. Then, reverse the motion back to the starting position.
- Repeat 10 reps.

Key Notes/Common Faults:

- Pain/discomfort/straining of any kind.
- Faulty breathing pattern.
- Loss of Full Spinal Control.
- One of the most common faults during overhead activity is loss of pelvic neutral and increased lower back extension. This is usually due to a lack of mobility (tight lats) in the shoulder joint. Do not allow the lumbar spine to extend.
- Any stressing or straining of any kind, especially in the face and neck, should not be allowed.

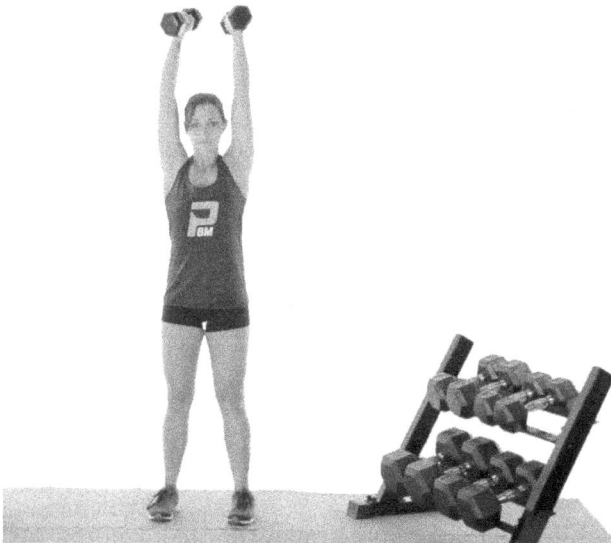

Overhead Press (Bilateral) Movement Position

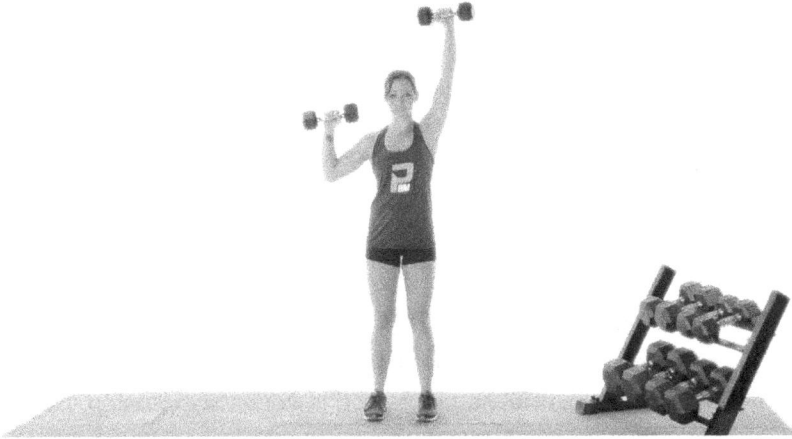

Overhead Press (Unilateral) Movement Position

Overhead Press (Unilateral)
  Goal/Purpose:

- Further progression of the shoulder pressing motion to overhead activity. Pressing weight/objects overhead is one of the most difficult activities the human body is asked to do, yet many daily tasks require overhead motions.

Beginning Position:

- Standing in a very slight Hip Hinge position with Full Spinal Control.
- Arms flexed at the elbow to allow one to hold dumbbell weights at the side of one's shoulder on either side of the head.

Movement/Action:

- While maintaining Full Spinal Control, perform an overhead press, pressing one weight up directly overhead one arm at a time. Then, reverse the motion back to the starting position.
- Repeat ten reps, alternating sides with each rep.

Key Notes/Common Faults:

- Pain/discomfort/straining of any kind.
- Faulty breathing pattern.
- Loss of Full Spinal Control.
- One of the most common faults during overhead activity is loss of pelvic neutral and increased lower back extension. This is usually due to a lack of mobility (tight lats) in the shoulder joint. Do not allow the lumbar spine to extend.

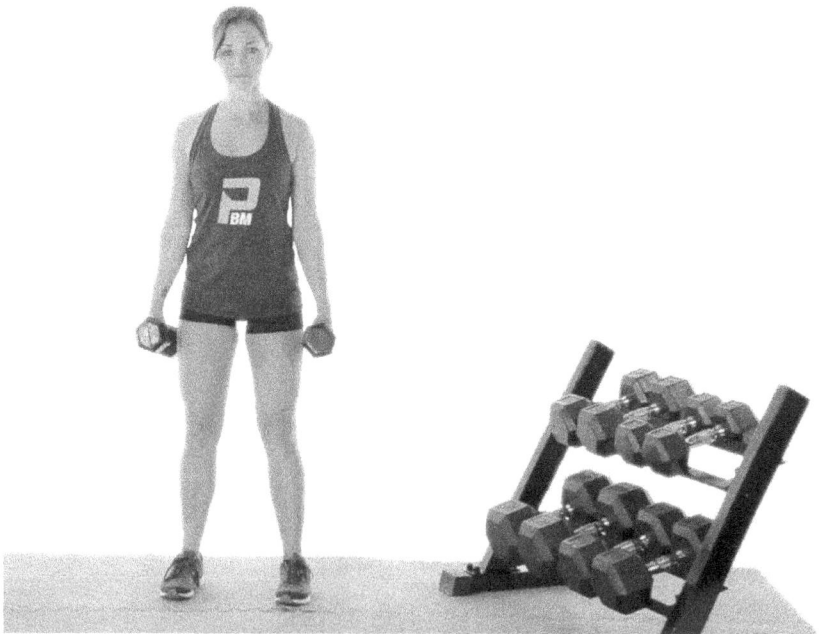

Curl and Press Beginning Position

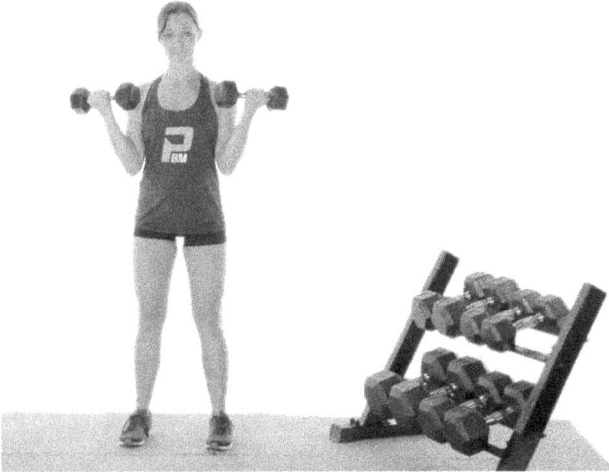

Curl and Press Movement Position I

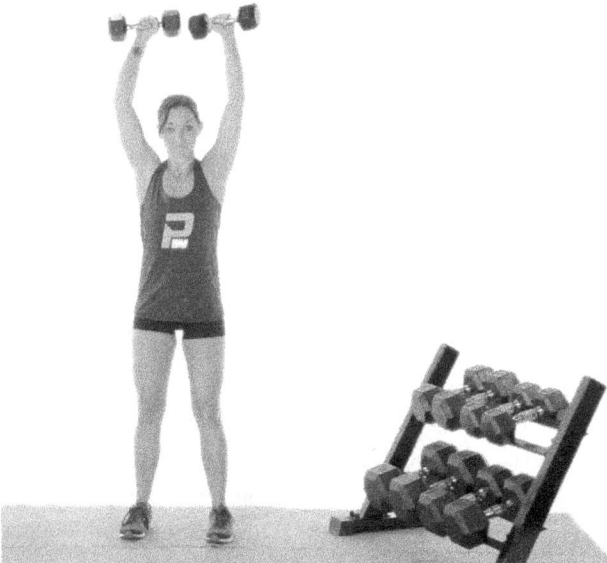

Curl and Press Movement Position II

Curl and Press
Goal/Purpose:

- Further progression of the shoulder pressing motion to overhead activity. This exercise is about as functional as it gets, simulating lifting an object at a low height all the way up overhead.

Beginning Position:

- Standing in a very slight Hip Hinge position with Full Spinal Control.
- Arms down at one's sides holding dumbbell weights.

Movement/Action:

- While maintaining Full Spinal Control perform first a bicep curl by lifting the weights by way of elbow flexion to achieve the starting position of an overhead press. Then perform an overhead press by pressing the weights up directly overhead. Reverse the motion back to the starting position
- Repeat 10 reps.

Key Notes/Common Faults:

- Pain / discomfort / straining of any kind.
- Faulty breathing pattern.
- Loss of Full Spinal Control.
- One of the most common faults during overhead activity is loss of pelvic neutral and increased lower back extension. This is usually due to a lack of mobility (tight lats) in the shoulder joint. Do not allow the lumbar spine to extend.
- Any stressing or straining of any kind, especially in the face and neck, should not be allowed.

[Image: SIDE BY SIDE: Label Overhead Press Unilateral AND Curl and Press – Image Overhead Press Unilateral movement position AND Curl and Press movement position]

Remember, just as with all exercises and movements learned, no pain should be experienced. All the same pathologies and pain generators explained throughout the Pressing Series may be accentuated here and must be kept in mind. The shoulder joint will be advancing in movement and control difficulty throughout this series. Special attention should be given to the set scapular position because if the scapular position is faulty, increased stress is commonly transferred to the GH joint.

Remember, one very common mistake made when pressing weight overhead is an extension in the lower back due to loss of pelvic neutral. This transfers much of the loading stress that the core musculature should take up and places it on the facet joints of the lumbar spine. Suppose pain is present in any part of the body at any time, and no correction attempts are successful at eliminating the pain. In that case, this particular exercise is beyond the limit capacity at this point in time and thus should not be done. Remember that pressing weight overhead is one of the most difficult movements to ask of the human body. If certain pathologies and injuries are present, this movement may be beyond the abilities of some. [932, 940, 941, 942, 943, 944, 945, 946, 947]

FUNCTIONAL HUMAN MOVEMENT EXERCISE PROGRAM

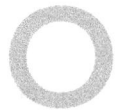

Once all biomechanical control series progressions have been completed through Level I, II, and the beginning of Level III, the trainee is ready to apply everything he has learned about the human body, its movement, and the control of that movement. Not only has the trainee learned correct human biomechanics, but he has also learned these mechanics on an individual basis according to his own unique human structures (anatomy) and physical abilities. This knowledge is now ready to be applied to a full body basic strength and conditioning exercise program, allowing the trainee not only to be able to perform his or her newly found mechanics but also give the trainee the strength and endurance needed to perform these mechanics throughout the day and throughout other physical activities.

The dynamics of training change with this basic functional strength program. The most efficient way to train full body mechanics in an exercise training fashion takes advantage of the three major motions of the body. The pace of training should increase to a conditioning level. With that being said, the quality of movement learned should never be sacrificed. **The quality of movement should never be sacrificed.** Throughout the entire program, we have built up piece by piece, with each preceding piece being added to, never disappearing. This does not stop now that the basic fitness level has been reached. We are now adding another piece, just as we have done time and time again. This next piece is the conditioning pace and strength program organization parameters.

The workout should progress to a high, nonstop pace with minimal rest between sets in a compound set exercise strategy, as in circuit training. This fatigues the entire body all at once, burns the most calories, and promotes physiologic, metabolic, hormonal, and body composition improvements. It will also promote good cardiovascular health and conditioning and tone the body. All this is done while keeping your body safe, stabilized, functional, and out of pain.

The three major motions of the body, Hip Hinging, pulling, and pressing, are performed in a cyclical manner. Trainees perform three exercises consecutively one from each category, cycling through with no rest in between. Three sets of each exercise, all interlaced (compound-set) together, should be done as fast as correct mechanics will allow. For example, you might select squats, bent-over rows, and push-ups for your three-way circuit. Do a set of squats, immediately followed by a set of rows, immediately followed by a set of push-ups, then immediately back to squats, then rows, etc., until all sets of exercises are complete.

After this, a new compound set of three exercises, one from each category again, will be performed in the same manner. Keep doing this for 30 to 40 minutes, and you will have a great, fun, and exciting workout. It will be different every time so you will never get bored or lazy. As you can imagine, you should be breathing hard the entire time.

The weight is moderate to begin, around 65% of 1 rep max for each exercise, and progression is according to the trainee's specific goals. The rep range is, on average, 10 reps per set for each exercise, and 3 sets are done for each exercise. A simple way to think about the weight is to make it challenging, staying in your 10-rep range. If you can't get 10 reps, it is too heavy. If you get 10 reps and are not tired yet, it is too light. You should not necessarily be going to complete muscular failure here. This will come in higher levels.

Keep in mind that failure is defined as no longer having the ability to correctly perform the movement within the biomechanically correct patterns learned throughout this program. Many times, people force out a few last reps, but these are compensated reps performed with incorrect mechanics. Therefore, you are no longer training what you are attempting to train, and you are most likely placing your body at risk by transferring loading stress to passive structures. Always remember to never sacrifice quality for quantity in the number of reps or amount of weight used.

Just as in all progressions, pain should not be experienced. By now, if the trainee has progressed through the program correctly by completing Levels I and II, all the holes in the biomechanical system should be corrected. Suppose the trainee has a true structural deficit, and a particular movement pattern is beyond the structural limitations of the trainee's body. In that case, this should also be evident by the time he or she has reached the Functional Human Movement Exercise Program of Level III. This gives the trainee the knowledge to train safely and effectively for the rest of his or her life.

Now, in Level III, it is time to apply this knowledge and make it effective in a full-body functional workout routine. Suppose a particular movement pattern or angle of motion is beyond the structural limits of the individual and thus unsafe. In that case, all exercises utilizing this particular angle of movement should be simply left out of the full body program, therefore leaving only non-pain generating, safe, and effective modes of training for each individual, based on the individual's own unique body structure.

If the trainee is an athlete utilizing this program to improve athletic performance, pain may not be the issue, although the athlete's own individual holes in the biomechanical system will still be learned by the time the athlete achieves Level III. This allows the athlete to use this knowledge to correct the holes, strengthen his or her weaknesses, and become a better, more complete athlete. It may also serve to reduce injury risk by correcting any and all biomechanical faults that may have predisposed this athlete to injury before.

Once this final exercise-conditioning piece is applied to everything learned thus far throughout the program, and is mastered, The PREMIER Body Method's human movement education course will be complete. As long as each progressing step of the program is followed correctly, a complete, functional human being will have been built from the ground up. All the holes in the system, whether causing pain and dysfunction, or hidden, possibly predisposing one to future injury, are found and filled in, leaving only biomechanically correct movement. The trainee will have learned how to move his or her body on an individual basis determined by his or her own unique physical abilities. This not only gives the knowledge and power to overcome injury and pain but improves health, fitness, and athletic performance. It may also serve to prevent mechanical dysfunction, pain, and injury in the future. By training efficient tissue-sparing movement, this program is also, in many ways, teaching anti-aging mechanics, in that the passive tissues of the body are spared as much as humanly possible. This gives the body longevity as we age, holding off the processes of degenerative joint disease created by mechanical stress. It also gives the athlete longevity. How many athletes have been forced to end their careers early due to pain and injury?

Once Level III of The PREMIER Body Method's human movement education is complete, higher-level performance athletes will be ready to return to higher levels of sports performance training with the confidence and knowledge of understanding how to use their God-given physical talents to the best of their ability. For the rest of us, you will be ready to move on to the next level – the sport of life.

PASSIVE MOTION, ACTIVE MOTION, AND LOADED MOTION

We need to keep in mind that the movement of the human body can be classified in three ways depending on how we are moving: Passive Motion, Active Motion, and Loaded Motion.

Passive Motion occurs when a joint (or body part) moves without its own effort. Specifically, it refers to the movement of a joint or limb without any voluntary effort or muscle contraction, where movement takes place due to an external force applied to the body. For example, if someone is stretching you, such as a therapist or trainer, and you are completely relaxed while they move your leg to stretch your hamstring. In my view, this concept also applies to posture. Remember, posture is merely a freeze frame of movement (biomechanics), and movement is essentially posture in action. We may refer to it as passive posture, such as when using a back brace to support the postural position of your spine, or how your body is artificially positioned by relaxing in a comfortable chair.

• • •

The second type of motion is *Active Motion*. Active Motion refers to the movement of a body part or joint using your own power through muscular contraction. Whenever you move independently, you are using active motion. This is the kind of movement we are all familiar with, and this is the primary movement type we have been discussing and will continue to discuss throughout this book.

The third type of motion is *Loaded Motion*. Loaded Motion is Active Motion with an additional external load or force beyond your own body. For instance, if you stand up from a chair by yourself, you are using Active Motion; however, if you stand up from that chair while holding a heavy box, you are demonstrating Loaded Motion.

Understanding the distinctions between these types of motions is crucial concerning everything we are teaching here. The movement and biomechanical strategies discussed throughout this book and the teachings of the PREMIER Body Method primarily focus on both Active Motion and Loaded Motion. The PBM provides ideal movement mechanics and postural strategies to keep your body safe (tissue sparing) and performing (functioning) at a highly effective level during your own physical movement and body control. This significantly aids in maintaining the health and safety of your joints, ligaments, tendons, and overall physical anatomy during exercise. The PBM approach to movement also fosters the most efficiently correct movement patterns, giving you the greatest advantage in utilizing your physical body. If you aim to reduce the risk of injury, promote longevity for your physical body, enhance fitness training results, boost sports performance, and function at your best physically, then the PREMIER Body Method is for you.

All that being said, one thing the PREMIER Body Method movement strategy is not necessarily for is Passive Motion, although it can still apply at times. Let's explain: One question I have been asked before is,

"So it is really unhealthy to move your spine at all, huh?" It seems like almost a silly question to me; however, if you are truly paying attention and genuinely embracing what the PBM is teaching, it may imply that the spinal column, including the scapula and pelvis, should never really move. This is correct for both Active Motion and even more so for Loaded Motion. However, movement, in general, is extremely important for all joints in the body, including those of the spine. Joint movement provides the mechanism for much of the fluid and nutrient exchange for the joint and the surrounding anatomy. To keep joints healthy, they need to move. Passive Motion for all joints, within the joint's correct range of motion, is healthy and safe.

The same cannot be said for Passive Posture, depending on the static position. If the static passive postural position is non-threatening, meaning it does not cause harm, then it should be considered safe and healthy for the joint(s). However, if the static passive postural position is compromised and harmful to the joint, then it should be deemed unsafe, and the person needs to be more aware of their artificial static position and strive to create a better one. Especially as the joint(s) become more compromised (injured or degenerated).

For example, getting a better chair that positions your body in a better static position. This allows you to rest in a safe position, and rest is important too. It is unrealistic to expect your body to always engage in Active Motion to keep you in the correct positions. The body and muscles need time to rest, and it is during those times that the teachings of the PBM need to be considered when placing the body in a passive static position. How many times have you woken up with a stiff neck or low back and thought, "Geez, I must have slept wrong?" This is exactly what happens. Your body—or parts of it—were placed in a non-ideal position statically (passive posture) for an extended period while you slept, and now you are facing the consequences. A better pillow, mattress, or sleeping position will most likely be a big part of the solution.

Active motion, performed correctly—slowly and gently—can be healthy and safe for all joints, including those of the spine. However, this assumes that the joint is structurally sound (without injury, pathology, or degenerative changes) and that the movement is highly controlled. If the joint involved in Active Motion is compromised, it may pose a greater risk of further injury and/or increased pain. This does not necessarily mean that the compromised joint should never engage in movement again, but one should lean toward caution, and the compromised joint(s) would likely be better off on the side of Passive Motion, staying closer to the PBM for Active Motion. Loaded Motion, in my opinion, should always follow the PBM strategy of movement, especially as the load increases.

To simplify this concept, consider the importance of PBM postures and movement strategies for all three movement types. Passive Motion is the least risky to apply (and, in some cases, may actually be inappropriate), while Loaded Motion is the most crucial to apply. Along with this, the more structurally damaged the anatomy is, the more essential it is to adhere to the rules.

FINAL THOUGHTS

The subject of human biomechanics and movement is fascinating. Human biomechanics is defined as the study of structure and function pertaining to biology. It describes the application of engineering mechanics in relation to biological systems. There are so many complexities to life, anatomy, biology, and physics. This simple book barely scratches the surface in terms of the underlying science behind all that is written, but going into the science is not its purpose. The true purpose of this text is to provide the practical application of all this science. It is to be able to teach and train human movement from the most basic level all the way to a high level of function and beyond.

We have learned about the practical side of structure by realizing the physical capability limits of that structure. We have learned the practical side of the function of structure as it pertains to movement mechanics. We have done this in a systematic, stepwise fashion that can be useful to anyone. We began with the basic fundamental pieces of movement, added those pieces together to create a large functional motion, and then applied strength and endurance to that motion to allow us to maintain correct biomechanics in any situation. We built a fully functional human who understands his own unique mechanics based on the specific structures (anatomy) of his individual body. This functional human is now trained to move well, minimize stress to the joints, cartilage, ligaments, and tendons of the body, control past injuries and chronic pain, and minimize the risk of future injury and excessive degenerative stress. This functional human is physically fit and can stay fit for the rest of his life. This functional human can continue to train his body to maintain the level achieved by the end of Level III of the PREMIER Body Method or can easily transition to higher levels of training and/or sports performance. We have succeeded in applying years of scientific knowledge from so many brilliant people before us.

I have seen this system work time and time again for so many people. I have seen injured people heal. I have seen people debilitated by chronic pain overcome that pain and train themselves to be fit and strong again. I have seen athletes reach levels of performance beyond what they thought was possible for them. So what is the problem? Let me ask another question. Do you know how many people who have completed The PREMIER Body Method have said to me, "I wish I had learned all this before I was hurt," or, "Why didn't someone teach me all this before I endured pain for years?" or, "Why didn't my coaches teach me this earlier in my athletic career so I could have been better?" Practically every single one of the people who have completed The PREMIER Body Method has said one of those things or something similar.

Despite all these successes, something still bothers me. It is the fact that these questions are being asked in the first place. It is troubling that so many people still suffer through pain, and we rarely stop to think, "How can we prevent or at least reduce the risk of pain and injury?" I am not saying that all injuries, traumas, pains, and degenerative processes are completely preventable, but if we learned how to move properly and how to take care of our bodies before doing major damage, we could prevent countless cases resulting from debilitating degenerative processes. How many compensation patterns that form following injury and then predispose us to further future injury and pain could be avoided if we just understood how to control our physical bodies?

We must keep in mind that structural change or damage to the anatomy of our bodies creates a mandatory compensation. Compensation results when the Law of 100% Motion is unbalanced, forcing some structures to perform at a greater capacity than they can handle. The longer these compensatory mechanisms persist, the more damage is done, the more degeneration occurs, and the more pain is suffered. The snowball effect of declining health prevails, including pain, loss of fitness, and emotional consequences. This scenario is all too common and largely accepted as inevitable. I cannot tell you how many times I have thought in my own mind about a patient, "If you only had come to me sooner." **The fact that so many of these very patients say the exact same thing to me once they have gone through the program tells me it must have something of value.**

I have long thought that if only there were a system designed to teach and train human movement in a simple and practical manner, people could use this system to teach and train themselves and each other before the damage was done. We teach ourselves everything else, with children learning to read, add, and look both ways before crossing the street as essential parts of growing up. Why not learn how to use our bodies correctly? Imagine for a moment what would happen if we taught our children from a young age how to physically control and use their bodies. It should be part of education in school, just like math, science, language, reading, and writing. I guess you would call it physical education, but not quite the PE that teaches us to play kickball and dodgeball. Beyond these games, whose benefits can include establishing healthy habits and learning motor skills, I am talking about real physical education using The PREMIER Body Method. Simpler versions for children of younger ages would be used of course, depending on age and level of education needed; however, you get the idea.

Outside of school, parents should teach their children proper movement, like they teach them how to tie their shoes and brush their teeth. The information and concepts in this book should be common knowledge, just like everyone, whether or not they majored in nutrition in college, knows that eating candy is unhealthy. Likewise, people should know that allowing a faulty pelvic position is not healthy.

344 YOUR LIFE, PAIN-FREE

Remember our example of the boy who sprained his ankle at age 12 and suffered from chronic pain and poor health by the end of another 50 years? This story ended fifty-plus years later with the man suffering from chronic pain and poor health. It sounded crazy at first to think that the simple ankle sprain at the age of twelve could have been related to the chronic back pain this person suffered throughout the majority of his adult life, leading him down a path of continuing health decline. Still, when we understand the mechanics and how to apply them, it becomes not only possible but also extremely logical.

There's another possible, more positive scenario to consider. What if this boy, his parents, his doctors, and teachers had understood this process from the time of the injury at 12 years and had dealt properly with the simple physical (mechanical) issues from the very beginning? The story might have a very different ending. Proper response to the injury, including better neural retraining and avoiding devastating compensation patterns, could have led to a happier outcome that didn't involve chronic pain and disability.

Many years ago, we needed doctors to tell us to clean and bandage wounds to prevent infection, allow for proper healing, and prevent permanent damage or even death. Now, proper wound care is common knowledge. If you cut yourself, you clean it and put some Neosporin and a Band-Aid on it without thinking twice. You know this because you were taught to do this from an early age.

In my opinion, taking care of our physical bodies, through the simple understanding of the way we are designed to move as humans, should also be common knowledge. It should be part of our culture and our upbringing. It should be a normal part of our lives, not something that is forced upon us after the fact once it is too late and the damage has been done. You should not need a doctor to tell you to set your scapula so your shoulder impingement pain can go away. You should not need to be told to prevent your knee from caving in during squatting movements so your meniscus damage can stop getting worse. You should not need to be told to maintain a neutral pelvic position so your back pain will go away. You should just know these things. We all should know these things.

It is not that complicated. Is there a lot to it? Maybe there is, to some extent. It takes a lot of practice, especially at first. But it's not that complicated. **When it comes down to it, there are really only a handful of basic fundamentals. Understand Full Spinal Control, which consists of pelvic neutral, a set scapular position, and a DNF neck position (core-shoulder-neck). Understand how to activate core stability to help you maintain Full Spinal Control no matter what you are physically doing. Understand basic Hip Hinging mechanics by keeping the weight through your heels, sitting your hips back so they do the work, keeping your legs apart, and maintaining Full Spinal Control. Understand the basics of pulling and pressing motions. That's really it! If you just did that throughout all movement, you would have pretty darn close to perfect mechanics. Just master the fundamentals and apply them to the things you do!**

If we all started to learn it now, and passed it along to our children in and out of school, and our children passed it along to future generations, we soon would all just know it. Within a few generations, it would be part of our culture. We can only imagine how drastically different the health of our species could be within just two or three generations.

The majority of people now experience low back pain in their lifetime. Low back pain is the leading cause of musculoskeletal pain in the US. Degenerative joint disease, disc disease, and arthritis are rampant among us. Countless people suffer every day from hip, knee, shoulder, neck, and other types of pain. On top of the pain, there are the risks of the "treatments:" addictions to painkillers, muscle relaxants, anxiety medications, and sleep aids; poor mental and physical health from avoiding physical activity; and complications of surgeries. This would be no more. Would these things still exist? Of course, but they could be potentially dramatically reduced in both prevalence and severity. The quality of life as we know it could be significantly improved.

This is my dream: a world free from unnecessary pain, degeneration, and reduced quality of life. It is a world where true physical health is common knowledge. It is a world with increased physical ability and performance. It is possible. It starts with the knowledge, the desire, and the willingness to try. It starts with you. It starts with The PREMIER Body Method.

APPENDICES

INJURY SPECIFIC SERIES

The Injury Specific Series provides additional training and exercise for smaller, more specific body regions such as the knee, foot, ankle, elbow, hand, and wrist. Once your body's large gross scale mechanics are sound, depending on the individual, more attention may be needed for some of the smaller, more local body regions to allow these areas to be corrected and to overcome certain specific injuries. If you are someone who has or has had injury, pathology, or other concerns in any of these particular body regions, then adding in some or all of these additional and supplemental exercises may be of great benefit to you.

LEVEL I KNEE-SPECIFIC SERIES

The Knee-Specific Series offers additional training for the lower extremity, specifically for the knee joint. Certain injuries or conditions specific to the knee may require more extensive training beyond the basic full-body biomechanical training. That does not mean that the basic fundamental mechanics can or should be overlooked. Quite the opposite. The more serious or complicated the injury or pathology is, typically, the more important the fundamentals become. That being said, adding in other supplemental training in addition to the basic fundamentals for certain types of knee injuries can have great value. This Knee-Specific Series reviews the basics of beginning knee-specific rehabilitation to help give additional support, control, mobility, strength, and stability to this area of the body.

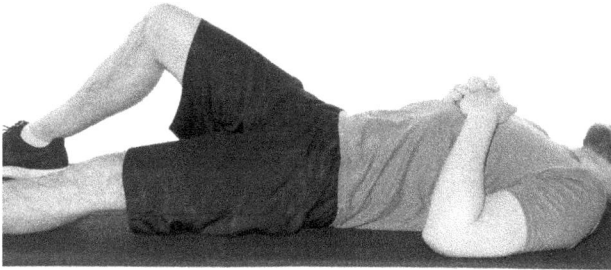

Active Straight Leg Raise Beginning Position

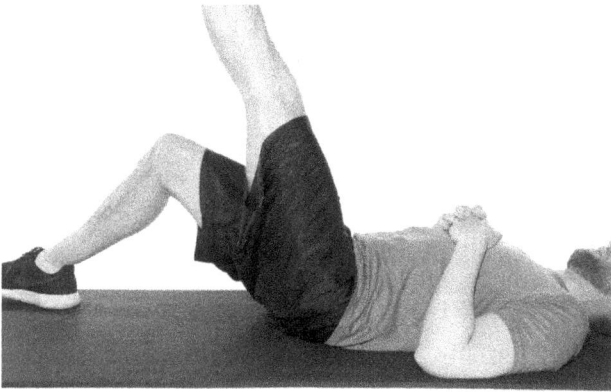

Active Straight Leg Raise Movement Position

Active Straight Leg Raise (SLR)
Goal/Purpose:

- This exercise is specific rehabilitation for certain knee pathology and is utilized for quad and hip flexor strengthening without knee movement.

Beginning Position:

- Supine (face up).
- Pelvic neutral.
- One leg is flexed, with the knee up and the foot flat on the ground. The other leg is straight and lying flat.
- Attention to Scapular and C/S neutral.

Movement/Action:

- The trainee will turn the core on and off in accordance with extremity movement.
- Activate core stability "on" by way of Core Bracing I, lift the straight left off the ground by way of hip flexion as high as comfort will allow, then lower the leg back to the starting position, and then relax core stability "off."
- Repeat 10 reps, and then switch to the opposite side.

Key Notes/Common Faults:

- Pain/discomfort/straining of any kind.
- Faulty breathing pattern.
- Loss of pelvic neutral position is seen as rotational disconnect, tilting, hiking, and/or <u>low back arching</u>.
- Other body region compromise.

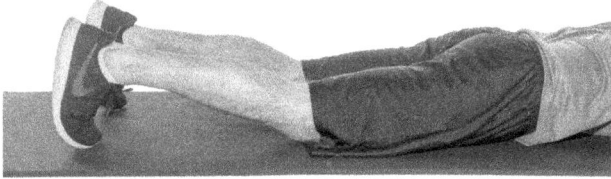

Prone Hip Extension Beginning Position

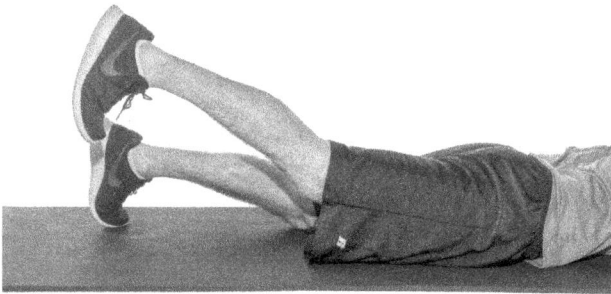

Prone Hip Extension Movement Position

Prone Hip Extension
Goal/Purpose:

- This exercise is specific rehabilitation for certain knee pathology and is utilized for glut and hamstring strengthening without knee movement.

Beginning Position:

- Prone (face down).

- Pelvic neutral (use bolster assistant if necessary).
- Attention to C/S neutral.

Movement/Action:

- The trainee will turn the core on and off in accordance with extremity movement.
- Activate core stability "on" by way of Core Bracing I, lift one leg off the ground by way of hip extension as high as comfort will allow, then lower the leg back to the starting position, and then relax core stability "off."
- Repeat 10 reps, and then switch to the opposite side.

Key Notes/Common Faults:

- Pain/discomfort/straining of any kind.
- Faulty breathing pattern.
- Loss of pelvic neutral position is seen as rotational disconnect, tilting, hiking, and/or low back arching.
- It is easy to allow the lower back to extend with the leg extension if one overdoes it. Do not allow this.
- Other body region compromise.

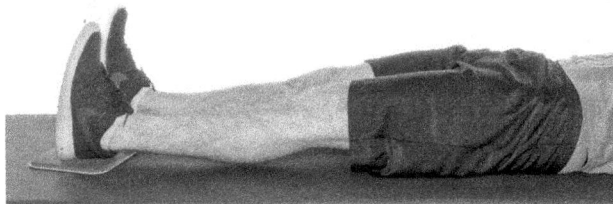

Heel Slide/Heel Push Beginning Position

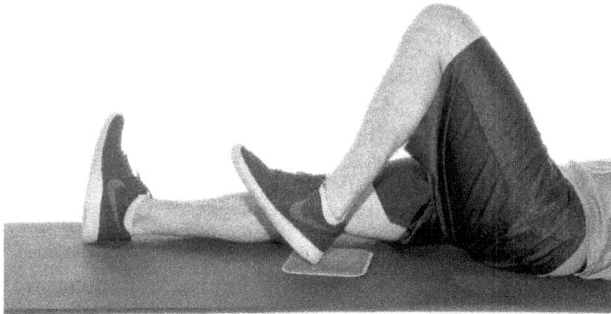

Heel Slide/Heel Push Movement Position

Heel Slide/Heel Push
Goal/Purpose:

- This exercise is specific rehabilitation for certain knee pathologies and is utilized to increase knee range of motion after injury.

Beginning Position:

- Supine (face up).
- Pelvic neutral.
- The non-affected knee/leg is flexed with the knee up and foot flat on the ground, while the injured knee/leg is straight and lying flat.
- Attention to Scapular and C/S neutral.

Movement/Action:

- The trainee will turn the core on and off in accordance with extremity movement.

- Activate core stability "on" by way of Core Bracing I, pull-slide the heel of the straight injured leg up towards the buttock by way of knee flexion and hip flexion as far as comfort will allow, then push-slide the heel by straightening the knee back to the starting position, and then relax core stability "off."
- Repeat 10 reps.

Key Notes/Common Faults:

- Pain/discomfort/straining of any kind.
- Faulty breathing pattern.
- Loss of pelvic neutral position, seen as rotational disconnect and/or tilting and/or hiking and or low back arching.

LEVEL II KNEE-SPECIFIC SERIES

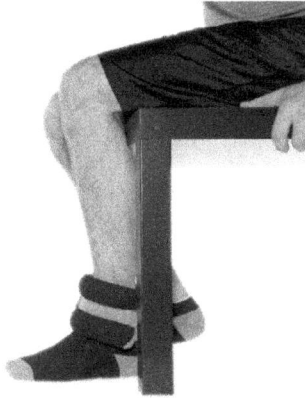

Seated Knee Extension Beginning Position

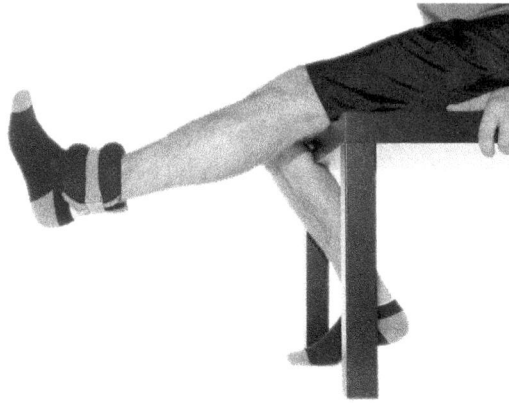

Seated Knee Extension Movement Position

Seated Knee Extension
Goal/Purpose:

- This exercise is specific rehabilitation for certain knee pathologies and is utilized to increase knee range of motion, quad strength, and stability.

Beginning Position:

- Seated with feet off the ground (open chain).
- Pelvic neutral.
- Attention to Scapular and C/S neutral.

Movement/Action:

- While maintaining Full Spinal Control, perform a seated knee/quad extension by way of knee extension by lifting the lower leg up as far as possible.
- Increase weight/resistance by adding an ankle weight as tolerated.
- Repeat 10 reps. Then, switch to the other side.

Key Notes/Common Faults:

- Pain/discomfort/straining of any kind.
- Moving beyond pain-free range of motion.
- Moving up in weight too quickly.
- Faulty breathing pattern.
- Loss of spinal control.

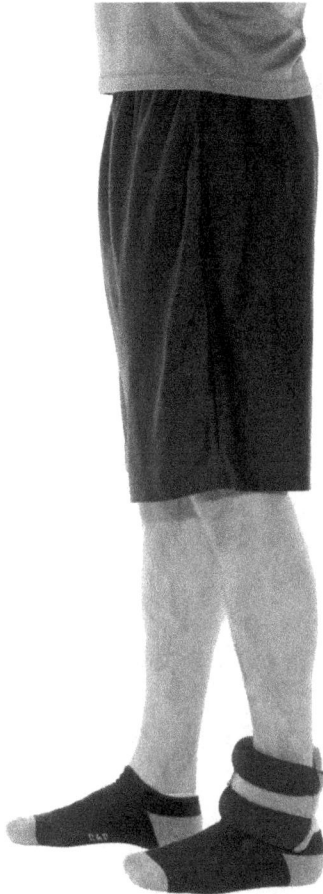

Standing Knee Flexion Beginning Position

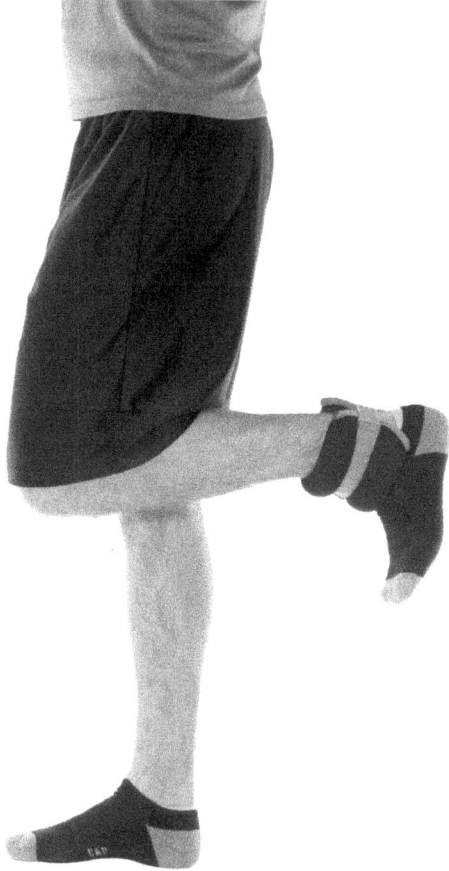

Standing Knee Flexion Movement Position

Standing Knee Flexion
  Goal/Purpose:

- This exercise is specific rehabilitation for certain knee pathologies and is utilized to increase knee range of motion, quad strength, and stability.

Beginning Position:

- Standing with the front of the affected / injured side knee / thigh against a wall or counter.
- Pelvic neutral.
- Attention to Scapular and C/S neutral.

Movement/Action:

- While maintaining Full Spinal Control, perform a standing knee / hamstring curl by way of knee flexion by lifting the lower leg up (heel towards butt) as far as pain-free range will allow.
- Increase weight / resistance by adding an ankle weight as tolerated.
- Repeat 10 reps. Then, switch to the other side.

Key Notes/Common Faults:

- Pain / discomfort / straining of any kind.
- Moving beyond pain-free range of motion.
- Moving up in weight too quickly.
- Faulty breathing pattern.
- Loss of spinal control.

LEVEL I ANKLE-SPECIFIC SERIES

The Ankle-Specific Series offers additional training for the lower extremities, specifically for the foot and ankle. Certain injuries or conditions specific to the foot and / or ankle may require more extensive training beyond the basic full-body biomechanical training. Again, just as discussed in the Knee-Specific Series, this does not mean that the basic fundamental mechanics can or should be overlooked. Remember, the more serious or complicated the injury or pathology is, typically, the more important the fundamentals become. This Ankle-Specific Series reviews the basics of beginning ankle-specific rehabilitation to help give additional support, control, mobility, strength, and stability to this area of the body.

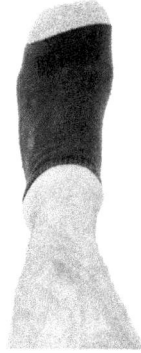

Ankle Alphabet Beginning Position

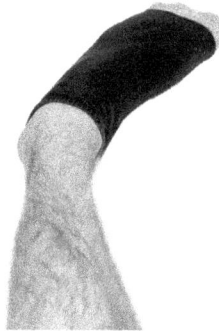

Ankle Alphabet Movement Position

Ankle Alphabet
  Goal/Purpose:

- This exercise is specific rehabilitation for certain ankle pathologies and is utilized to increase ankle range of motion and fine motor control post-injury.

Beginning Position:

- Seated.
- Pelvic neutral.
- The affected/injured ankle should be propped up in free space.
- Attention to Scapular and C/S neutral.

Movement/Action:

- Without moving the entire leg, write the alphabet with the big toe of the injured ankle. Only foot and ankle motion should be occurring.
- Only move the ankle within a pain-free range of motion.
- Perform several times a day or as directed by your healthcare practitioner.

Key Notes/Common Faults:

- Pain/discomfort/straining of any kind.
- Moving beyond pain-free range of motion.
- Faulty breathing pattern.
- Loss of spinal control

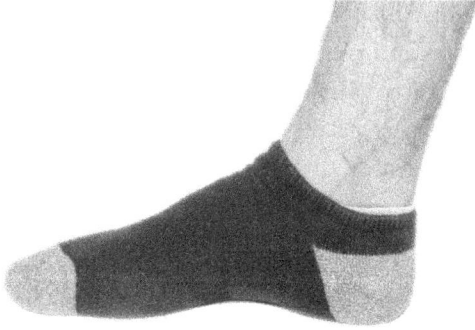

Small Foot Beginning Position

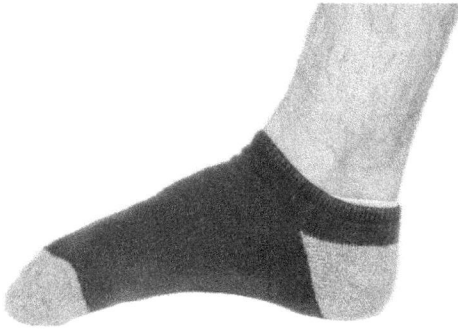

Small Foot Movement Position

Small Foot
Goal/Purpose:

- This exercise is specific rehabilitation for certain foot / ankle pathology and is utilized for increasing intrinsic foot muscle strength, coordination, and stability.

Beginning Position:

- Seated.
- Pelvic neutral.
- The affected/injured foot/ ankle should be securely on the flat ground.
- Attention to Scapular and C/S neutral.

Movement/Action:

- Without moving the ankle, flex the mid-arch of the foot by squeezing the ball of the foot back towards the heel. It is like performing a tiny foot crunch.
- The toes, however, should not crunch during the arch activation. There is not much movement here, so don't overdo it.
- Repeat 10 reps.

Key Notes/Common Faults:

- Pain/discomfort/straining of any kind.
- Excessive curling crunching of the toes.
- Moving beyond pain-free range of motion.
- Faulty breathing pattern.
- Loss of spinal control

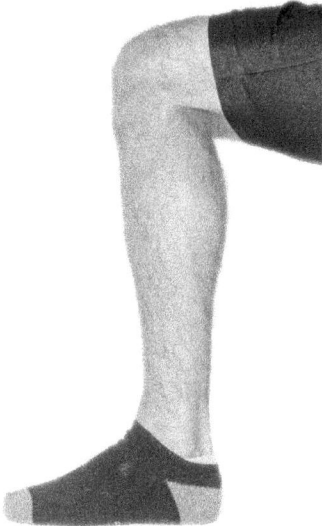

Seated Calf Raises Beginning Position

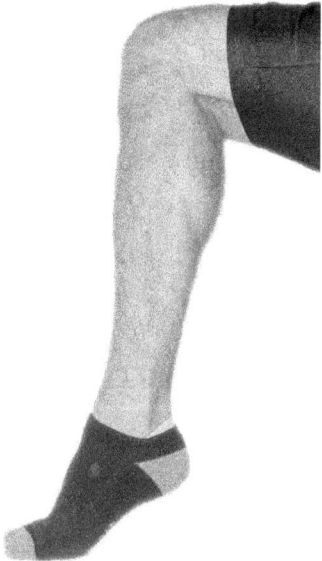

Seated Calf Raises Movement Position

· · ·

Seated Calf Raises
  Goal/Purpose:

- This exercise is specific rehabilitation for certain foot/ankle pathology and is utilized for increasing ankle range of motion, coordination, and stability.

Beginning Position:

- Seated.
- Pelvic neutral.
- The affected/injured foot/ankle should be securely flat on the ground.
- Attention to Scapular and C/S neutral.

Movement/Action:

- Without moving the entire leg, perform a seated calf raise by way of ankle plantar flexion by pressing the ball of the foot down into the ground with enough force to raise the heel off the ground.
- Direct the line of force through the first (big toe) and second toes as the calf raise motion is performed.
- Only move the ankle within a pain-free range of motion.
- Repeat 10 reps.

Key Notes/Common Faults:

- Pain/discomfort/straining of any kind.
- Moving beyond pain-free range of motion.
- Faulty breathing pattern.
- Loss of spinal control

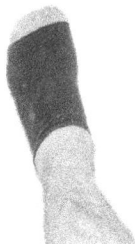

Peanut Butter Spread Beginning Position

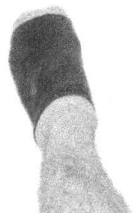

Peanut Butter Spread Movement Position I

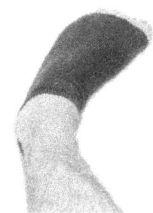

Peanut Butter Spread Movement Position II

Peanut Butter Spread
Goal/Purpose:

- This exercise is specific rehabilitation for certain foot/ankle pathologies and is utilized for increasing foot/ankle strength (Tibialis Posterior specifically), coordination, and stability.

Beginning Position:

- Seated.
- Pelvic neutral.
- The affected/injured foot/ ankle should be securely on the flat ground.
- Attention to Scapular and C/S neutral.

Movement/Action:

- Without moving the entire leg, perform a peanut butter spread by scraping the ball of the foot across the ground from lateral to medial (outside to inside), as if one were trying to spread peanut butter across the ground with the ball of the foot.
- Repeat 10 reps.

Key Notes/Common Faults:

- Pain/discomfort/straining of any kind.
- Moving beyond pain-free range of motion.
- Faulty breathing pattern.
- Loss of spinal control

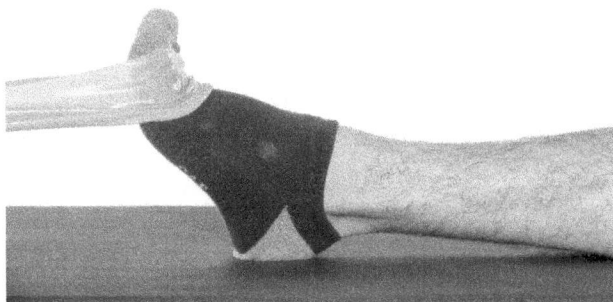

Theraband Tibialis Anterior Beginning Position

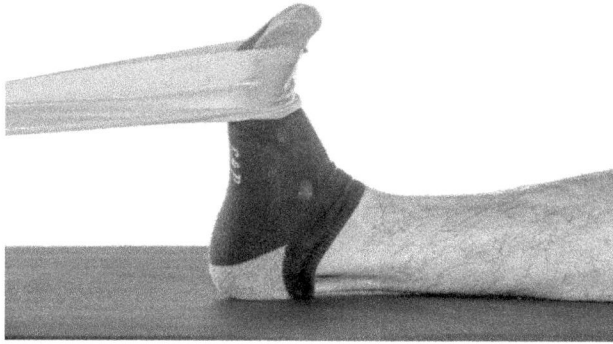

Theraband Tibialis Anterior Movement Position

Theraband Tibialis Anterior

Goal/Purpose:

- This exercise is specific rehabilitation for certain foot/ankle pathology and is utilized for increasing foot/ankle strength (Tibialis Anterior specifically), coordination, and stability.

Beginning Position:

- Seated.
- Pelvic neutral.
- The affected/injured ankle should be propped up in free space with a Theraband securely attached around the foot, pulling the foot downward into plantar flexion (toes pointed down).
- Attention to Scapular and C/S neutral.

Movement/Action:

- Without moving the entire leg, pull the foot up into dorsiflexion against the resistance of the Theraband.

- Repeat 10 reps.

Key Notes/Common Faults:

- Pain/discomfort/straining of any kind.
- Moving beyond pain-free range of motion.
- Faulty breathing pattern.
- Loss of spinal control

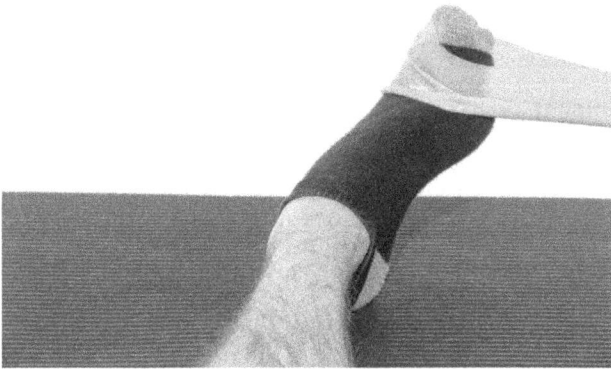

Theraband Peronei Beginning Position

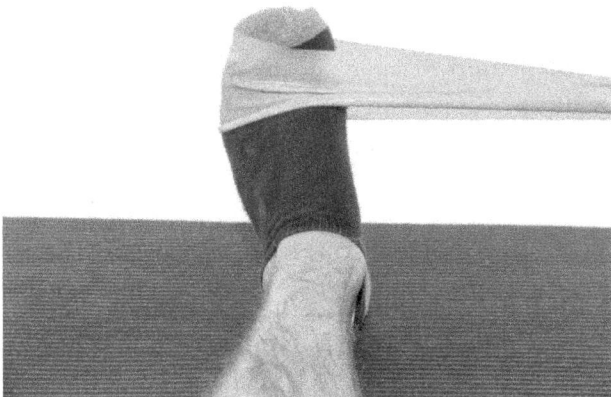

Theraband Peronei Movement Position

Theraband Peronei
Goal/Purpose:

- This exercise is specific rehabilitation for certain foot/ankle pathologies and is utilized to increase foot/ankle strength (specifically Peronei), coordination, and stability.

Beginning Position:

- Seated.
- Pelvic neutral.
- The affected/injured ankle should be propped up in free space with a Theraband securely attached around the foot, pulling the foot inward into inversion and slight supination (toes pointed in and down).
- Attention to Scapular and C/S neutral.

Movement/Action:

- Without moving the entire leg, pull the foot up and out into dorsiflexion and eversion against the resistance of the Theraband.
- Repeat 10 reps.

Key Notes/Common Faults:

- Pain/discomfort/straining of any kind.
- Moving beyond pain-free range of motion.
- Faulty breathing pattern.
- Loss of spinal control

LEVEL II ANKLE-SPECIFIC

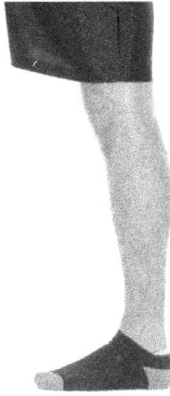

Standing Calf Raises Beginning Position

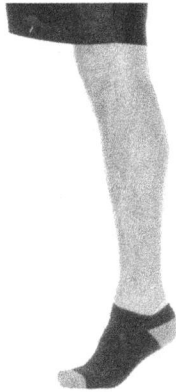

Standing Calf Raises Movement Position

Standing Calf Raises
  Goal/Purpose:

- This exercise is specific rehabilitation for certain foot/ankle pathology and is utilized for increasing ankle strength, coordination, and stability.

Beginning Position:

- Standing on the edge of at small step.
- Pelvic neutral.
- The affected / injured foot / ankle should be securely on a step with the heel off the step.
- Attention to Scapular and C/S neutral.

Movement/Action:

- While maintaining Full Spinal Control, perform a calf raise by way of ankle plantar flexion by pressing the ball of the foot down into the ground (step) with enough force to raise the heel up as far as comfortably possible.
- Direct the line of force through the first (big toe) and second toes as the calf raise motion is performed.
- Repeat 10 reps. (The goal is 25 reps for this exercise)
- Repeat with the opposite ankle

Key Notes/Common Faults:

- Pain / discomfort / straining of any kind.
- Faulty breathing pattern.
- Loss of spinal control.
- If you have difficulty performing this exercise with one leg or ankle at a time, begin with both ankles at the same time.

SHOULDER-SPECIFIC

The Shoulder-Specific Series offers additional training for the upper extremity, specifically for the shoulder. Certain injuries or conditions specific to the shoulder may require more extensive training beyond the basic full-body biomechanical training. The shoulder joint is one of the most complex joints in all of the human body. Providing extra support and training can be a great idea for anyone. Still, for persons coming back for a specific shoulder injury, one of the most important things to consider is the range of motion and mobility of the shoulder. Again, as discussed, this does not mean that the basic fundamental mechanics can or should be overlooked. Remember, the more serious or complicated the injury or pathology is, typically, the more important the fundamentals become. This Shoulder-Specific Series reviews the basics of beginning shoulder-specific rehabilitation to help give additional flexibility and mobility to this area of the body.

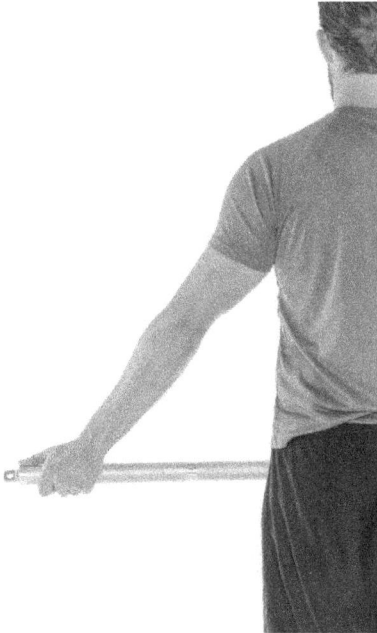

Wand Mobility Beginning Position

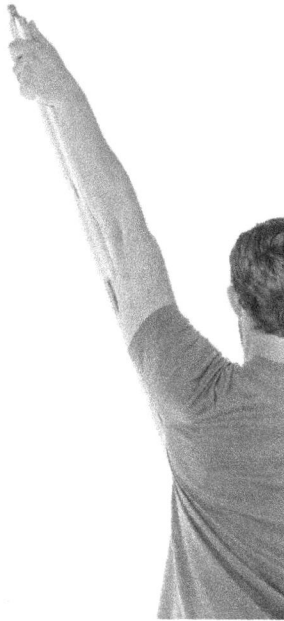

Wand Mobility Movement Position

Wand Mobility
Goal/Purpose:

- This exercise is specific rehabilitation for certain shoulder pathologies and is utilized to increase the shoulder (GH Joint) range of motion following trauma/injury.

Beginning Position:

- Standing with Full Spinal Control.
- Pelvic neutral.
- The hand of the affected/injured side shoulder grasps the end of a dowel (stick/broom handle) with an underhand grip. The non-affected/non-injured side hand holds the other side of the dowel with an overhand grip.

- Attention to Scapular and C/S neutral.

Movement/Action:

- While maintaining Full Spinal Control, perform a wand mobility lift by using the non-affected arm to push the affected side arm/shoulder up into should flexion and abduction as far as pain-free range will allow. Then, slowly lower the arm back down.
- The shoulder/arm on the affected side should do none of the lifting work. The non-affected side needs to do all the work to use the dowel to push the injured side up.
- Repeat 10 reps.

Key Notes/Common Faults:

- Pain/discomfort/straining of any kind.
- Moving beyond pain-free range of motion.
- Faulty breathing pattern.
- Loss of spinal control.

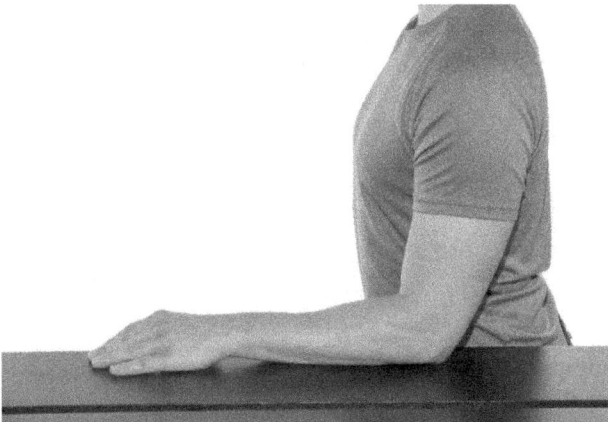

Table Walk Beginning Position

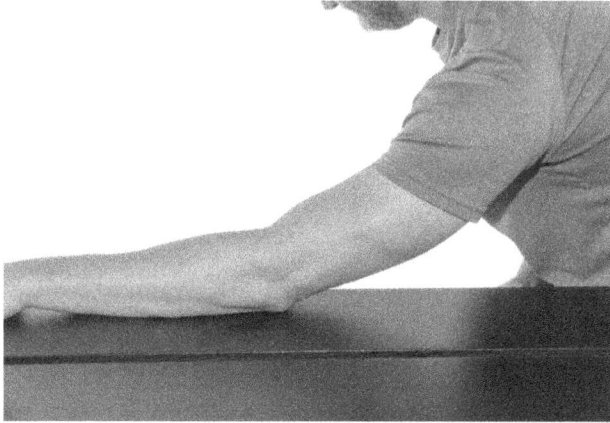

Table Walk Movement Position

Table Walks
Goal/Purpose:

- This exercise is specific rehabilitation for certain shoulder pathologies and is utilized to increase the shoulder (GH Joint) range of motion following trauma / injury.

Beginning Position:

- Seated next to a table.
- Pelvic neutral.
- The affected / injured side shoulder towards the table with this arm lying on / supported by the table.
- Attention to Scapular and C/S neutral.

Movement/Action:

- Without actively moving the shoulder, perform a table slide by leaning with the body to slide the arm up on the table to create passive shoulder flexion and / or abduction.
- Repeat 10 reps.

Key Notes/Common Faults:

- Pain/discomfort/straining of any kind.
- Moving beyond pain-free range of motion.
- Faulty breathing pattern.
- Loss of spinal control

ELBOW/WRIST/HAND-SPECIFIC

The Elbow/Wrist/Hand-Specific Series offers additional training for the upper extremity, specifically for the elbow, hand, and wrist. Certain injuries or conditions specific to these areas may require more extensive training beyond the basic full-body biomechanical training. There are many joints, ligaments, muscles, and tendons in the elbow, hand, and wrist, which can lead to complications during training. Providing extra support and training in these areas can help tremendously. Again, as discussed, this does not mean that the basic fundamental mechanics can or should be overlooked. Remember, the more serious or complicated the injury or pathology is, typically, the more important the fundamentals become. This Elbow/Wrist/Hand-Specific Series reviews the basics of beginning rehabilitation specific to these areas to help give additional support, control, mobility, strength, and stability to these areas.

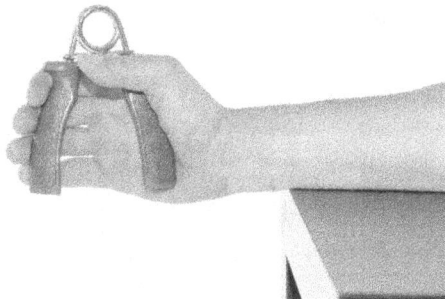

Grip Strength Beginning Position

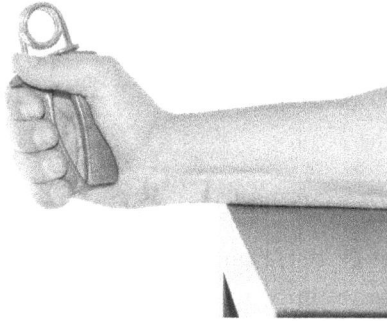

Grip Strength Movement Position

Grip Strength
Goal/Purpose:

- This exercise is specific rehabilitation for certain elbow and/or wrist and/or hand pathologies and is utilized to increase the strength of the wrist and hand flexor muscles.

Beginning Position:

- Standing or Seated.
- Pelvic neutral.
- The affected/injured side hand is grasping a grip vice.
- Attention to Scapular and C/S neutral.

Movement/Action:

- Without loss of Full Spinal Control, squeeze the grip strength vice by way of finger/ hand flexion.
- Repeat 25 reps.

Key Notes/Common Faults:

- Pain/discomfort/straining of any kind.
- Moving beyond pain-free range of motion.
- Faulty breathing pattern.
- Loss of spinal control

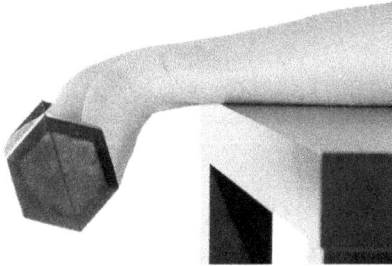

Wrist Flexion Beginning Position

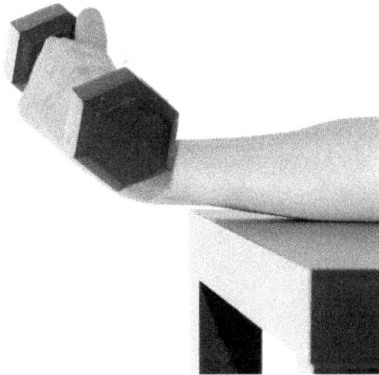

Wrist Flexion Movement Position

Wrist Flexion
  Goal/Purpose:

- This exercise is specific rehabilitation for certain elbow and/or wrist and/or hand pathology and is utilized for increasing the strength of the wrist and hand flexor muscles.

Beginning Position:

- Standing or Seated.
- Pelvic neutral.
- The affected/injured side hand is grasping a grip vice.
- Attention to Scapular and C/S neutral.

Movement/Action:

- Without loss of Full Spinal Control, squeeze the grip strength vice by way of finger/ hand flexion.
- Repeat 25 reps.

Key Notes/Common Faults:

- Pain/discomfort/straining of any kind.
- Moving beyond pain-free range of motion.
- Faulty breathing pattern.
- Loss of spinal control

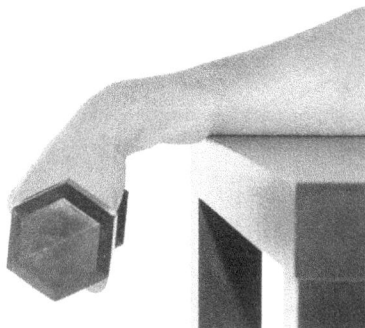

Wrist Extension Beginning Position

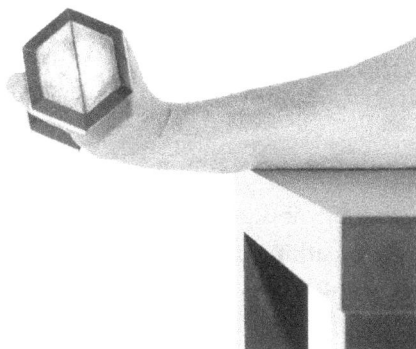

Wrist Extension Movement Position

Wrist Extension
   Goal/Purpose:

- This exercise is specific rehabilitation for certain elbow
  and/or wrist and/or hand pathology and is utilized for
  increasing the strength of the wrist and hand extensor
  muscles.

Beginning Position:

- Standing or Seated.
- Pelvic neutral.
- The affected/injured side hand/lower arm is supported by a
  table or bench with the hand off the edge with the palm
  down (pronated), holding a light dumbbell weight.
- Attention to Scapular and C/S neutral.

Movement/Action:

- Without loss of Full Spinal Control, allow the weight to sag
  down as the wrist is flexed down towards the ground. Then

curl the wrist and hand up into wrist extension as far as pain-free range will allow.

- Repeat 10 reps.

Key Notes/Common Faults:

- Pain/discomfort/straining of any kind.
- Moving beyond pain-free range of motion.
- Faulty breathing pattern.
- Loss of spinal control

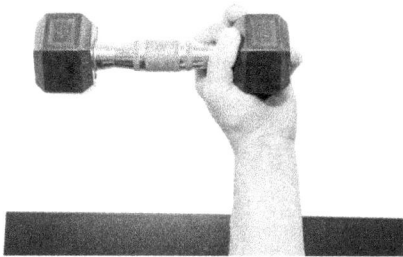

Wrist Pronation + Supination Beginning Position

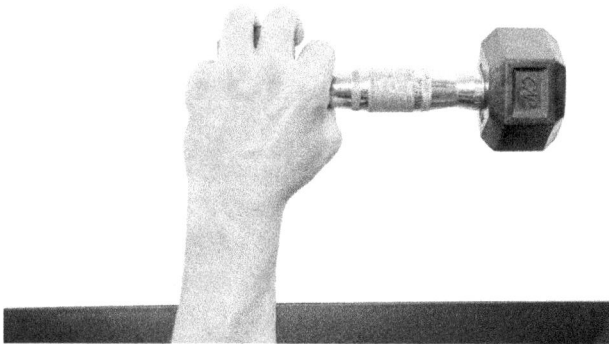

Wrist Pronation + Supination Movement Position

Wrist Pronation + Supination

Goal/Purpose:

- This exercise is specific rehabilitation for certain elbow and/or wrist and/or hand pathologies and is utilized to increase the strength of the wrist/forearm pronator and supinator muscles.

Beginning Position:

- Standing or Seated.
- Pelvic neutral.
- The affected/injured side hand/lower arm supported by a table or bench with the hand off the edge with the palm up, holding a light dumbbell weight at one edge (holding a short 2-4 foot long dowel can also work well for this exercise).
- Attention to Scapular and C/S neutral.

Movement/Action:

- Without loss of Full Spinal Control, rotate the weight/dowel over by way of forearm pronation to achieve a palm-down (pronated) position. Then, rotate the wrist/forearm back to the starting palm-up (supinated) position by way of forearm supination.
- Repeat 10 reps.

Key Notes/Common Faults:

- Pain/discomfort/straining of any kind.
- Moving beyond pain-free range of motion.
- Faulty breathing pattern.
- Loss of spinal control

RECOVERY STRETCHING SERIES

T he Recovery Stretching Series presents a basic yet well-rounded and complete series of static, self-stretching, and mobility exercises to help assist the biomechanical rehabilitative training process. Remember, we said that if your mechanics are 100% perfect 100% of the time throughout your entire life, then there would be no need for these static stretches. While theoretically this may be true, in reality it is more of a bit of a joke, as it is basically impossible to be 100% mechanically correct 100% of your life. So, as discussed before, taking advantage of some basic stretching and mobility procedures can help tremendously in terms of aiding, speeding up, and smoothing out the biomechanical re-training process.

COOL DOWN MOBILITY STRETCHES

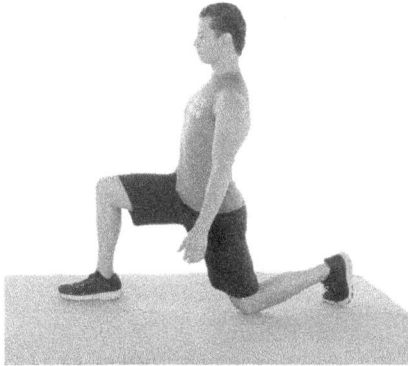

Hip Flexors Beginning Position

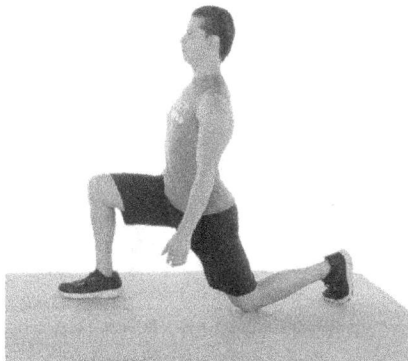

Hip Flexors Movement Position

Hip Flexors
Goal/Purpose:

- Gaining functional hip range of motion to help achieve and maintain pelvic neutral, utilized for either therapeutic purposes, intelligent compensation purposes, and/or training beyond normal human functional range for alternative performance goals.

Beginning Position:

- Single-leg kneeling position with Full Spinal Control.
- The down leg will be the stretch leg.

Stretch Position:

- While maintaining Full Spinal Control, especially pelvic neutral, bring the body slightly forward as if you were going to drag your back knee on the ground.
- One should feel stretch in the hip flexor down the front of the down-leg thigh.
- Hold the stretch position for at least 30-45 seconds.

Key Notes/Common Faults:

- Pain/discomfort/straining of any kind.
- The major key is to maintain pelvic neutral. This is often a neglected detail, but it is critical.
- Faulty breathing pattern.
- Loss of Full Spinal Control.
- Any stressing or straining of any kind, especially in the face and neck, should not be allowed.
- An alternative position of a split stance may be used if the kneeling position does not work for whatever reason. All the other details remain the same.

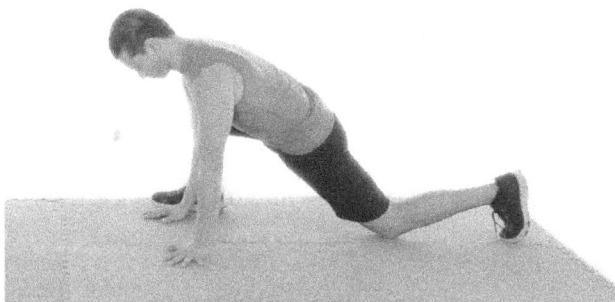

Glute Stretch Beginning Position

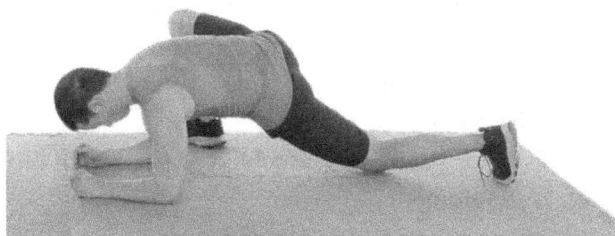

Glute Stretch Movement Position

. . .

Glute Stretch
Goal/Purpose:

- Gaining functional hip range of motion to help achieve and maintain pelvic neutral, utilized for either therapeutic purposes, intelligent compensation purposes, and/or training beyond normal human functional range for alternative performance goals.

Beginning Position:

- Single-leg kneeling position with Full Spinal Control.
- The down leg will be the stretch leg.

Stretch Position:

- While maintaining Full Spinal Control, especially pelvic neutral, bring the body slightly forward as if you were going to drag your back knee on the ground.
- One should feel stretch in the hip flexor down the front of the down-leg thigh.
- Hold the stretch position for at least 30-45 seconds.

Key Notes/Common Faults:

- Pain/discomfort/straining of any kind.
- The major key is to maintain pelvic neutral. This is often a neglected detail, but it is critical.
- Faulty breathing pattern.
- Loss of Full Spinal Control.
- Any stressing or straining of any kind, especially in the face and neck, should not be allowed.
- An alternative position of a split stance may be used if the

kneeling position does not work for whatever reason. All the other details remain the same.

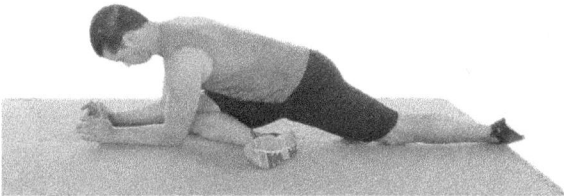

Hip Rotators Beginning Position

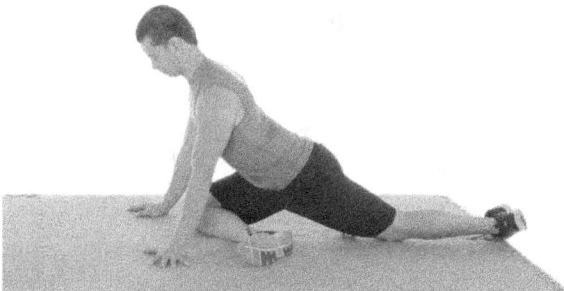

Hip Rotators Movement Position

. . .

Hip Rotators
Goal/Purpose:

- Gaining functional hip range of motion to help achieve and maintain pelvic neutral, utilized for either therapeutic purposes, intelligent compensation purposes, and / or training beyond normal human functional range for alternative performance goals.

Beginning Position:

- Single-leg kneeling position with Full Spinal Control.
- The down leg will be the stretch leg.

Stretch Position:

- While maintaining Full Spinal Control, especially pelvic neutral, bring the body slightly forward as if you were going to drag your back knee on the ground.
- One should feel stretch in the hip flexor down the front of the down-leg thigh.
- Hold the stretch position for at least 30-45 seconds.

Key Notes/Common Faults:

- Pain / discomfort / straining of any kind.
- The major key is to maintain pelvic neutral. This is often a neglected detail, but it is critical.
- Faulty breathing pattern.
- Loss of Full Spinal Control.
- Any stressing or straining of any kind, especially in the face and neck, should not be allowed.
- An alternative position of a split stance may be used if the

kneeling position does not work for whatever reason. All the other details remain the same.

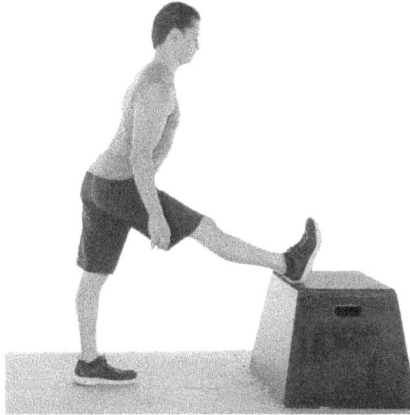

Hamstring With Nerve Floss Beginning Position

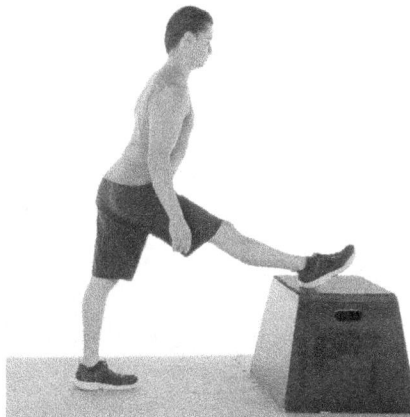

Hamstring With Nerve Floss Movement Position

Hamstrings With Nerve Floss
   Goal/Purpose:

- Gaining functional hip range of motion to help achieve and maintain pelvic neutral, utilized for either therapeutic purposes, intelligent compensation purposes, and / or training beyond normal human functional range for alternative performance goals.

Beginning Position:

- Single-leg kneeling position with Full Spinal Control.
- The down leg will be the stretch leg.

Stretch Position:

- While maintaining Full Spinal Control, especially pelvic neutral, bring the body slightly forward as if you were going to drag your back knee on the ground.
- One should feel stretch in the hip flexor down the front of the down-leg thigh.
- Hold the stretch position for at least 30-45 seconds.

Key Notes/Common Faults:

- Pain / discomfort / straining of any kind.
- The major key is to maintain pelvic neutral. This is often a neglected detail, but it is critical.
- Faulty breathing pattern.
- Loss of Full Spinal Control.
- Any stressing or straining of any kind, especially in the face and neck, should not be allowed.
- An alternative position of a split stance may be used if the kneeling position does not work for whatever reason. All the other details remain the same.
- An alternative kneeling position may be utilized if need be.

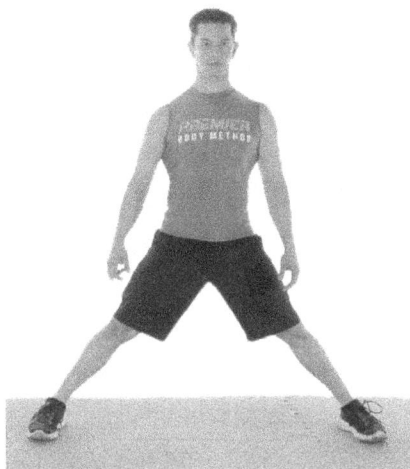

Lateral Groin Beginning Position

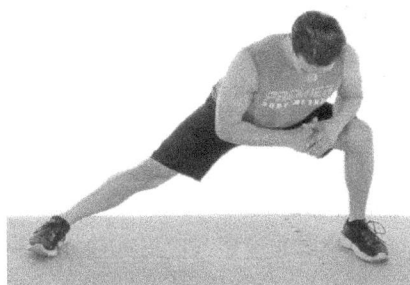

Lateral Groin Movement Position

Lateral Groin
  Goal/Purpose:

- Gaining functional hip range of motion to help hip mechanics, utilized for either therapeutic purposes, intelligent compensation purposes, and/or training beyond the normal human functional range for alternative performance goals.

Beginning Position:

- Standing in a wide stance position with Full Spinal Control.
- The groin inside of the hip (hip adductor muscle group) will be stretched.

Stretch Position:

- While maintaining Full Spinal Control, perform a lateral squat motion to one side to the desired amount of stretch tension.
- One should feel stretch in the straight leg groin, not the squatting leg.
- Hold the stretch position for at least 30-45 seconds.

Key Notes/Common Faults:

- Pain/discomfort/straining of any kind.
- Make sure to maintain and follow all mechanical rules for the lateral squat position.
- Loss of Full Spinal Control.
- Any stressing or straining of any kind, especially in the face and neck, should not be allowed.
- An alternative position of seated performing a butterfly stretch can be utilized. However, it should be noted that this position will take out the stretch of one of the hip adductor muscles (the Gracilis) due to the knee being bent.

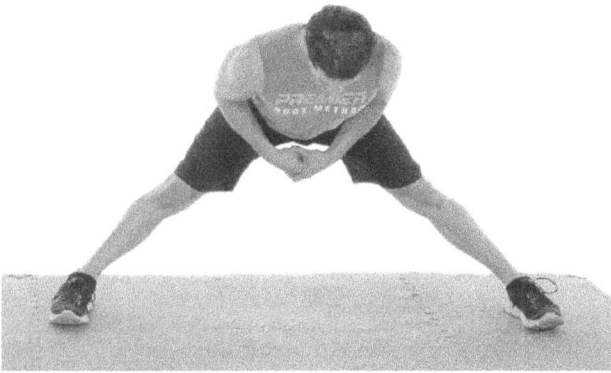

Straddle

Straddle
  Goal/Purpose:

- Gaining functional hip range of motion to help hip mechanics, utilized for either therapeutic purposes, intelligent compensation purposes, and / or training beyond the normal human functional range for alternative performance goals.

Beginning Position:

- Standing in a wide stance position with Full Spinal Control.

- The medial hamstring and groin inside of the hip (hip adductor muscle group) will be stretched.

Stretch Position:

- While maintaining Full Spinal Control, hinge from the hips by pushing the hip back to the desired amount of stretch tension (keep the knees straight).
- One should feel stretch in the back inside to the thighs in both legs.
- Hold the stretch position for at least 30-45 seconds.

Key Notes/Common Faults:

- Pain / discomfort / straining of any kind.
- Make sure to maintain and follow all mechanical rules for Hip Hinging.
- Loss of Full Spinal Control.
- Any stressing or straining of any kind, especially in the face and neck, should not be allowed.
- An alternative position of seated performing the same straddle stretch can be utilized. All details are basically the same.

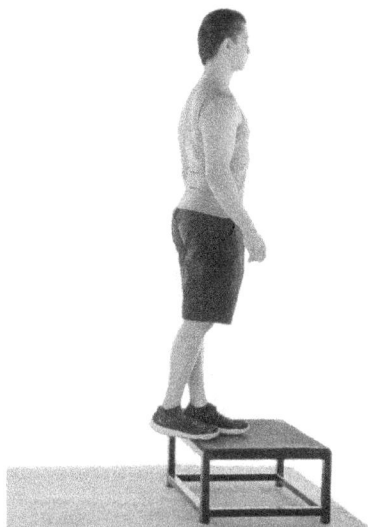

Calf Two-Way Beginning Position

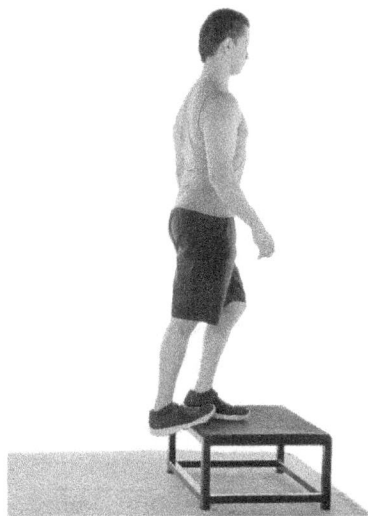

Calf Two-Way Movement Position I

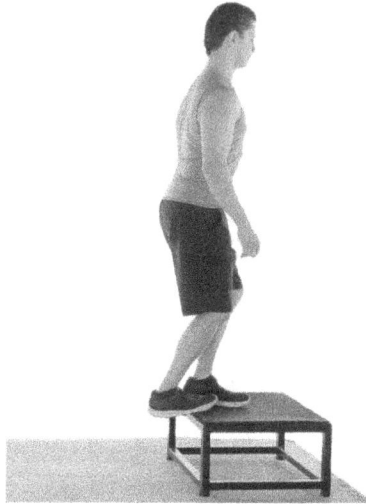

Calf Two-Way Movement Position II

Calf Two-Way
Goal/Purpose:

- Gaining functional ankle range of motion to help hip-hinging mechanics, utilized for therapeutic purposes, intelligent compensation purposes, and/or training beyond the normal human functional range for alternative performance goals.

Beginning Position:

- Standing on the edge of a step of vertical ramp with Full Spinal Control.
- The calf muscles in the back of the lower leg will be stretched.

Stretch Position:

- While maintaining Full Spinal Control, lower one heel off the back of the step or vertical ramp to the desired amount of stretch tension.
- This should be done two ways: once with the knee straight and again with the knee bent.
- Hold each stretch position for at least 30-45 seconds.

Key Notes/Common Faults:

- Pain / discomfort / straining of any kind.
- Loss of Full Spinal Control.
- Any stressing or straining of any kind, especially in the face and neck, should not be allowed.
- An alternative position of a quadruped position can be utilized if no step / vert. ramp is available.

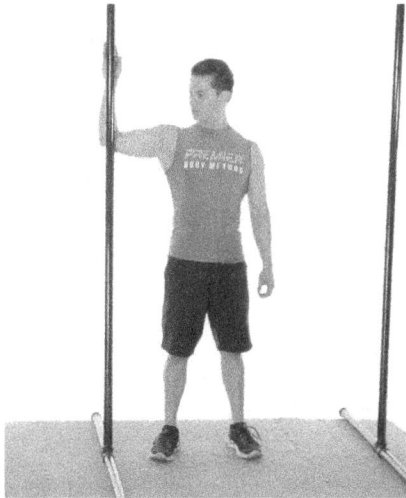

Pecs Beginning Position

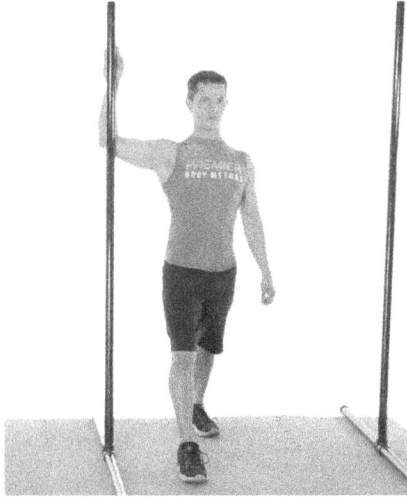

Pecs Movement Position

Pecs

Goal/Purpose:

- Gaining functional shoulder range of motion to help achieve and maintain the set scapular position, utilized for either therapeutic purposes, intelligent compensation purposes, and/or training beyond the normal human functional range for alternative performance goals.

Beginning Position:

- Standing with one arm/elbow up on a doorway or corner wall with Full Spinal Control.
- The pec muscles in the front of the shoulder and chest will be stretched.

Stretch Position:

- While maintaining Full Spinal Control, step the body forward to the desired amount of stretch tension.
- Hold the stretch position for at least 30-45 seconds.

Key Notes/Common Faults:

- Pain/discomfort/straining of any kind.
- Loss of Full Spinal Control.
- Do not rotate the body away, as this can torque the spine. Just move straight forward to the desired stretch tension.
- Any stressing or straining of any kind, especially in the face and neck, should not be allowed.
- An alternative position of bilateral arm can be utilized to stretch both sides and the same time.
- It should be noted that the height of the arm/elbow on the wall can be varied to achieve a greater variety of stretch through the tissues.

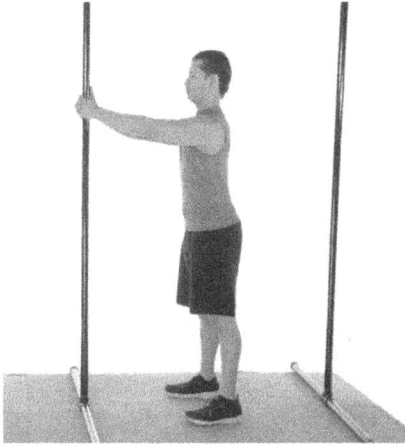

Lats Beginning Position

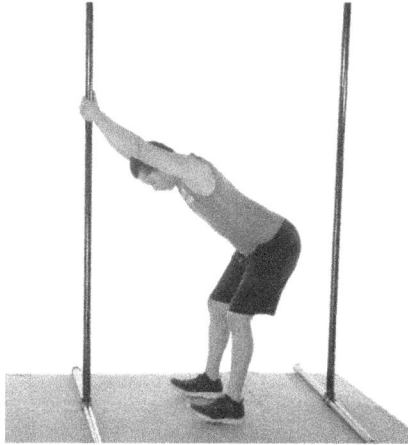

Lats Movement Position

Lats

Goal/Purpose:

- Gaining functional shoulder range of motion to help achieve and maintain the set scapular position, utilized for either therapeutic purposes, intelligent compensation purposes, and/or training beyond the normal human functional range for alternative performance goals.

Beginning Position:

- Standing with arms reaching up on a wall with palm or thumbs up, with Full Spinal Control.
- The lat muscles in the back underneath the region of the shoulder and back will be stretched.

Stretch Position:

- While maintaining Full Spinal Control, step the body

backward and hinge the hips to the desired amount of stretch tension.

- Hold the stretch position for at least 30-45 seconds.

Key Notes/Common Faults:

- Pain/discomfort/straining of any kind.
- Loss of Full Spinal Control.
- Any stressing or straining of any kind, especially in the face and neck, should not be allowed.
- An alternative position on a counter can be utilized.

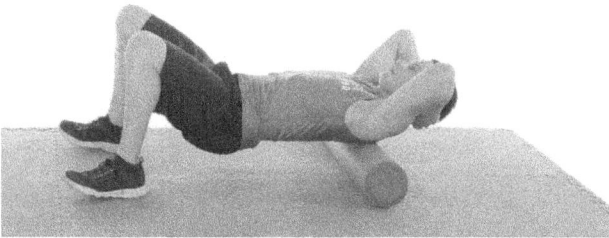

T/S Foam Roller Mobilization Beginning Position

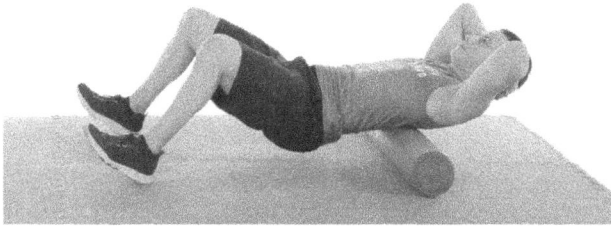

T/S Foam Roller Mobilization Movement Position

T/S Foam Roller Mobilization
   Goal/Purpose:

- Gaining functional thoracic spine range of motion to help achieve and maintain the set scapular position and spinal control, utilized for therapeutic purposes, intelligent compensation purposes, and/or training beyond the normal human functional range for alternative performance goals.

Beginning Position:

- Supine lying over a foam roller crosswise with the roller across the upper back (T/S), with Full Spinal Control.
- Make sure to support the head and neck with the arms/hands.

Stretch Position:

- While maintaining Full Spinal Control, arch the upper back (T/S) over the foam roller to the desired amount of stretch tension.
- Gently roll up and down the foam roller through the T/S range only. Do not arch the lower back.
- Hold the stretch position for at least 30-45 seconds.

Key Notes/Common Faults:

- Pain/discomfort/straining of any kind.
- Loss of Full Spinal Control.
- Any stressing or straining of any kind, especially in the face and neck, should not be allowed.
- An alternative position on a back bridge arch support can be utilized if the foam roller is too aggressive.

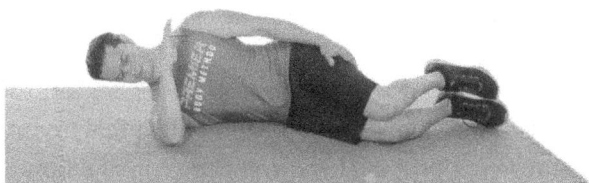

Posterior GHJ (Shoulder) Capsule Beginning Position

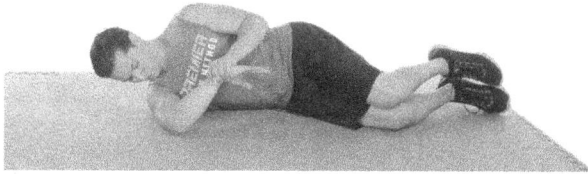

Posterior GHJ (Shoulder) Capsule Movement Position

Posterior GHJ (Shoulder) Capsule
Goal/Purpose:

- Gaining functional GH joint range of motion mainly for throwing athletes, utilized for either therapeutic purposes, intelligent compensation purposes, and/or training beyond the normal human functional range for alternative performance goals.

Beginning Position:

- Side-lying with the down-side arm shoulder flexed to 80 degrees with the elbow bent up, with Full Spinal Control.
- Make sure to support the head and neck with a pillow.

Stretch Position:

- While maintaining Full Spinal Control, roll over slightly onto the down-side arm and use the up-side arm to rotate the down-side arm into the internal rotation to the desired amount of stretch tension.
- The stretch should be felt deep in the back of the down-side shoulder.
- Hold the stretch position for at least 30-45 seconds.

Key Notes/Common Faults:

- Pain/discomfort/straining of any kind.
- Loss of Full Spinal Control.
- Any stressing or straining of any kind, especially in the face and neck, should not be allowed.

GLOSSARY

PHYSICAL CAPABILITY LIMITS: The limits of one's functional movement range of motion based on anatomical structure and how that structure may have changed due to true structural injury, pathology, and/or degeneration. Example: if an individual had 35 degrees of lumbar spine extension at age 20, but then suffered years of repetitive stress to the facet joints of the lumbar spine causing the degenerative adaptive change of facet arthropathy, now this individual at age, let's say 40, now only has the ability to go 20 degrees into lumbar spine extension.

FULL SPINAL CONTROL: The ability to position the spinal collum, pelvis, scapula, and skull correctly and maintain those correct positions during active motion/movement of the human body.

HIP HINGING MOTIONS: A motion of the hip joint utilizing mainly the hip, thigh, and spinal control/core musculature, as the pelvis, spinal column, and torso are levered forward and back in the sagittal plane with the hip joint as the axis of rotation. The hip hinge motion is the single most functional motion the human body is capable of producing.

PULLING MOTIONS: Any motion in which weight or resistance is pulled in towards the body's center of mass.

PRESSING MOTIONS: Any motion in which weight or resistance is driven away from the body's center of mass.

ANABOLISM: The synthesis of complex molecules in living organisms from simpler ones together with the storage of energy; constructive metabolism; tissue building. Anabolic processes promote increased muscular development, tissue healing, energy, and a general sense of well-being.

CATABOLISM: The breakdown of complex molecules in living organisms to form simpler ones, together with the release of energy; destructive metabolism; tissue wasting. Catabolic processes decrease muscle development, decrease energy, and may cause a poor sense of well-being.

FLEXIBILITY: Refers to the elasticity in the soft tissue structures of the body, particularly muscles.

MOBILITY: The range of motion capable of a particular region of the body, particularly a joint and the connective tissue structures associated with that joint, i.e., the joint capsule, ligaments, and fascia.

THERAPEUTIC PURPOSES: Refers to any form of physical body care, including but not limited to movement, exercise, stretching, mobilization, physical therapy modalities, massage, or other body care, for the purpose of aiding the body's pursuit of health and homeostasis.

LUMBOPELVIC CONTROL: The ability to control one's pelvic, hip, and spinal posture and position, both static and during movement, in order to maintain the correct individual pelvic neutral position. This is achieved through proper core stability activation.

SCAPULOTHORACIC CONTROL: The ability to control one's scapula, thoracic spine, and shoulder girdle position/posture static and during movement for the purpose of maintaining the correct shoulder and spinal neutral position.

CERVICAL SPINE NEUTRAL CONTROL: The ability to control one's head and neck position/posture static and during movement in order to maintain the correct Cervical Spine Neutral position.

FRONTAL/CORONAL PLANE: A vertical plane that divides the body into ventral/anterior and dorsal/posterior (front and back) sections.

TRANSVERSE PLANE: A horizontal plane that divides the body into superior and inferior (top and bottom) sections.

SAGGITAL PLANE: A vertical plane that divides the body into left and right sections.

PELVIC NEUTRAL POSITION: Anatomical pelvic neutral is defined as the center of a range of motion between all three planes of motion (Coronal, Sagittal, and Transverse) for the pelvic bone. Individual-specific pelvic neutral is then fine-tuned from the anatomical pelvic neutral position based on one's individual anatomy.

SET SCAPULAR POSITION: Anatomical set scapular position is defined as the center of range of motion between all three planes of motion (Coronal, Sagittal, and Transverse) for the scapula (shoulder blade). The individual-specific set scapular position is then fine-tuned from the anatomical set scapular position based on one's individual anatomy.

SUPINE: A face-up position.

PRONE: A face-down position.

VALSALVA: A technique of creating pressure in one's abdominal cavity, thoracic cavity, and spinal column, thus increasing intra-abdominal pressure and intra-thecal pressure.

MOTOR LEARNING ABILITY: The rate at which an individual can transition from conceptually understanding a new movement or physical skill, to then actually being able to physically apply and perform that new movement/physical skill.

REFERENCES AND CITED WORKS

Please refer to https://premierbodymethod.com/research for a bibliographic list of references to this text.

ABOUT THE AUTHOR

CONNECT WITH ME!

Thank you for reading *Your Life, Pain-Free*! You have already taken the first step towards a pain-free life. I would love to stay in touch with you and hear about your progress throughout this journey. Pain-free living is attainable, and I hope that you will find the methodologies described in this book useful.

All reader feedback is welcome—I'd love to hear what was helpful, what was hard, and what impacted you the most! I would greatly appreciate it if you would post a review for this book on Amazon and Goodreads. Every reader review goes a long way in helping make books like this more accessible to others.

Not only is the PREMIER Body Method the methodology described in this book, but my clinic's treatment is centered around it as well. If you'd like to learn more, follow the links below:

Visit us on the web at: premierbodymethod.com

instagram.com/premierbodymethod
facebook.com/premierbodymethod

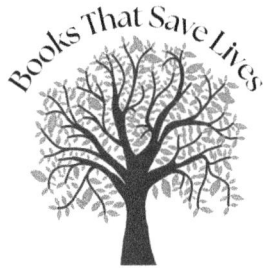

Books That Save Lives

Books That Save Lives came into being in 2024 when the editor and publisher, Brenda Knight, heard directly from readers and authors that certain self-help, grief, psychology books, and journals were providing a lifeline for folks. We live in a stressful world where it is increasingly difficult not to feel overwhelmed, worried, depressed, and downright scared. We intend to offer support for the vulnerable, including people struggling with mental wellness and physical illness as well as people of color, queer and trans adults and teens, immigrants and anyone who needs encouragement and inspiration.

From first responders, military veterans, and retirees to LGBTQ+ teens and to those experiencing the shock of bereavement and loss, our books have saved lives. To us, there is no higher calling.

We would love to hear from you! Our readers are our most important resource; we value your input, suggestions, and ideas.

Please stay in touch with us and follow us at:
www.booksthatsavelives.net
Instagram: @booksthatsavelives

www.ingramcontent.com/pod-product-compliance
Lightning Source LLC
Chambersburg PA
CBHW050558270326
41926CB00012B/2099